ADVANCES IN DANCE/MOVEMENT THERAPY

Theoretical Perspectives and Empirical Findings

Edited by

Sabine C. Koch & Iris Bräuninger
Foreword by Robyn Flaum Cruz

λογος

Bibliografische Information Der Deutschen Bibliothek

Die Deutsche Bibliothek verzeichnet diese Publikation in der Deutschen
Nationalbibliografie; detaillierte bibliografische Daten sind im Internet über
http://dnb.ddb.de abrufbar.

ISBN 3-8325-1237-3

Logos Verlag Berlin
Comeniushof, Gubener Str. 47,
10243 Berlin
Tel.: +49 030 42 85 10 90
Fax: +49 030 42 85 10 92
INTERNET: http://www.logos-verlag.de

CONTRIBUTORS

Silvia B. Birklein, Ph.D, MA, ADTR, LPC, NCC, CMA, received her Ph.D. in Clinical Psychology from the New School University in New York, and her M.A. in Dance Therapy and Counseling Psychology from Antioch University. She studied Psychology at Freie University in Berlin, trained as a dance therapist (FPI), certified movement analyst (Laban/Bartenieff Institute for Movement Studies) and as a dancer (Regina Baumgart) in Germany. She is currently a postdoctoral fellow at the William Alanson White institute for psychoanalysis in New York, an adjunct professor for clinical technique at Montclair State University, and is involved in nonverbal behavior research and in teaching of the Kestenberg Movement Profile. She maintains a private practice for psychotherapy, dance therapy and supervision in New York and continues to teach and present nationally and internationally. Correspondence should be addressed to: sbirklein@mail.com

Eva Bojner Horwitz, Ph.D., Registered Physiotherapist (specialized in psychosomatic medicine) and Registered dance/movement therapist. She is researching at Uppsala University, Sweden (Public Health and Caring Sciences) on method development in Creative Arts in stress related disorders, and working in Stockholm in a private clinic with chronic pain patients (Fibromyalgia) and stress prevention. In 2004 she completed her thesis (for the degree of Doctor of Philosophy from the Faculty of Medicine) and is teaching at the University of Uppsala and at the University College of Dance in Stockholm. Correspondence concerning her chapter should be addressed to: Department of Public Health and Caring Sciences, Uppsala Science Park, Uppsala University, SE-751 83 Uppsala Sweden, eva.bojner@telia.com

Iris Bräuninger, Dr. rer.soc. (University of Tübingen, Dept. of Clinical and Physiological Psychology), European Certificate for Psychotherapy (ECP), former board member and acknowledged DMT trainer of the German DMT association BTD, Dance Therapist Registered (DTR) of ADTA, M.A. in DMT from Laban Centre/City University London, KMP Notator. She is currently the deputy head of Physio-, Dance-, and Movement Therapy Departement/Psychiatric University Hospital Zurich, Switzerland. Research emphases: DMT efficacy studies, stress management, quality of life, KMP and movement analysis in relation to emotion, interaction, and psychopathology. Correspondence should be addressed to: tanztherapie@swissonline.ch

Meg Chang, Ed.D., NCC, ADTR has worked as a dance-movement therapist in psychiatric facilities, medical and wellness settings, and in private practice since 1979; former faculty at Pratt Institute, NY. and Lesley College, Cambridge, MA, and currently teaching in the Creative Arts Certificate Program at The New School, New York, NY. Doctoral research in aesthetic adult education at Teachers College Columbia University was conducted in Seoul, Korea. Prior publications include "Mobilizing Battered Women: A Creative Step Forward", in Fran Levy (1995) *Dance and Other Expressive Art Therapies*. A staff teacher at the Center for Mindfulness at the University of Massachusetts Medical Center, now combining mindfulness-based stress reduction with dance-movement therapy in medical settings and as a consultant to organizations. Contact: MHChang@aol.com.

Sharon W. Goodill, Ph.D., ADTR, NCC, LPC, is Associate Professor and Director of the Hahnemann Creative Arts in Therapy Program, at Drexel University, Philadelphia, PA, USA. She has taught dance/movement, art, and music therapy graduate students for 15 years, and served on the Board of Directors of the American Dance Therapy Association for 10 years. She was awarded one of the first national research grants into complementary and alternative medicine to study DMT for adults with cystic fibrosis. Her current clinical focus is on patients with chronic medical illness (including cancer) and their families. Correspondence should be addressed to: sg35@drexel.edu.

Heather Hill, PhD, M.Ed, B.A., Grad. Dip. Movement and Dance, Grad. Cert. Dance Therapy, Professional Member of the Dance Therapy Association of Australia. She has worked for 20 years as a dance therapist, focussing particularly on the area of aged care and dementia. She has had articles on dementia and book chapters published. Her book "Invitation to the Dance: Dance for people with dementia and their carers" was published in 2001. She currently works in the disability field, teaches and supervises creative arts therapy and dance therapy students and is working on a person-centred dementia care curriculum for nurses. Correspondence concerning her chapter should be addressed to: heatherhill@hotkey.net.au

Sabine C. Koch, Ph.D., Psychologist, M.S.W., M.A., DTR, studied psychology at the University of Heidelberg, Germany, and Madrid, Spain (UAM). She completed the dance/movement therapy program at MCP Hahnemann University, Philadelphia, PA, USA, on a Fulbright grant. DMT experience with diverse populations. Specialized in Kestenberg Movement Profiling (KMP), its use in research, and education, KMP Notator. She did her Ph.D. in a national research project at the Psychology Department of the University of Heidelberg in microanalysis of verbal and nonverbal communication patterns in groups, where she currently works in gender and communication research. Correspondence should be addressed to: sabine.koch@urz.uni-heidelberg.de

Maria E. Lacour, Medical Doctor, Dance/Movement therapist and Immunologist, is specialized in immunology and allergy as a medical doctor and organic illness as dance therapist. She studied at Medicine University in Buenos Aires, Argentina, and at the Buenos Aires Immunology and Allergy Association. She has done a 3-year-professional training in DMT with Graciela Vella in Argentina and has been a DMT dancer for 15 years now (with Maria Fux, Graciela Vella, and multiple local and international DMTs). Currently she is a Dance/ Movement Therapist in a public hospital (Hospital Tornu, Argentina), working with oncology patients and other organic illnesses. She is a board member of the Argentine Association of Dance Therapists (AADT), member of the DMT Investigation and Study Group (GAD), Argentina, and invited teacher in the new postgraduate program on DMT in Argentina. She does DMT and Tango workshops for social recovery of chronic patients in Argentina and neighboring countries. Correspondence should be addressed to: melacournur@yahoo.com.ar

Malvern Lumsden has an M.A. and a Ph.D. in Psychology from the University of Edinburgh, Scotland, and an M.A. in Dance Movement Therapy from New York University, USA. He was head of the programme in DMT at the Norwegian College of Dance, Oslo, Norway, from 1998–2002 and is now Associate Professor in Mental Health, Faculty of Sports and Health Sciences, Agder University College, Arendal, Norway. He can be contacted at: malvern.m.lumsden@hia.no

Elana G. Mannheim, ECP (European Certified Psychotherapist), D/MT, is trained in movement-teaching at the Dore-Jacobs-School, Essen/Germany, studied New Dance at the University of Arts, Amsterdam/Netherlands, and is trained in depth-psychological breath-therapy in Stuttgart/Germany. Freelance teacher in institutes of education for adults and in applied universities and colleges. Specialized in work with cancer-patients, her research interests are evidence-based research in the field of D/MT in psycho-oncology. Correspondence should be addressed to: Tumor Biology Center, Breisacher Str. 117, D- 79106 Freiburg/Germany, mannheim@tumorbio.uni-freiburg.de

Claire Moore, BA (Hons.) in Psychology (Open University London), MA in Dance Movement Therapy and Movement Analysis (Laban Centre/City University London); training in Traumatherapy (New York, Hannover) and Thought Field Therapy & Emotional Freedom Technique (New York, London). Extensive work experience in industry, schools, psychiatric care (hospitals, day centres), women's refuge, research projects. Fellow researcher at the Fachhochschule (University of Applied Sciences) Oldenburg/Ostfriesland/Wilhelmshaven. She is currently completing her Ph.D. at the C.v.O. Universität Oldenburg; co-leader, organizer and therapist in project against domestic violence. Correspondence concerning her chapter should be addressed to: c.moore@freenet.de

Päivi Pylvänäinen, M.A., DTR, is a Finnish psychologist. She completed her DMT degree at MCP Hahnemann University, Philadelphia, as a Fulbright scholar. In Finland she has worked in vocational rehabilitation and adult outpatient psychiatry. She is also starting her private practice. When writing the present chapter, she was living in Tokyo with her family, mothering her two sons and studying butoh. Correspondence should be addressed to: paivi.pylvanainen@tanssiterapia.fi.

María Gabriela Sbiglio, MCAT, DTR, is a dancer, licensed psychologist, and psychotherapist from Argentina. She graduated with a Masters Degree in dance/ movement therapy from MCP Hahnemann University, Philadelphia, USA. Clinical and research activities she developed in Argentina in the times frame going from 1994-1997/1999-2001 include: working with parents-children- groups in a center for rehabilitation of neurological impaired children; collaborating in government projects for prevention of family violence and running different groups for people with eating disorders, psychosomatic, and post-traumatic stress disorders in private practice. She is currently working in a multidisciplinary clinical setting with neurological and psychological impaired children and teenagers in private practice in Italy, where she lives with her family. Correspondence should be addressed to: gabrielasbiglio@hotmail.com

K. Mark Sossin, Ph.D. is Associate Professor of Psychology at Pace University (NYC), and Clinical Associate Professor of Psychology at the Derner Institute for Advanced Psychological Studies at Adelphi University. He is a clinical psychologist and a child/adolescent- and adult-psychoanalyst. Special areas of interest include early development, nonverbal behavior, and applications of the KMP. He teaches in the post-analytic program in Parent/Infant Toddler Psychotherapy at the New York Freudian Society, and he is a Director of the Parent-Infant/Toddler Research Nursery at Pace. He serves on the editorial boards of the *Journal of Early Childhood and Infant Psychology* and the *Journal of Infant, Child, and Adolescent Psychotherapy*. Coauthor of *The Meaning of Movement: Developmental and Clinical Perspectives of the Kestenberg Movement Profile* (1999). He maintains a private practice in New Hyde Park, NY. Correspondence should be addressed to ksossin@pace.edu

Joachim Weis, Ph.D., is trained in psychology and cognitive behavioral therapy. Head of Department of Psychooncology, Tumor Biology Center Freiburg, Head of the Association for Psychooncology (PSO) of the German Cancer Society (DKG). Member of national and international scientific societies. Work areas: Psychotherapy and research in psycho-oncology, medical psychology, art therapy, rehabilitation, education and training programs for students and medical staff. Correspondence should be addressed to: mannheim@tumorbio.uni-freiburg.de

Helle Winther is Associate Professor and currently completing her Ph.D. at the Institute of Exercise and Sport Sciences, University of Copenhagen. She is a Life Energy Process® group leader in the dance therapy form Dansergia®. Her research focuses on movement psychology, dance therapy, and movement communication. She is also a teacher of dance, movement, communication, and body psychology. Correspondence concerning her chapter should be addressed to: hwinther@ifi.ku.dk.

CONTENTS

FOREWORD

Dance/movement therapy (DMT) has officially come of age -- and this volume edited by colleagues, Sabine C. Koch and Iris Bräuninger, is truly the harbinger of the profession's newest developmental phase. It is an exciting time for the profession as DMT practitioners now span the globe, working with individuals with many conditions, disabilities, and illnesses, as well as, individuals interested in prevention and wellness. In 1972, Bartenieff described DMT as recapturing and reviving the vital role dance played in ancient cultures when community cohesion and the marking of important life transitions were achieved through communal dance.

Modern DMT with its attendant theorizing and training began relatively recently during the last half of the 20th century. In fact, the professionalization of DMT in the U.S. celebrates 40 years in 2006. Considering the recency of the profession, its remarkable international impact offers testament to the continued universal appeal of dance as communication, underscoring Bartenieff's (1972) earlier interpretation. DMT has the power to move individuals to better health and functioning by harnessing the symbolic and communicative essence of dance for individual transformation. Dance is the language of the soul -- the core of our human experience, and in the hands of professionally trained dance therapists, it is an absolutely unique psychotherapy. Because dance/movement therapists are immersed in the language of the body rather than focusing solely on the verbal, their work has characteristics that set it apart from other types of psychotherapy.

Until recently, research in DMT had not kept pace with its development in other areas such as, the proliferation of its applications. The neglect of DMT research is a fact frequently mentioned over the years (Chaiklin, 1968; Politsky, 1995; Berrol, 2001; Higgins, 2001). Happily, this volume demonstrates that research is beginning to bloom in many creative forms via the labors of dance therapists around the world! Contributors to this volume hail from countries as distant from one another as Argentina, Australia, and Denmark, and their equally diverse approaches to research enhance and enrich the literature in DMT. Truly, DMT is embarking on a new phase in which research will play a central part in developing new knowledge and firming its time honored foundations.

There are of course, many arguments that can be put forth about why research is important to dance therapy. These include building a base of evidence to support, inform, or refute theory as mentioned, and providing evidence-based practices to promote better care for clients that can also be used by healthcare administrators to create and maintain access to therapists for clients. Probably the most persuasive argument lies in the challenge dance therapists face every day -- striving to serve their clients to the best of their abilities in environments that may not be ideal for either client or therapist. It requires great focus and dedication to practice DMT. Frequently, healthcare administrators must be convinced that DMT is "real" psychotherapy, and DMT practitioners struggle for recognition within their settings. But dance/movement therapists also must struggle to stay current with developments in the understanding of normal and abnormal human systems. And most importantly, they must continually examine the epistemologies, knowledge, and theories they use. While dance therapists frequently fall into the trap of thinking that research is the key to recognition and job survival (Cruz & Hervey, 2001), it is actually practice that can be most enriched by increased DMT research and dance therapists who bring research thinking to their work.

Dance therapists, like other clinicians, face hazards that can affect their practice by limiting its effects and usefulness. Williams and Irving (1999) described these hazards as: (a) relying on personal knowledge that is not shared and thus difficult to judge for validity; (b) relying on beliefs or emotionally held ideas to the exclusion of facts to the contrary; (c) using constructs loosely rather than using them within a defined theoretical framework; (d) tending to work within a theory and defend it regardless of other evidence; and (e) seeing evaluation or evaluative thinking about practice and theories as criticism.

The real value in DMT research then, is in its potential to change how dance therapists conceptualize and inform their work -- in its potential to reach and inspire practicing dance therapists so that they guard against these hazards to clinical effectiveness. Thinking and feeling clinicians continually strive for valid and reliable therapeutic practices that enrich the lives of clients. Of course, therapists who take an active and involved approach to research are also better armed to support their survivability in changing and competitive healthcare arenas around the world.

I have great respect and hope for this volume that so fully ushers in a new age of global DMT development. My respect is for the dance therapist contributors who have already recognized the value of research to their practices and forged new territory so engagingly presented here. My hope is that this volume entices, interests, and motivates dance/movement therapists around the world to new levels of excitement about and participation in the interface of DMT practice and research.

Robyn Flaum Cruz

REFERENCES

Berrol, C., F. (2000). The Spectrum of Research Options in Dance/Movement Therapy. *American Journal of Dance Therapy, 22(1),* 29-46.

Bartenieff, I. (1972). Dance therapy: A new profession or a rediscovery of an ancient role of the dance? *Dance Scope, Fall/Winter, 6-18.*

Chaiklin, H. (1968). Research and the development of a profession. In *Proceedings of the third annual American Dance Therapy Association conference* (pp. 64-74). Columbia, MD: American Dance Therapy Association.

Cruz, R. F., & Hervey, L. W. (2001). The American Dance Therapy Association research survey. *American Journal of Dance Therapy, 23(2),* 89-118.

Higgins, L. (2001). On the value of conducting dance/movement therapy research. *The Arts in Psychotherapy, 28(3),* 191-195.

Politsky, R. H. (1995). Toward a typology of research in the creative arts therapies. *The Arts in Psychotherapy, 22(4),* 307-314.

Williams, D. I., & Irving J. A. (1999). Symposium: Why are therapists indifferent to research? *British Journal of Guidance & Counseling, 27,* 367-376.

INTRODUCTION

This completely peer reviewed edited volume was born out of a fruitful cooperation of two DMT researchers from Germany.[1] It presents a collection of recent empirical research as well as advances in theoretical work in the field of dance movement therapy (DMT). It compiles research projects that reflect the present state-of-the-art research in dance/movement therapy world wide. This volume joins researchers from five continents and eleven countries. Many of the chapter authors have completed their doctoral dissertation on a DMT-related project and report part of their results in this volume. Others work in research projects of hospitals and universities. Some do both. Most of these projects have been presented at the *1st International Research Colloquium in Dance/Movement Therapy* of the BTD (Berufsverband der Tanztherapeutinnen Deutschlands, e.V.; German Dance Movement Therapy Association) in Hannover, Germany, in February 2004. The great majority of the authors are DMT practitioners and do DMT research in their "spare time". All of them contribute to the state-of-the-art research in dance movement therapy, and thus advance DMT in their field of investigation. Conducting DMT research still means doing pioneering work. It is of special importance to compile ongoing DMT research projects, as they readily contribute to the field's body of knowledge and reveal current trends and developments in the professional field.

Such developments are for instance DMT's advances into the field of somatic medicine, i.e. the work with patients with a medical condition such as cancer, AIDS, or chronic pain, next to the classical fields of application in psychosomatic and psychiatric medicine (Goodill, 2005). Goodill who did her doctoral dissertation on this development and on defining DMT's role within somatic medicine has written an introductory chapter within this framework. The chapters of Bojner Horwitz, Lacour, and Mannheim are directly related to this development and exemplify work with single groups of cancer and pain patients (fibromyalgia).

Another development can be seen under the broader terms of DMT philosophy and theory: DMT and phenomenological approaches have much to contribute to one another (Hill, 2004; Koch, in press; Winther, this volume). Recent interdisciplinary embodiment approaches do relate to DMT-theory in many aspects (Payne, 2006). After many decades under Cartesian doctrine, they acknowledge the central role of body and movement in cognitive and emotional development - ontogenetically and phylogenetically. Likewise, applied fields such as nursing care have much to contribute to DMT and vice versa (Kierr, 2004).

A further trend can be related to research on trauma and trauma treatment. Body psychotherapies have much to offer to trauma treatment. The role of the body and body memory is increasingly emphasized by the most renowned trauma researchers (e.g., van der Kolk, 2003). The chapter of Lumsden provides the theoretical background, the chapters of Sbiglio, and Moore are directly related to trauma treatment. Bräuninger, and Birklein and Sossin worked on stress with subclinical samples.

[1] We would like to thank Robyn F. Cruz for bringing the two of us in contact, facilitating contact to other contributing authors of this volume, for statistical advice and support, and for her continued encouragement of our identities as DMT researchers. We would like to thank Sherry W. Goodill for facilitating contact with other international DMT researchers who have contributed to this edited volume. We would like to thank our families for their patience and support in times of increasing late computer working hours to get this volume together.

The fourth recent trend is an intense learning from developmental processes and research: Nonverbal communication starts when we have not yet even been born. Expression in movement follows its own rules within developmental processes. In DMT, these rules have been made explicit in the work of Judith Kestenberg, who provided a comprehensive system to developmental movement analysis (Kestenberg, 1975, Kestenberg-Amighi et al. 1999). The Kestenberg Movement Profile (KMP) is the most differentiated tool for DMT movement observation and assessment and, due to its high degree of systematization, naturally lends itself to research. An example is the research by Lotan and Yirmiya (2002) on nonverbal-sleeping patterns of toddlers and interaction patterns when parents were present. A number of researchers who contributed to this volume have used the KMP in their work (Birklein & Sossin, Koch, Bräuninger, Mannheim, and Moore, all this volume). And a further trend related to development is the work at the other end of the life span spectrum, i.e. DMT and old age. Hill provides a positive outlook on work with dementia patients showing what is possible in movement therapy when growth had already been given up.

Yet another development is the birth of idiosyncratic research methods rising from DMT creative work, born out of DMT as a living art (Hervey, 2004; Meekums, 1993). Such forms of artistic inquiry are used by Pylvänäinen, Hill, and Winther. Cultural awareness is another trend as exemplified in the chapter of Chang.

There are more international trends and common themes that we invite the reader of this volume to discover while making their way through the book. Publishing this volume to us has two important meanings: it signals to others where we are standing as DMT researchers and where we move towards. It also may signal to other dance/movement therapists that it is not too hard and definitely worth while to do research about their inspiring work with diverse populations in order to advance the field. We hope this volume will reach both aims.

Advances in Dance/Movement Therapy, Theoretical Perspectives and Empirical Findings is divided into four major categories: Part A. Advances in Theory and Fields of Investigation provides a theoretical frame of four chapters serving as advance organizers for subsequent chapters. Part B. Advances in Empirical Studies consists of five chapters that introduce a broad variety of empirical and clinical research projects. Part C. Advances in Nonverbal Child-Parent-Interaction highlights the potential of DMT in nonverbal interaction research from two different perspectives, and Part D. Advances in Single Case and Group Case Studies expands the scope of case studies in innovative areas and contexts. All chapters of this volume have been completely peer reviewed.

The chapter by Sabine C. Koch (Germany) offers insights into the evolving interdisciplinary perspective of embodiment approaches. Embodiment approaches start from the body as the central capacity in cognition (thought/intellect), affect (emotion/mood), and behavior. Embodiment research is based on phenomenological philosophy (Merleau-Ponty, 1960), is empirically anchored in a growing number of scientific disciplines, and is closely related to neuro-scientific evidence and perspectives.

The second chapter focuses on the affective Self and affect regulation. Starting from trauma research literature, Malvern M. Lumsden (Norway) gives an overview on how our self is a body self, and how affect and affect regulation are two central capacities in normal development that can be deeply affected by trauma. Lumsden argues that recent progress in developmental neuroscience and traumatology offers a new theoretical basis for the value of dance movement therapy (DMT). Trauma with complex somatic, emotional, cognitive, and social symptoms, requires complex therapies such as DMT which includes the body level, emotional and aesthetic expression, social interaction, symbol and metaphor. DMT builds upon an extensive training in non-verbal expression and attunement which is invaluable in relating to the core self of the client, an idea which is reflected in many if not all other chapters.

The third chapter by Paivi Pylvänäinen (Finland/Japan) introduces the tripartite model of body-image with its central components of (a) image-properties, (b) body-self, and (c) body-memory (Pylvänäinen, 2003). Image-properties are the subjectively perceived appearance of body. Body-self is the experiencing, and emotional core-self. Body-memory stores the lived experiences and serves as a background for online evaluations of present experiences. The contents of body-memory and image-properties tune the action that the body-self carries out. Together, they constitute the body image and shape it continuously. In an application of artistic inquiry (Hervey, 2004), Pylvänäinen related the model to her own experience in Butoh.

The chapter by Sharon W. Goodill (USA) provides an overview on the use of DMT in treatment of patients with a medical diagnosis, other than psychiatric or psychosomatic. Goodill focuses on the five concepts of vitality, coping (primarily relationship-focused), self-efficacy, body image of illness, and mood (Goodill, 2005) that can serve as important dependent variables in Creative Arts Therapies research designs. Findings suggest that DMT has an important effect on these variables. Goodill explores these concepts from a biopsychosocial and holistic perspective with linkages to and extensions of the existing theory and practice of DMT.

The fifth chapter, the first of part *B. Advances in Empirical Studies,* is contributed by Elana G. Mannheim and Joachim Weis (Germany), who demonstrate with their groups of cancer patients how DMT can be used to reduce depression and anxiety and increase personal well-being and quality of life. The authors discuss dance/movement therapy as a clinical intervention method in oncology rehabilitation in a multi-treatment context (Mannheim & Weis, 2004). Results show significant improvements in quality of life, reduction of anxiety and depression, and increased self-esteem. Even though the results may not be attributed to DMT alone, the qualitative assessments of interviews clearly showed that DMT had a positive influence on coping processes.

In the sixth chapter, Eva Bojner Horwitz (Sweden) introduces DMT research with fibromyalgia patients. She conducted a multi-measure randomized control trial presenting hormonal, emotional, physical and visual status changes in thirty-six female fibromyalgia patients (FMS) who participated in a six months dance movement therapy group. Measurement included biological factors, verbal self-ratings scales, the video interpretation technique (VIT) and self-figure drawings. Results suggest that DMT improved the psychological and physiological function. The VIT and self-figure drawings captured treatment effects that were not evident from verbal scales or reflected in hormone levels. Effects on treatment outcome because of using different assessment techniques were discussed. Bojner Horwitz suggests that the body has its own language and is probably more alert in signalling changes over time, before changes are evident in inner biological hormonal systems after DMT (Bojner Horwitz, 2004).

The following chapter by Iris Bräuninger (Switzerland/Germany) provides an analysis of the group process in twelve short-term DMT groups (N = 97) in order to identify common themes and phases present across all groups. The ten sessions of short-term group DMT programs were closely monitored as part of a major research project, which compared the treatment groups to a wait-listed control condition regarding the improvement of quality of life and the reduction of stress (Bräuninger, 2006). Qualitative data on the group processes were gained from the Intervention-Checklist 2 (ICL2). Bräuninger's findings suggest that across all DMT groups included in the study, there is a correspondence of phases and group process to the group phase model of Bender (2001).

Claire Moore (Germany/United Kingdom) follows with another multidisciplinary research project that evaluated Dance Movement Therapy as a method for the treatment of traumatized clients. She investigated DMT effects on women and children who had experienced domestic violence by analysing questionnaires and documentation, and comparing movement parameters, session notes, and psychometric test results before and after therapy. Moore introduces concepts of body memory and body expression on the basis of a neurophysiological understanding of the body's reactions to trauma. Her study suggests that DMT can positively influence the specific symptoms of abuse because of the body's central capacity in memorizing traumatic incidents.

The ninth chapter by Sabine C. Koch (Germany) investigated the use of rhythms and movement qualities in team communication at the workplace depending on gender and leadership. Her findings suggest that female team leaders differ from male team leaders in use of running-drifting (men > women) and jumping rhythms (women > men), assessed with the Kestenberg Movement Profile (KMP). Female leaders showed more direct and particularly more indirect movement qualities than male leaders. Some findings were not in accordance with the predictions from KMP-theory, such as the higher use of fighting qualities in women. Expectations and double standards theories help explain these counterintuitive findings. Reliability assessment brought mixed results, but enough encouragement for continued research.

Chapter ten of *part C. Advances in Nonverbal Child-Parent-Interaction* by Silvia Birklein and K. Marc Sossin examines nonverbal indices of stress in parent-child interaction patterns with the Kestenberg Movement Profile (KMP) and the connections to established indices of parental stress. The authors focus mainly on three of the KMP diagrams the ones that are most associated with affective experiences, namely tension-flow attributes, bipolar shape-flow and unipolar shape-flow. By this they survey relations among affect-related KMP movement patterns in each parent, each child, and each dyad. Three standardized self-reporting stress questionnaires pertaining to life-, event-, and parenting-stress were additionally presented to assess parents' stress levels. Results give a differentiated insight into the complex relationship between stress and movement for the parent, the child, and each of the 26 parent-child dyads (N=52).

The nonverbal assessment of family violence is the topic of chapter eleven by Maria Gabriela Sbiglio (Italy/Argentina). She applied the Dulicai Nonverbal Assessment of Family Systems to domestic violence prevention in parent child interaction, comparing two sets of families, one with a history of violence and one without a history of violence. The comparison illustrates that the families without a history of violence, shows a wide range of behaviors and more options in their interactions. Families with a history of violence presented more blocking and bonding behaviors. Bonding was not necessarily positive, its valence rather depended on the movement quality used (the "how" of the movement). The results suggest that nonverbal assessment can be a low cost and non-invasive method that may contribute to secondary and tertiary prevention of family violence. Future studies need to develop assessment scales especially designed to detect movement patterns linked to violence in larger and more culturally diverse samples.

Part D. on *Advances in Single Case and Group Case Studies* starts with the chapter by Helle Winther (Denmark) which combines theoretical considerations on movement as primary language with an illustrative case study. Winther discusses body language and expressive energy based on the dance therapy form Dansergia. Using a phenomenological research method, the project explores the potential of movement for personal development and its application to therapy.

Chapter thirteen by Heather Hill (Australia) introduces the reader into dance therapy's experiential meaning for people with dementia. She integrates DMT into the context of dementia care, specifically person-centered care. Movement-, verbal-, and video-based analyses of four individual dance therapy sessions illustrate Hill's theoretical considerations. Hill expands the purely biomedical view of dementia and its impact on the person by means of adding the dimension of the "lived body" concluding that DMT can contribute to maintain and strengthen personhood in person-centered care.

Maria Eugenia Lacour (Argentina) presents a report of a 3-year dance movement therapy work with adult cancer patients in chapter fourteen. She integrates quantitative and qualitative methods. The first part depicts a long-term intervention process of 3 years during the treatment time when DMT was provided to the patients with the aim to improve quality of life (QoL), immune system (IS), and to ease patients' way through the crisis. The second part of the chapter focuses on a short-term intervention of 9 weeks when DMT was offered to oncology patients after treatment as a useful resource for social recovery. The author concludes that more dance therapists are needed to offering their skills and knowledge of the body-mind connection to the growing population of cancer patients. The study suggests that DMT is an effective resource for oncology patients during and after treatment, providing enhancement of quality of life, of adherence to treatment and, in remission stage, of social recovery. A somatically and expressively oriented psychosocial intervention, DMT is an important rehabilitation tool for a program of comprehensive patient care in oncology treatment.

The chapter by Meg Chang (USA) reflects on the cultural, ethnic, and racial identity of dance movement therapists and their clients, and the implications for DMT training. She discusses how clinicians' intercultural empathy with clients from diverse backgrounds could be enhanced in practical DMT work. Focusing on the relationships among intercultural education, and personal and social identity, Chang critically examined the educational and psychological theories that underlie DMT practice.

This book presents a truly international scope on DMT research. Authors from five continents have participated and shared their research findings and methods here. We hope to inspire others to follow up on this research collection. To do a dissertation in dance movement therapy is a stony path. To date, there are still no official genuine PhD studies anywhere in the world in DMT. Thus, people with a scientific passion for DMT research mostly do a PhD in psychology, educational science, medicine, or related field. Many of them "get lost" to new fields of research on this way. Some return. Some never leave and stay with their initial research questions, shaping and differentiating them on the way. All know: The field's body of knowledge and scientific advances need to be made explicit and readily available. This is a beginning.

Sabine Koch, Heidelberg (Germany)
& Iris Bräuninger, Zürich (Switzerland)

REFERENCES

Bender, S. (2001). Lasst die Gruppe tanzen, Teil 2[Let the group dance, Part 2]. *Zeitschrift für Tanztherapie, 8(13)*, 3-11.

Bojner Horwitz, E., Theorell, T., & Anderberg, U.M. (2004). New technique for assessment of clinical condition in fibromyalgia -- a pilot study by video-interpretation. *The Arts in Psychotherapy, 31*, 153-164.

Bräuninger, I. (2006). *Tanztherapie. [Dance Therapy].* Weinheim, Germany: Beltz / PVU.

Goodill, S.W. (2005). *An Introduction to Medical Dance/Movement Therapy: Health care in motion.* London: Jessica Kingsley.

Hervey, L.W. (2004). Artistic Inquiry in Dance/Movement Therapy. In R. Cruz & C. Berrol (Eds.). *Dance/Movement Therapists in action. A working guide to research options* (pp. 181-205). Springfield, IL: Charles C. Thomas.

Hill, H. (2004). *Talking the talk but not walking the walk. Barriers to person centred care in dementia.* Online publication of dissertation, available at http://www.lib.latrobe.edu.au/thesis/public/adt-LTU20041215.100826/index.html

Kestenberg, J.S. (1975). *Parents and Children. Psychoanalytic studies in development.* New York: Jason Aronson.

Kestenberg-Amighi, J., Loman, S., Lewis, P., & Sossin, K. M. (1999). *The meaning of movement. Developmental and clinical perspectives of the Kestenberg Movement Profile.* Amsterdam: Gordon and Breach.

Kierr, S. (2004). Dance Movement Therapy and Nursing Care. In C.L. le Navenec & L. Bridges (Eds.). *Creating connections between nursing care and the creative arts therapies: expanding the concept of holistic care.* Springfield, IL: Charles C. Thomas.

Koch, S.C. (in press). Theoretical Perspectives in Dance/Movement Therapy: A Vision for the Future. In Brooke, S.L. (Ed.). *Handbook of the Creative Arts Therapies: History, theories, methods and applications.* Springfield, IL: Charles C. Thomas.

Lotan, N. & Yirmiya, N. (2002). Body movement, presence of parents and the process of falling asleep in toddlers. *International Journal of Behavioral Development, 26*(1), 81-88.

Mannheim, E., & Weis, J. (2004). Dance/Movement Therapy as a clinical intervention method in oncological rehabilitation. First results of an evaluation of treatment effects. *Journal of Cancer Research and Clinical Oncology, Supplement to Volume 130*, Scientific Proceedings (Abstracts), p. 23, Heidelberg: Springer.

Meekums, B. (1993). Research as an act of creation. In H. Payne (Ed.). *Handbook of inquiry in the art therapies. One river, many currents* (pp. 130-137). London: Jessica Kingsley.

Merleau-Ponty, M. (1962). *Phenomenology of perception.* London: Routeledge.

Payne, H. (2006). *Dance Movement Therapy. Theory, Research and Practice* (2nd ed.). London: Routledge.

van der Kolk, B.A. (2003). Posttraumatic stress disorder and the nature of trauma. In M. F. Solomon & D. J. Siegel (Ed.). *Healing trauma. Attachment, mind, body, and brain* (pp. 168–195). New York & London: Norton.

INTERDISCIPLINARY EMBODIMENT APPROACHES. IMPLICATIONS FOR CREATIVE ARTS THERAPIES

Sabine C. Koch

The chapter introduces interdisciplinary embodiment approaches from anthropology, linguistics, and psychology and relates them to creative arts therapies. It particularly focuses on the role of the body proper, body motion, basic dimensions of movement, body memory, and gender, fields that lie at the intersection of cognitive sciences and dance/movement therapy. It is argued that the body may be the place where the usefulness of the computer metaphor ends. The potential and limitations of the embodiment perspective in relation to the creative arts therapies are discussed.

Keywords: Embodiment, human movement, body memory, creative arts therapy research, dance/movement therapy

"Well, what do you think you understand with? With your head? Bah!" (from Nikos Kazantzakis'
"Zorba the Greek", cited after Andy Clark, 1997, p. 9)

Creative arts therapies (CATs), i.e. dance, music, art, drama, and poetry therapy, have acquired increasing acceptance and application in recent years. The professional fields are prospering internationally, accompanied by numerous qualitative research studies and a smaller number of outcome studies, which altogether almost unanimously support CATs' effectiveness. CATs work well for all clients for whom the verbal channel is not the primary means of expression. In dance/movement therapy (DMT) for example, if indicated, "assessment and therapy can proceed entirely in the nonverbal realm of movement, touch, rhythm, and spatial interaction" (Goodill, 2005, p. 16). It has, however, continuously been emphasized that it remains unclear how exactly creative arts therapy interventions work. New findings in neuroscience and cognitive science increasingly shed light on the mechanisms underlying CAT. Some embodiment approaches go so far as to proclaim a paradigmatic change in favour of the inclusion of the phenomenal, lived, subjective body into behavioural sciences' major theorizing.

RECONCILIATION OF BODY AND MIND

Creative arts therapists have always assumed the union of body and mind as a basic underlying principle of their work (e.g., Loman & Brandt, 1992), even though -- lacking a more adequate vocabulary -- they still have been talking about the two realms as two separate capacities. On the basis of their clinical practice, for them self and world are interconnected, and the mind speaks through the body in numerous ways. Conversely, only now are the cognitive sciences on the verge of reconciling the body and the mind. This new trend is reflected in the emerging embodiment approaches.

Descartes (1596-1650) most clearly formulated the separation of body and mind for the sake of the emerging bio-medical sciences being able to do research on and with the body, expelling the mind from "the hard sciences" to the realm of philosophy and theology. The heritage of Cartesian dualism has taught us to think in dichotomies, and to value them as scientific ways of looking at life. Scientific psychology has adapted much of this belief to develop its own theories and methods. Finally, at the turn of the millennium, the body-mind problem has reached cognitive psychology as a serious topic of empirical investigation. Ever since Merleau-Ponty's groundbreaking work on the ontological and epistemological meaning of the body for our human condition (Merleau-Ponty, 1962), the reconciliation of body and mind emerged in many scientific disciplines. Merleau-Ponty (1962) wanted us to start from the experience of authentic perception. Asking where perception begins, he then answered, in the body. The body is in the world from the beginning and phenomenology as the descriptive science of existential beginnings leads Merleau-Ponty to describe the body as a "general power of inhabiting all the environments, which the world contains." (Merleau-Ponty, 1962, p.311). In philosophy the problem of embodiment has further been treated by Richard Zaner (1964; reflecting on the philosophical contributions of Marcel, Sartre, and Merleau-Ponty) and lately by Fuchs (2000) and Hurley (1998).

This chapter provides an overview of the interdisciplinary embodiment theories that have developed in the tradition of Merleau-Pontys philosophical-phenomenological approach. With them, a more holistic, and systemic thinking came into the sciences. Embodied theories have their roots in philosophy, neurosciences, medical anthropology and cognitive linguistics, but nowadays also include artificial intelligence research, arts and art-related research, communication research, dynamic systems approaches, educational sciences, linguistics and language-related research, psychology, robotics, sociology, sports, and other fields. One of the main characteristics of embodiment theories is that they take the body as the existential ground for perception and action; they collapse such dualisms as body and mind, subject and object (Sax, 2002), perception and conception (e.g., Lakoff & Johnson, 1999), and perception and action (e.g., Hurley, 1998; v. Weizsäcker, 1940/1996). They assume a perceptual, modality-specific way of knowledge representation (as opposed to an abstract, symbolic way), a way that leads via the sensory-motor system and uses this system for thinking through embodied simulations (Barsalou, 1999; Barsalou, Niedenthal, Barbey, & Ruppert, 2003; Gallese, 2003; Glenberg, 1997). Embodiment approaches are furthermore closely related to approaches of situated cognition (e.g., dependency of cognition on cultural context) and dynamic systems approaches (e.g., Thelen, 1995) in fact overarching literature speaks of humans as situated, embodied, dynamical agents (cf. Beer, 2000). Whether embodiment approaches offer a simple shift in cognitive psychology or a full paradigmatic change remains to be determined (cf. Clark, 1999).

This chapter focuses on theoretical developments in anthropology, linguistics, and psychology. Within psychology it introduces the subdisciplines where embodiment approaches presently emerge, and addresses connections to and future directions in creative arts therapies research.

EMBODIED COGNITION: EMBODIMENT APPROACHES IN ANTHROPOLOGY AND COGNITIVE LINGUISTICS

Anthropological Perspectives: Human Nature and Culture are Grounded in the Body

"The locus of the sacred is the body, for the body is the existential ground of culture." (Csordas, 2002, p.87).

One of the early precursors of embodiment theories was Margret Lock's and Nancy Scheper-Hughes' widely quoted article "The mindful body" (1987), transmitting a medical anthropological analysis in order to "problematize the body (...) by investigating the lived experience of the individual body-self and its interwovenness with the social and the political body" (Lock & Scheper-Hughes, 1987; p.6).

Shortly after Lock and Scheper-Hughes, Thomas Csordas published his influential article "Embodiment as a Paradigm for Anthropology" (1988; here quoted from the reprint in 2002). To successfully confront the "hard sciences", in his view, it is necessary to formulate a "science of subjectivity" (and he quotes Shweder, 1986; p.178, here) "the real world it seems is populated with subject-dependent and object-like subjectivity, two types of phenomena for which there is no place in the mutually exclusive and exhaustive realms of the symbol-and-meaning-seeking hermeneuticist and the automated-law-seeking positivist." (Csordas, 2002, p.86). Csordas suspects that "embodiment has paradigmatic scope" for example for the dissolution of dichotomies, such as cognition and emotion. Andrew Strathern in "Body Thoughts" (1996) continues this line of thought. Strathern (1996) asserts that the term embodiment has reached the status of a major concept in cultural analysis. Yet, in his view it is not enough to switch from one side of the Cartesian dichotomy to the other. It might, however, be a necessary step in the process to a more adequate conceptualization. Creative arts therapies work within and between body/mind. For instance, in searching with the patient for an adequate metaphor as an anchor that allows them to work toward health.

Linguistic Perspectives: Concepts and Language are Grounded in the Body

„Our ability to move in the ways we do and to track the motions of other things gives motion a major role in our conceptual system. The fact that we have muscles and use them to apply force in certain ways leads to the structure of our system of causal concepts. What is important is not just that we have bodies and that thought is somehow embodied. What is important is that the peculiar nature of our bodies shapes our very possibilities for conceptualization and categorization". (Lakoff & Johnson, 1999, p.19)

In their 1999 book "Philosophy in the Flesh" Lakoff and Johnson define an embodied concept as "a neural structure that is actually part of, or makes use of, the sensorimotor system of our brains. Much of the conceptual inference is, therefore, sensorimotor inference" and not just preceded by or followed by sensorimotor inference (Lakoff & Johnson, 1999, p. 20). They state that the embodied mind hypothesis radically undercuts the distinction between perception and conception. In an embodied mind, the same neural systems engaged in perception or in motion play a central role in conceptualization and reasoning. This implies that *movement is a direct part of reasoning*. Lakoff and Johnson emphasize that replacing traditional disembodied with embodied concepts is a gain for science, and how it is in line with the most recent neuroscience and cognitive findings. In their view, traditional scientific thought misses that *"what has always made science possible, is our embodiment, not our transcendence of it, and our imagination, not our avoidance of it."* (Lakoff & Johnson, 1999, p.93). It is exactly the human embodiment, the human experience, and the use of metaphor and imagination that makes science possible. The authors' theory on metaphor as a central human capacity could benefit from creative arts therapists knowledge on how metaphor on a nonverbal body-level and art-related level is part of that capacity.

TABLE I: OVERVIEW OF MAJOR EMBODIMENT THEORIES

Major Embodiment Approaches (Overview)		
Philosophy	Merleau-Ponty, 1962 Hurley, 1998	Perception is grounded in the body Unity of perception and action
Anthropology	Lock & Scheper-Huges, 1987	The phenomenal body

	Csordas, 1988, 2002	Culture is grounded in the body
Linguistics	Lakoff & Johnson, 1999	Concepts are grounded in the body Language/metaphor is grounded in the body Unity of perception and conception
Neurosciences	Gallese, 2003	Embodied Cognition/Simulation
Artificial Intelligence	Clark, 1997	Intellect/being is grounded in the body
Psychology	Varela, Thompson & Rosch, 1991	The embodied mind
Social Psychology	Barsalou, Niedenthal et al., 2003 Niedenthal et al., 2005	Cognition is grounded in the body Attitudes/emotions are grounded in the body
Memory Research	Glenberg, 1997	Memory is grounded in the body
Developmental Psych.	Thelen, 1995; 2000	Development is grounded in the body Primacy of Motion

THE ROLE OF BODY AND MOVEMENT: EMBODIMENT APPROACHES IN PSYCHOLOGY

Cognitive Psychology and Neurosciences: Cognition and Emotion are Grounded in the Body

"We explicitly call into question the assumption -prevalent throughout cognitive science- that cognition consists of the representation of a world that is independent of our perceptual and cognitive capacities by a cognitive system that exists independently of the world. We outline instead a view of cognition as embodied action". (Varela, Thompson, & Rosch, 1991, p. XX)

Varela, Thompson and Rosch (1991) were the first authors to introduce embodiment approaches into cognitive psychology. Their approach is revolutionary. They state that cognitive science has hardly brought forth any applicable knowledge, and therefore it was time to change this trend. Since their original work, embodied mind theories gain influence in the context of explaining situated social cognition and behavior (e.g., Jeannerod, 1997; Niedenthal, Barsalou, Winkielman, Krauth-Gruber, & Ric, 2005). Action simulation is an integral part of embodiment theorizing. Empirical evidence for action simulation comes from Rizzolatti, Fadiga, Fogassi, & Gallese (2002) study on "mirror neurons" and subsequent research into similar "hard wired evidence". Rizzolatti et al. (2002) have shown that in apes observation of a grasping movement, led to the same activation in motor centers that in the individual that was actually performing the grasp, just less strong. Hormonal and endocrinal findings also suggest convergent evidence for the central relevance of the body as an organ of perception, internal communication, memory, and other human capacities (cf. Pert, 1997). Meanwhile a strong body of convergent evidence has accumulated in favor of cognitive simulations while perceiving motor activity (Barsalou, 1999), of the interconnectedness between perception and action (Hurley, 1998), on the sensory-motor qualities of thought, shown by the activation of the same sensory-motor pathways while thinking about the activity as if actually performing the activity (Gallese, 2003; Rizzolatti et al., 2002). For CATs this means evidence for functional mechanisms in relaxation and mental imagery exercises.

Developmental Psychology: Human Development is Grounded in the Body

The notion that development is grounded in the body is not new, ever since Piaget's influential work, it is the state-of-the-art knowledge and the ground that cognitive developmental psychology builds upon. However, there have been a number of outstanding theorists lately whose names are related to the new embodiment approaches, particularly: Ester Thelen. Thelen describes the dynamics and situatedness of human development and human motion in infant stepping ability (Thelen and Smith, 1994; Thelen, 1995; 2000; similarly, Kelso, 1996, for adult rhythmic finger motions). She found evidence for the influence of motor behavior on the cognitive and affective development of the young infant. She writes about rhythms as fundamental properties of infant movement. Nava Lotan a DMT researcher from Israel adapted Thelen's new approaches for her work on behavior patterns of small children with the Kestenberg Movement Profile (Lotan & Yirmiya, 2002).

Additionally, Barbara Tversky (2002) points out that bodies are special kinds of categories integral to all our perceptions. She reports own and other's findings that support the critical function of the body and of body motion in human development. Bryant, Tversky, and Franklin (1992) hypothesized that reaction times would be correlated with the degree of mental rotation needed to face an object. The results, however, were contrary to the hypothesis. Subjects responded fastest to objects located on the head/feet axis, followed by the front/back axis, followed by the left/right axis. Tversky argues that these results follow from using a "spatial framework" that is sensitive to environmental asymmetries (such as gravity) and perceptual asymmetries (we generally look and attend to the front). In other words, retrieval processes seem to be sensitive to how we use our bodies, and in this case related to the movement planes.

In a similar vein, Pauen and Träuble (2002), two developmental psychologists specialized in early infant cognition, describe the *primacy of motion* in human cognitive development. Motion perception is a basic cognitive process. The ability to distinguish animate from inanimate objects is one of the first cognitive functions we acquire in life (Pauen & Träuble, 2002). To recognize intention from motion is psychologically and evolutionarily important at the most elementary level of social cognition (Blythe, Todd, & Miller, 1999; Krämer, 2001). Motion is a major cue to infer intentions and motivations, and to make causal attributions (Heider, 1958; Heider & Simmel, 1944).

Social- and Language-Psychology: Social Cognition, Emotion, and Interaction are Grounded in the Body

"Ago ergo cogito – I act, therefore I think" (Glenberg, 2005)

Preverbal motor development does not happen in the individual space, but in the interpersonal space. We are social beings and social psychology has contributed a new line of body-based research culminating in the *social embodiment approach* of Barsalou, Niedenthal, Barbey, and Ruppert (2003). By *embodiment* Barsalou et al. (2003) mean that "states of the body, such as postures, arm movements, and facial expressions, arise during social interaction and play central roles in social information processing" (Barsalou et al., 2003, p. 43). Social information processing means cognitive processing (or thinking) related to social situations. Four types of embodiment effects have been reported by social psychologists. First, perceived social stimuli next to cognitive states produce bodily states as well. Second, perceiving bodily states in others produces bodily mimicry in the self. Third, bodily states in the self produce affective states. Fourth, the compatibility of bodily states and cognitive states modulates performance effectiveness (Barsalou et al., 2003). Movement therapists might be strongly reminded of the empathy theory of Theodor Lipps (1903; cf. Wallbott, 1991) for the first three types of findings. The social embodiment approach bundles single empirical results and other body-based research strings and propose an alternative theoretical account for the workings of mind and memory with reference to recent results in the neurosciences. Embodiment theories offer a new view on knowledge representation. While traditional theories assume that a symbolic system "redescribes" sensory, motor, and introspective states, resulting in amodal descriptions, embodied theories of cognition proclaim the following:

> "embodied theories represent knowledge as partial simulations of sensory, motor, and introspective states (...). When an event is experienced originally, the underlying sensory, motor, and introspective states are partially stored. Later, when knowledge of the event becomes relevant in memory, language, or thought, these original states are partially simulated. Thus, remembering an event arises from partially simulating the sensory, motor, and introspective states active at the time. (...) Depending on the situation, embodiment may range from simulation, to traces of execution, to full-blown execution. (...) these embodiments are not merely peripheral appendages (...) of social information processing - they constitute the core of it. (Barsalou et al., 2003, p. 44).

Most embodiment effects are unconscious and occur automatically (Dijksterhuis & Bargh, 2001). Wilson (2002) and Niedenthal et al. (2005) distinguish online and offline embodiment. Online embodiment refers to a present situated embodiment effect where cognitive activity operates directly on real-world environments or vice versa. Offline embodiment refers to effects from memory, where cognitive activity that is de-coupled from real-world environments. For example, sitting in the classroom being called upon by the teacher and not knowing the answer to any of her questions might cause cold sweat, a dry throat, gaze aversion, and an increased heart rate (online). Imagining this situation may have the same bodily effects (offline). This distinction has implications for CAT work with traumatized patients.

A theory of embodied memory has been suggested by Arthur Glenberg (1997). Glenberg started from the open research question of how language conveys meaning and suggests that linguistic meaning is grounded in bodily activity. Glenberg and Kaschak (2002) found that participants were faster at judging the meaning of a sentence when it was compatible with the hand movement required for the response (e.g., "close the drawer" with forward movement; "open the drawer" with backward movement). This action-sentence compatibility effect occurred even when the sentences referred to abstract actions that involved directional communication (i.e., participants were fastest in judging the sentence "You told Liz the story" with a forward movement and the sentence "Liz told you the story" with a backward movement). These findings are consistent with the claim that language comprehension is grounded in bodily action, and are inconsistent with abstract symbol theories of meaning.

Clinical Psychology and Psychotherapy: Healing is Grounded in the Body

Clinical practice is increasingly involved with nonverbal techniques, basically without being conversant of their explicit way of working (e.g., EMDR, NLP, body feedback, mirroring, passing, etc.). Authors such as Damasio (1994/1999), LeDoux (1996), and Schore (1994) have indicated important directions in clinical thinking. There is, however, no explicit embodiment approach in clinical psychology and psychotherapy research. Even though the saluto-genetic approach (Antonovsky, 1997) and trauma-related approaches (e.g., van der Kolk, 2003) are closely linked to concerns in embodiment and creative arts therapies (Koch, in press). CAT research could be contributing to understand the common principles at work behind all therapies by looking at the therapeutic intervention techniques applied by therapists of any school, and organizing them along the lines of embodiment theories.

Evidence for clinical relevance of embodiment research is presently again coming from social psychological research: Piotr Winkielmann from the University of California St. Barbara compared autistic subjects to typical subjects (Winkielman, 2005). On the basis of the mirror neuron theory and the amygdala theory to explaining autism, he finds that particularly social mirroring is impaired in autists (McIntosh, Reichmann-Decker, Winkielman, & Wilbarger, 2005). The treatment implied by this research is the use of mirroring interventions to create reciprocity, interventions dance therapists have been using ever since they worked with autists (Adler, 1969). This DMTs specific autism treatment is now finally science based.

Three Examples for Research Applications

1. Embodiment and Basic Dimensions of Motion

Social psychology has just started to investigate basic embodiment dimensions and their psychological meaning. The *movement planes* for example have been addressed in latest psychological research by Schubert (in press) in which the vertical plane is related to power, and by Boroditsky (2001) in which the sagittal plane is related to time.

The *bi-directionality of affect/cognition and motor behavior* has been investigated since research on the *body feedback hypotheses* suggested that the incorporation of distinct facial expressions or postures leads to distinct emotions or evaluations (see Hatfield, Cacioppo, & Rapson, 1994). This line of research supports that next to emotions and cognitions causing certain motor behaviors and bodily expressions, *certain motor behaviors cause certain emotions and cognitions.* The notion of bidirectionality of affect/cognition and motor behavior supports the basic maxim according to which CATs have been working from the beginning of the profession. Yet, only recently has research in social psychology rendered empirical evidence that confirms this assumption.

Research working on the specific embodiment effect of *approach and avoidance motor behavior* on attitude formation (Cacioppo, Priester, & Berntson, 1993; Neumann & Strack, 2000) can be directly related to the DMT concept of *Shape* and *Shape-Flow.* Cacioppo, Priester and Berntson (1993) placed participants at a table and asked them while studying arbitrary Chinese signs (written in Chinese script) to either activate the flexor or the extensor of their arm muscles by pressing against their table either from below or from above (from the table surface). The resulting movement was thus either an approach or an avoidance movement, either towards the body or away from the body. Those signs that had been studied while pulling the arms towards the body were later judged as significantly more positive, than the signs that had been studied while pushing against the table. This finding is consistent with other "motor congruency effects" (Förster & Strack, 1996). For a dance/movement therapist, parallels to shape-flow and shaping stand out (Laban, 1960; Laban & Lawrence, 1974). The findings of

Cacioppo et al. (1993) are directly supporting KMP theory about unipolar shape flow (Kestenberg-Amighi, Loman, Sossin, & Lewis, 1999; Kestenberg & Sossin, 1979; Kestenberg, 1995) that offers a classification system for attraction and repulsion motion toward and away from objects.

2. Body Memory

Merleau-Ponty (1962) has almost entirely spared the issue of body memory from his otherwise very exhaustive discussion of the body's role in perception. The philosopher who has taken on the challenge of treating the topic of body memory was Edward T. Casey (1987; cf. Pylvänäinen, 2003, and this volume). Casey defines body memory as "memory that is intrinsic to the body, to its own ways of remembering: how we remember in and by and through the body." He emphasizes the tacit and non-deliberate nature of such memory. In fact, body memory is so much part of the ground of our experience that the topic has been ignored from the ancient Greeks to Kant. Casey distinguishes habitual body memory, traumatic body memory, and erotic body memory. Habitual body memory becomes salient when it is disrupted, such as when one gets a new keyboard for the typewriter and finds oneself in a "state of disorientation" at first. What Casey calls habitual body memory has much in common with what cognitive psychology calls implicit memory. For Casey body memory is located both in the objective, material body (fibers and tissues; cf. Pringer, 1995/2005) and in the phenomenal, lived body (after *Leib* in Husserl). "Because it re-enacts the past, it need not represent it; (…) body memory includes its own past by an internal osmotic intertwining with it." (Casey, 1987, p.88). As Fuchs (2004) writes

> "*body memory mediates the basic experience of familiarity and continuity in the succession of events. It unburdens us from the necessity to constantly find our bearings again. Bodily learning means to forget what we have learned or done explicitly, and to let it sink into implicit, unconscious knowing. By this we acquire the skills and dispositions of perceiving and acting that make up our very personal way of being in the world. We might also say: What we have forgotten has become what we are. (Fuchs, 2004, p.3).*

In contrast to memory categories of cognitive psychology, such as autobiographic memory only representing the past as the past, body memory mediates the living presence of the past. It is therefore the essential basis of the self. As such it can be found entirely intact in dancing, singing, or sculpting with a demented patient. Fuchs notes *"Freedom and art are essentially based on the tacit memory of the body." (Fuchs, 2004, p.3).*

Evidence in neuroscientific research is accumulating that active remembering, such as the recall of representations or mental imagery, activates sensory (e.g., Wheeler, Peterson, & Buckner, 2000) as well as motor responses (e.g., Nyberg, Pertersson, Nilsson, Sandbloom, Aberg, & Ingwar, 2001), and that in fact, sensory and motor processing is more intimately linked than ever assumed (Tucker & Ellis, 1998).

3. Embodiment and Gender

Research is just starting to explore what differential implication embodiment views have on the cognition and affect of men and women. Warren Lamb has worked on gender differences in motion (Lamb, 1965; Davies, 2001). Recent findings from embodiment research suggest, for instance, power related differences. Schubert (2004) found that making a fist had different implications on cognition and emotions of women and men. It influenced their automatic processing of words related to the concept of power.

Embodiment theories are closely related to gender issues. As we increasingly investigate embodiment we will also increasingly move to an understanding on the different forms of embodiment in men, women, gays, transsexuals, etc. Development of sex roles is necessarily intertwined with cognitive development, and both are grounded in the body. It remains up to future research to start looking at the implication gender has on embodiment (and vice versa). An example of recent research relating gender and artificial intelligence comes from Alison Adam (2002). Starting out to investigate the role of the body in the generation of knowledge, Adam offers a critique of artificial intelligence research and embodiment in artificial life. She points out that the specificities of gender (and other embodied variations; the author) cannot be adequately addressed with methods such as computer simulations.

Outstanding Questions

Is the world centerless and is it just we searching for a center, an inner organizer (that some may call god, some may call theory, some may call metaphor, some may call psyche, some may call mind). Is it just we in search of sense and meaning (cf. Heider, 1958), contingency, and predictability, that is not objectively there but merely constructed (by categorization, dichotomization, attribution)? Or is the existential ground given in form of our bodies?

Does this existential ground bereave us humans of our special position in the universe?

Can we explain all perceptual and memory phenomena on the grounds of embodiment or are embodiment theories just a constraint for specific cases? I.e., is the sensory-motor simulation occurring in all cases or are there still other forms of processing information and of being? Is embodiment a new paradigm that will replace cognitive science or will it find its place as a part of it?

In the progression from cognitive sciences to embodied sciences, the mind is increasingly viewed as part of the body. There are at present many attempts to find the neurological, endocrinological, hormonal, etc. traces of the mind or consciousness. Is this the return to a disenchanted view on life? Or is it, on the contrary, a reconciliation of the century-long analytical separation of body, mind, and world?

CONCLUSIONS

Embodiment approaches offer new scientific perspectives for creative arts therapies. Most embodiment approaches compile empirical results that are suited to support CAT practice, to stimulate CAT research, and to explain how CAT work. Particularly, the cognitive science model of modality specific knowledge representation (Barsalou et al., 2003) lays a foundation for CAT theory development and provides a rationale for CATs functioning. Topics of CAT relevance that thus far have been standing isolated such as body memory, basic movement dimensions, or body and gender can be tied to embodiment theories and find their place in a broader scientific framework.

Embodiment approaches claim that the typical partition of the cognitive system into a variety of neural or functional subsystems is often misleading. It blinds us to the possibility of alternative, more explanatory categories that cut across the traditional body/mind/world division (cf. Clark, 1997). For cognitive science this means that researchers need to critically rethink their subject matter. For creative arts therapists with their more holistic approach their task will be to diligently and thoroughly formulate their embodiment ideas and make them available to other scientific communities and outlets. The potential is a better visibility and a more explicit formulation of CATs theory in the light of a new paradigm. The danger of the embodiment view is a too explicit and one-sided focus on the body as mentioned above. Nevertheless, all cognition and affect can be conceptualized as embodied and grounded in the body and is describable in terms of its functions. Mind and body are not two entities related to each other but a living inseparable whole.

Embodiment approaches strengthen the theoretical underpinnings of the bodily basis of thought and affect. Theories of embodied cognition attribute new scientific value to experience-based approaches and validate major theoretical assumptions in DMT and CATs. In turn, DMT and CATs can offer their well-developed assessments and experience-based knowledge to provide these theories with a higher degree of exactness and differentiation. One starting point is the investigation of basic dimensions of motion and their dynamic feedback on cognition and affect. This research will be relevant to our fields wherever the manipulation of movement is intended for the promotion of health, improvement of symptoms, or freedom from symptoms. This applies to DMT, all other creative art therapies, all forms of body psychotherapies, and physiotherapy. All of them work with the body as an instrument of resonance and central relevance.

REFERENCES

Adam, A. (2002). Gender/Body/Machine. *Ratio, 15,* 354-389.

Adler, J. (1969). *Looking for me.* A film documenting Adler's work with autistic children. Center for Media and Independent Learning, 2000 Center Street, Berkely, CA, 94704.

Antonovsky, A. (1997). *Salutogenese: zur Entmystifizierung der Gesundheit* [Salutogenesis: The demystification of health]. Tübingen: DGVT.

Barsalou, L.W., Niedenthal, P.M., Barbey, A.K., & Ruppert, J.A. (2003). Social Embodiment. In B. H. Ross (Ed.), *The psychology of learning and motivation: Vol. 43* (pp. 43-92). San Diego, CA: Academic Press.

Barsalou, L.W. (1999). Perceptual symbol systems. *Behavioral and Brain Sciences, 22,* 577-660.

Beer, R.D. (2000). Dynamical Approaches to cognitive sciences. *Trends in Cognitive Sciences, 4,* 91-99.

Blythe, P.W., Todd, P.M., & Miller, G.F. (1999). How motion reveals intention. Categorizing social interactions. In G. Gigerenzer, P. Todd, & the ABC Research Group (Eds.). *Simple heuristics that make us smart* (pp. 256-285). Oxford: Oxford University Press.

Boroditsky, L. (2001). Does language shape thought? Mandarin and English speakers' conceptions of time. *Cognitive Psychology, 43,* 1-22.

Bryant, D. J., Tversky, B., & Franklin, N. (1992). Internal and external spatial frameworks for representing described scenes. *Journal of Memory and Language, 31,* 74–98.

Cacioppo, J.T., Priester, J.R., & Berntson, G. (1993). Rudimentary determinants of attitudes II: Arm flexion and extension have differential effects on attitudes. *Journal of Personality and Social Psychology, 65,* 5-17.

Casey, E. S. (1987). *Remembering: A phenomenological study.* Bloomington: Indiana University Press.

Clark, A. (1997). *Being There. Putting brain, body and world together again.* Cambridge: MIT Press.

Clark, A. (1999). An embodied cognitive science. *Trends in Cognitive Science, 3,* 345-351.

Csordas, T.J. (2002). *Body Meaning Healing.* New York: Palgrave MacMillan.

Damasio, A.R. (1994). *Descartes' error: Emotion, reason, and the human brain.* New York: Putnam.

Damasio, A.R. (1999). *The feeling of what happens: Body and emotion in the making of consciousness.* Orlando, FL: Harcourt Brace.

Davies, Eden (2001). Beyond dance. Laban's legacy of movement analysis. London: Brechin.

Dijksterhuis, A., & Bargh, J.A. (2001). The perception-behavior expressway: Automatic effects of social perception on social behavior. In M.P. Zanna (Ed.), *Advances in Experimental Social Psychology: Vol. 33* (pp. 1-40). San Diego, CA: Academic Press.

Förster, J., & Strack, F. (1996). Influence of overt head movements on memory for valenced words: A case of conceptual-motor compatibility. *Journal of Personality and Social Psychology, 71,* 421-430.

Fuchs, T. (2000). *Leib Raum Person.* Stuttgart: Klett-Cotta.

Fuchs, T. (2004). *The Memory of the Body.* Unpublished Manuscript.

Gallese, V. (2003). The manifold nature of interpersonal relations. The quest for a common mechanism. *Philosophical Transcripts of the Royal Society of London, 358,* 517-528.

Glenberg, A.M. (1997). What memory is for. *Behavioral and Brain Sciences, 20*, 1-55.

Glenberg, A.M., & Kaschak, M.P. (2002). Grounding language in action. *Psychonomic Bulletin & Review, 9,* 558-565.

Glenberg, A. (2005). *Laboratory for embodied cognition. http://psych.wisc.edu/glenberg/glenberglab/GLindex. html* Retreived 05/03/05

Goodill, S.W. (2005). *An Introduction to Medical Dance/Movement Therapy. Healthcare in Motion.* Philadelphia: Jessica Kingsley Publishers.

Hatfield, E., Cacioppo, J.T., & Rapson, R.L. (1994). *Emotional contagion.* Paris: Cambridge University Press.

Heider, F. (1958). *The Psychologie of Interpersonal Relations.* New York: Wiley.

Heider, F., & Simmel, M. (1944). An experimental study of apparent behavior. *American Journal of Psychology, 57,* 243-259.

Hurley, S.L. (1998). *Consciousness in Action.* Cambridge: Harvard University Press.

Jeannerod, M. (1997). *The cognitive neuroscience of action.* Cambridge, MA: Blackwell Press.

Kelso, S.C. (1996). *Dynamic Patterns.* Cambridge: MIT Press.

Kestenberg, J.S., & Sossin, K.M. (1979). *The role of movement patterns in development, Vol. 2.* New York: Dance Notation Bureau Press.

Kestenberg, J.S. (1995). *Sexuality, body movement and rhythms of development.* Northvale: Jason Aronson. (Originally published in 1975 under the title *Parents and Children*)

Kestenberg-Amighi, J.K., Loman, S., Lewis, P., & Sossin, K.M. (1999). *The meaning of movement. Developmental and clinical perspectives of the Kestenberg Movement Profile.* Amsterdam: Gordon & Breach.

Koch, S.C. (in press). Theoretical Perspectives in Dance/Movemnet Therapy: A Vision for the Future. In S.L. Brooke (in press). *Handbook of the Creative Arts Therapies: History, theories, methods and applications.* Springfield, IL: CC Thomas.

Krämer, N.C. (2001). *Bewegende Bewegung. Sozio-emotionale Wirkungen nonverbalen Verhaltens und deren experimentelle Untersuchung mittels Computeranimation.* [Moving Movement]. Lengerich: Pabst.

Laban, R.v. (1960). *The mastery of movement.* London: MacDonald & Evans.

Laban, R.v., & Lawrence, F. C. (1974). *Effort: Economy in body movement.* Boston, MA: Plays. (Originally published in 1947)

Lakoff, G., & Johnson, M. (1999). *Philosophy in the flesh. The embodied mind and its challenge to Western thought.* New York: Basic Books.

Lamb, W. (1965). *Posture and Gesture.* London: Gerald Duckworth.

LeDoux, J. (1995). Emotions. Clues from the brain. *Annual Review of Psychology, 46,* 209-235.

Lipps, T. (1903). *Leitfaden der Psychologie (Kap. 14: Die Einfühlung,* pp. 187-201). Leipzig: Wilhelm Engelmann.

Lock, M.M. & Scheper-Hughes, N. (1987). The mindful body: A prolegomenon to future work in anthropology. *Medical Anthropology Quaterly, 1,* 6-41.

Loman, S.T., & Brandt, R. (Eds.). (1992). *The body-mind connection in human movement analysis.* Keene, N.H.: Antioch New England Graduate School.

Lotan, N. & Yirmiya, N. (2002). Body movement, presence of parents and the process of falling asleep in toddlers. *International Journal of Behavioral Development, 26*(1), 81-88.

McIntosch, D.N., Reichmann-Decker, A., Winkielman, P. & Wilbarger, J.L. (2005). When the Social Mirror Breaks: Deficits in Automatic, but not Voluntary Mimicry of Emotional Facial Expressions in Autism. *Manuscript under review.*

Merleau-Ponty, M. (1962). *Phenomenology of perception.* London: Routeledge.

Neumann, R. & Strack, F. (2000). Approach and avoidance: The influence of proprioceptive and exteroceptive cues on encoding of affective information. *Journal of Personality and Social Psychology, 79,* 39-48.

Niedenthal, P., Barsalou, L. W., Winkielman, P., Krauth-Gruber, S., & Ric, F. (2005). Embodiment in Attitudes, Social Perception, and Emotion. *Personality and Social Psychology Review, 9,* 184-211.

Nyberg, L., Pertersson, K.M., Nilsson, L.G., Sandbloom, J., Aberg, C., & Ingwar, M. (2001). Reactivation of motor brain areas during explicit memory for actions. *NeuroImage, 14,* 521-528.

Pauen, S., & Träuble, B. (2002, April). *Causal attribution of animate motion in 7-months-olds.* Paper presented at the biannual meeting of the International Conference on Infant Studies, Toronto, ON, Canada.

Pert, C. (1997). *The Molecules of Emotion: Why You Feel the Way You Feel.* Scribner, NY.

Pylvänäinen, P. (2003). Body Image: A tripartite model for the use in dance/movement therapy. *American Journal of Dance Therapy, 25,* 39-55.

Pringer, C. (1995/2005). *The fascia-memory project.* http://hometown.aol.com/bridge22/FasciaMem Project.html Retreived: 05/02/05

Rizzolatti, G., Fadiga, L., Fogassi, L., & Gallese, V. (2002). From mirror neurons to imitation: Facts and speculations. In A.N. Meltzoff & W. Prinz (Eds). *The imitative mind: Development, evolution, and brain bases* (pp. 247-266). New York: Cambridge University Press.

Sax, W. (2002). *Dancing the Self. Personhood and Performance in the Pandav Lila of Garhwal*. New York: Oxford University Press.

Schore, A. (1994). *Affect regulation and the origin of the self*. Hillsdale, NJ: Erlbaum.

Schubert, T.W. (2004). The power in your hand: Gender differences in bodily feedback from making a fist. *Personality and Social Psychology Bulletin, 30*, 757-769.

Schubert, T.W. (in press). Your highness: Vertical Positions as Perceptual Symbols of Power. *Journal of Personality and Social Psychology*.

Strathern, A.J. (1996). *Body Thoughts*. Ann Arbour: University of Michigan Press.

Thelen, E., & Smith, L. (1994). A dynamic systems approach to the development of cognition and action. Cambridge: MIT Press.

Thelen, E. (1995). Motor development -- A new synthesis. *American Psychologist 50*, 79-95.

Thelen, E. (2000). Grounded in the world: Developmental origins of the embodied mind. *Infancy, 1*, 3-28.

Tucker, M., & Ellis, R. (1998). On the relations between seen objects and components of potential actions. *Journal of Experimental Psychology: Human Perception and Performance, 24*, 830-846.

Tversky, B., Morrison, J.B., & Zacks, J. (2002). On bodies and events. In A.N. Meltzoff & W. Prinz (Eds). *The imitative mind: Development, evolution, and brain bases. Cambridge studies in cognitive perceptual development* (pp. 247-266). New York: Cambridge University Press.

van der Kolk, B.A. (2003). Posttraumatic stress disorder and the nature of trauma. In M. F. Solomon & D.J. Siegel (Ed.). *Healing trauma. Attachment, mind, body, and brain* (pp. 168–195). New York & London: Norton.

Varela, F.J., Thompson, E., & Rosch, E. (1991). The embodied mind. Cognitive Science and Human Experience. Cambridge: MIT Press.

Wallbott, H.G. (1991). Recognition of emotion from facial expression via imitation? Some indirect evidence for an old theory. *British Journal of Social Psychology, 30*, 207-219.

Weizsäcker, V.v. (1996). *Der Gestaltkreis. Theorie der Einheit von Wahrnehmen und Bewegen* (6te unveränderte Auflage). Stuttgart: Thieme. (Originally published in 1940).

Wheeler, M.E., Peterson, S.E., & Buckner, R.L. (2000). Memory's echo: Vivid remembering reactivates sensory-specific cortex. *Proceedings of the National Academy of Sciences of the United States of America, 97*, 11125-11129.

Wilson, M. (2002). Six views of embodied cognition. *Psychonomic Bulletin & Review, 9*, 625-636.

Winkielman, P. (2005). Embodied emotional responses as exemplified in impairments such as autism. Presentation at the Biannual Conference of the European Association of Experimnetal Social psychology (EAESP) 19.-23.July, in Würzburg, Germany.

Zaner, R.M. (1964). *The problem of embodiment. Some contributions to a phenomenology of the body*. Nijhoff: DenHaag.

Zajonc, R.B., & Markus, H. (1984). Affect and cognition: The hard interface. In C. Izard, J. Kagan, & R. B. Zajonc (Eds.). *Emotions, cognition and behavior* (pp. 73-102). Cambridge: Cambridge University Press.

THE AFFECTIVE SELF AND AFFECT REGULATION IN DANCE MOVEMENT THERAPY[2]

Malvern Lumsden

In this chapter, it is argued that recent progress in developmental neuroscience and traumatology offers a new theoretical basis for the value of dance movement therapy (DMT). Early childhood interactions influence the development of the brain, particularly with respect to affect regulation and the development of the self. Core facets of the self may be injured, or their development delayed, by short- or long-term trauma. "Complex trauma," experienced over a lifetime leads to complex somatic, emotional, cognitive, and social symptoms, and requires complex therapies. DMT is just such a complex therapy, involving the body level, emotional and aesthetic expression, social interaction, symbol, and metaphor. DMT builds upon an extensive training in non-verbal expression and attunement, which is invaluable in relating to the core self of the client. Dance and improvisational movement offers a scope for working with relational trauma at two levels: the *poeitic* and the *cathartic*. The poeitic level refers to a playful, creative exploration of new modes of being, enabling growth of the self (and probably neurogenesis) in a safe physical and social space. The cathartic level enables the working through of emotional trauma without freezing up in defence or collapsing.

Keywords: Self, affect-regulation, trauma, dance movement therapy.

INTRODUCTION

Dance movement therapy is a *complex* mode of therapy, combining a number of elements including movement, emotional expression, social interaction, and the use of symbol, metaphor, and narrative. Recent progress in developmentally-oriented affective neuroscience as well as in the study of complex relational trauma, added to an increased understanding of the role of movement in the development of the *brain* (the neurological substrate) and the *self* (the subjective experience), provide us with a sound theoretical basis for such a complex therapy.

First, the affective self and its roots in the body and in movement communication are described. Secondly, current thinking in the field of complex/relational development trauma, where the issue of affect-regulation is central, is discussed. This discussion builds on findings in neurobiology. Finally, the relevance of the primary operational modes of DMT in the treatment of complex relational trauma (whatever the associated diagnosis is), is highlighted.

THE AFFECTIVE SELF

Daniel Stern (1985) introduced the notion of an "affective self" as one of the core facets of self, developing in the period of approximately 2 to 6 months of age. The infant responds early in post-natal existence to both internal and external stimuli, sometimes with pleasure, sometimes with pain. These emotional reactions play an important role in triggering the empathic responses of the caretaker. Indeed, Bowlby (1971) concluded that these dyadic response patterns were crucial to the infant's survival and therefore a key to the evolution of the human species. The infant does not just learn to

---

[2] A short version of this paper was presented at the research seminar on dance at NTNU (Norwegian University of Science and Technology) in January 2004. This revision is also inspired by participation at the Art for All summer camp, Thailand, August 2004. The summer camp gathered some 500 disabled youngsters for a week of artistic activities, including a workshop run by *Child in Motion*, a group of former dancers based in the Netherlands.

master the movements of its body in space (another key to survival), it responds emotionally, and the emotion drives the movement. The emotionally-driven movement response, in turn, elicits a more or less appropriate emotionally-driven movement response in the caretaker, typically the mother. Most mothers are what Winnicott (1971) called "good-enough mothers" and are able by their own actions (timing, level of intensity, shaping of the body, etc.) to help the infant manage its emotional responses, sometimes giving increased stimulation, at other times damping/calming the infant's response levels. The Affective Self is thereby shaped in a dialogical, two-way process whereby the infant reacts to internal and external stimuli, and the "external world" of other individuals responds to the infant.

In this conception, the self is seen as a complex self-organising system of both cognitive and affective aspects of prior experience in a social world. The self may be "presented" in therapy just as in "everyday life" (cf. Goffman, 1959/1990) and reacts to what it sees in the "mirror" of other peoples' responses (cf. Cooley, 1902; Mead, 1934). The self may also be disordered, traumatised, shattered (Glass, 1993), and restored (Kohut, 1977). Therapists bring their own selves to the therapy (Rowan & Jacobs, 2002), the main reason why many schools of therapy emphasise the importance of personal therapy in their training programmes.

The self has multiple facets, which are central in dance movement therapy. It is *embodied* (see Koch, this volume), *acting* in *time* and *space*, and it is *affective*, engaging in social and sexual *relations* ("relational self," "engendered self"). Other facets of self include *language* and *narrative* selves, *moral* self, *creative* self and *spiritual* self (see Table I).

TABLE I: SUMMARY OF COMPONENTS OF THE SENSE OF SELF

(Lumsden, 2002; expanded from Stern, 1985)

The Embodied Self
Bodily coherence, sense of being nonfragmented, physical whole with boundaries and locus of integrated action, both while moving and when still. Loss or injury leads to: fragmentation of bodily experience, depersonalization, out-of-body experiences, de-realization, somatoform disorders (Stern, 1985).

The Affective Self
Self-affectivity, experiencing patterned inner qualities of feeling (affects) that belong together with other experiences of self. Loss leads to: anhedonia, dissociated states (Stern, 1985).

The Spatial Self
Sense of being an agent in space: locomotion, ability to manipulate objects. Basis of much cognitive processing. Loss leads to passivity, helplessness with respect to objects.

The Self in Time
Sense of coherent time, personal history, 'sense of enduring, of continuity with one's own past so that one 'goes on being' and can even change while remaining the same. Loss leads to: temporal dissociation, fugue states, amnesia, not "going on being" (Winnicott) (Stern, 1985).

The Self as Agent
Sense of authorship of one's own actions: having volition, control over self-generated action. Loss leads to: paralysis, sense of non-ownership of action, loss of control to external agents (Stern, 1985).

The Relational Self
Sense of belonging, participation, sense of sharing, and unity with another person. Loss leads to rootlessness, isolation, relational vagabonding.

The (En)gendered Self
Sense of self as male or female. Loss or injury leads to: fear of sexual relations, relationships, gender identity disorders, paraphilias, psychosexual dysfunction.

The Moral Self
Sense that one's actions are (or should be) influenced by social rules, collective rationality, or philosophical principles, rather than by immediate gains and losses. Lack of leads to deficient conscience, ruthlessness, (moral) disorientation.

The Verbal Self
Sense of 'ownership' of language and of relationship associated with membership in a particular language community. Lack of leads to limited speech competence, restricting verbal communication in relationships and impacts identity.

The Narrative Self
The self as a set of symbolic narratives. Lack of or injury to leads to lack of meaningful worldview, problems in social relationships.

The Creative Self
Sense of freedom and efficacy in transforming given forms, of dealing with chaos, and of expressing the self. Loss may lead to an impoverished life/world, helplessness in changing conditions, frustration and passivity.

The Spiritual Self
A sense of the transpersonal, of transcendence beyond the confines of the individual self. Loss may lead to existential crisis, and pathological states such as depression.

Movement is the key to the development and expression of many of these facets of self, involving both cognitive and affective areas of the brain. While Llinas (2000) argues that movement requires cognitive processing -- and therefore a brain -- psychiatrists such as Reich (1945/1972; see also Sharaf, 1983) and Schilder (1950) focused on the expressive aspects of movement. More recently, Stern (1973; 1985) has drawn attention to "vitality affects," or qualities of feeling. Stern sees vitality affects as "better captured by dynamic, kinetic terms such as 'surging,' 'fading away,' 'fleeting,' 'explosive,' 'crescendo,' 'decrescendo,' 'bursting,' 'drawn out,' and so on" (Stern, 1985, p. 54). These qualities will be familiar to the dance movement therapist from Rudolf von Laban's or Judith Kestenberg's movement analysis systems (Hodgson &
Preston-Dunlop, 1990; Bartenieff & Lewis, 1980; Preston-Dunlop, 1998; Kestenberg Kestenberg-Amighi, et al., 1999), in which most dance movement therapists have extensive training. This training makes dance/movement therapists particularly suited to working with "vitality affects" in therapeutic movement interactions.

There are thus two sides to the relationship between movement and emotion:

- Movement offers a means of emotional expression, and thereby of *autonomous* (monadic) affect regulation; Reich says, expressive movement comes from the inside out.

- Movement offers a means of communicating and relating, and thereby of *interpersonal* (dyadic) affect regulation.

Both aspects involve basic qualities of movement such as intensity, timing, shape, and spatial pathways, which are the media of the dance. Dance is an archetypal art form in which men and women express many aspects of human existence in abstract, narrative and ritual form. How can movement have such a profound impact? The dancer and choreographer Doris Humphrey (1958) offers the following suggestion: Dance, she says, communicates through *kinesthesis*, which means sensory responses to the movements of the dancers in the body/mind of the observer.[3]

---

[3] I am grateful to Sabine Koch for pointing out that this form of sensory response is now brought to the foreground in embodiment research (e.g., Niedenthal, et al., in press), and in the neurosciences, it has been recently been described in the context of "mirror neurons" (Gallese, Keysers, & Rizzolatti, 2004).

Recent developmental research is showing how the non-verbal parent-infant "dance" is crucial to the child's development and in the process offering a totally new understanding of ways in which dance-movement therapy "works."

AFFECT, ATTACHMENT AND ATTUNEMENT

Attachment theory (Bowlby, 1971; Ainsworth, et al. 1978; Mains & Solomon, 1986) focuses on the mother-child relationship, interpreting the behaviour of the child in response to the mother (child turns towards mother, turns away from, ignores, cries, etc.). The "classic" studies suggest that about 70% of children achieve secure attachment, the rest insecure, ambivalent, or disorganised. There is a huge literature on attachment and its various ramifications in later life. Studies of young adults who were originally observed at 12 months of age in the "strange situation" (Ainsworth, et al., 1978) show a high correlation between early attachment patterns and adult patterns, though with some discrepancies, largely related to the occurrence of traumatic stress later in development (Waters, et al., 2000).

Crucial in promoting attachment in interaction is kinesthesis and *attunement* (Kestenberg, 1975; Stern, 1985), which refers to the immediate relationship between two or more individuals:

> *"Affect attunement... is the performance of behaviors that express the quality of feeling of a shared affective state without imitating the exact behavioral expression of the inner state." (Stern, 1985, p. 142)*

Attunement refers to the degree to which infant and caregiver are able to match their "intensities, shapes, temporal patterns...," etc. Stern insists that the significance of early attuned interaction is a meeting of *selves*: "Interaffectivity may be the first, most pervasive, and most immediately important form of sharing subjective experiences." It is through the sharing of subjective experience that the infant develops a positive or negative *sense of self*.

Kestenberg points out that there can also be too much attunement in a relationship, that there is a role for clashing, so long as it is followed by the opportunity for repair of the relationship:

> *"Generally speaking attunement promotes symbiosis and clashing promotes separation. Exaggerated attunement fosters fears of engulfment and exaggerated clashing brings on excessive fears of separation. Too much attunement may lead to inhibition of independent functioning. Too much clashing enhances motor discharge as response to stress, but it may also lead to inhibition of function." (Kestenberg, 1975, p. 171)*

Finding the balance is the (difficult) key, both to good parenting and to good therapy. In dance a *pas de deux* is an archetype of attunement. The point that Kestenberg and Stern are making is that some parents (some teachers, psychologists, and psychiatrists) are not good at non-verbal attunement. Children may be subjected not only to maternal deprivation but to maternal depression. All too often they are neglected and abused. Although some children show "resilience", there is growing evidence that infant neglect and abuse contributes to a wide range of somatic, psychiatric, and social disturbance (for a detailed review see Sroufe, et al., 2000).

AFFECT REGULATION THEORY

Affect regulation theory makes important contributions to understanding psychopathology (Taylor, Bagby, & Parker, 1997; Bradley, 2000). Schore (1994, 2003a) focuses on how emotional regulation is affected by the maturing brain. This approach studies how the developing brain *is affected by the child's social interactions*. Schore follows in Bowlby's footsteps, adding important new perspectives, which have methodological, theoretical, and clinical significance. He writes that "coping [with stress] can occur either by autoregulation or by going to others for interactive regulation ... this adaptive ability ... is the product of our early attachments." (Schore, 2003a, p. xvii). Interactive regulation of affect involves the "resonance" of the two right brains of the "psychobiologically attuned mother-infant dyad" (Schore, 2003a, p. 51), something which also applies to the therapeutic context.

In its first year, the infant becomes increasingly activated as the sympathetic nervous system and its connections into the limbic system of the brain mature. The child may show joy, sadness, anger and other responses but has limited capacity to regulate these feelings until the "thermostat" of the later-developing parasympathetic system becomes more functional at around 18 months (Schore, 1994), followed by the integration of limbic system and cortex and right and left hemispheres. During infancy the right cerebral hemisphere is the dominant one, characterised by dealing more with global, "feeling" characteristics than the later-developing left hemisphere, more adapted to linear, rational decision-making, language, and mathematics (for a general overview, see Cozolino, 2002).

During the second-year hiatus the child is very much dependent upon the availability of an emotionally sensitive carer that can offer external support for containing emotion. Only later do the child's internal resources develop enough to cope. Where such an emotionally-attuned caretaker is unavailable (for whatever reason), the maturation of the brain may be held back and distorted resulting in weak connections within and between the two hemispheres. Indeed, the growth of the left hemisphere itself may be held back: "The right hemispheres of abused patients had developed as much as the right hemispheres of the control subjects, but their left hemispheres lagged substantially behind" (Teicher, 2002, p. 73).

The work of Allan Schore and others is groundbreaking in that it integrates the biological/neurological and the social and intrapsychical to mutual benefit. Recent technologies such as *in vivo* brain scans are making it possible to record the impact of optimal as well as less than optimal developmental conditions on brain development --and, theoretically, to study the impact of early or later therapeutic interventions accordingly. "Interpersonal neurobiology" (Cozolino, 2002), perhaps for the first time, integrates recent advances in neuroscience with modern developmental and clinical psychology, with an emphasis on the impact of social relationships on the *self* (Kohut, 1971, 1977; Stern, 1985; Stolorow, Atwood, & Brandchaft, 1994; Crossley, 1996).

The self, it is suggested, may be seen as the experience of integration of multiple facets of being. A lack of integration between the various levels of the brain and central nervous system can result in "disorders of the self", depending in part upon the age and circumstances of the "misattunement". When affected, some children become overtly passive, others uncontrollably active. Some passive children are not arroused, others are aroused but block the action, a pattern that can lead to psychosomatic problems in the long run (e.g. Reich 1945/1972).

CLINICAL IMPLICATIONS

These findings have many implications not only for parenting but also for the education, health, and social systems. Hyperactive and "hyperpassive" children are less able to cope with the academic programmes emphasised in most school systems. Consequently, such children tend to do poorly in school, leading to further deterioration of their sense of self and community. By contrast, they will likely have access to spatial and emotional resources, if only these could be put to constructive use in psychosocially-oriented educational programmes.

There is now a large amount of evidence supporting the general lines of this analysis and applying it to various mental disorders (Perry, et al. 1995). For example:

> *"Together these findings suggest an intriguing model that explains one way in which borderline personality disorder can emerge. Reduced integration between the right and left hemispheres may predispose these individuals to shift abruptly from left- to right-dominated states with very different emotional perceptions and memories... Moreover, limbic electrical irritability can produce symptoms of aggression, exasperation and anxiety." (Teicher, 2002, p. 75)*

Studies of *abused and traumatised* individuals show that they commonly present a range of symptoms and receive varying diagnoses (ADHD, borderline personality disturbance, depression, anxiety, chronic tension/pain, detachment, substance abuse, criminal behaviour, etc.; see e.g. van der Kolk, 2000). As a result, they are offered different treatments. McKenzie & Wright (1996) found that a high proportion of *schizophrenics* had siblings two years younger, suggesting another pattern of misattunement and traumatization, contributing to schizophrenia.

COMPLEX TRAUMA, COMPLEX THERAPY

Some recent work in traumatology is making a distinction between "simple" and "complex" trauma. Simple trauma, for want of a better term, refers to single traumatic episodes, for example when a "normal" adult suffers from a car accident or rape. The consequences may be dramatic and difficult to deal with but the assumption is that the "normal" person has the resources to deal with traumatic stress. Only about one-third of people subjected to a traumatic event develop "post-traumatic stress *disorders*" (PTSD).

Complex trauma, DESNOS (Disorders of Extreme Stress Not Otherwise Specified), or chronic developmental and relational trauma, refers to a *life-history* of trauma, not just a single incident.

> *"DESNOS is conceptualized as a constellation of chronic problems with the regulation of self, consciousness, and relationships that is not formally recognized as a diagnostic entity ... DESNOS is hypothesized to occur when extreme traumatization compromises the fundamental sense of self and relational trust at critical developmental periods (such as in child abuse; Herman, 1992; van der Kolk, McFarlane, & Weisæth, 1996), and therefore has been posited to be a set of "associated features" of PTSD linked to interpersonal childhood trauma." (Roth et al., 1997).*

DESNOS is formally defined by a set of seven criteria operationalized in the form of a "Structured Interview for Disorders of Extreme Stress" (SIDES) (Pelcovitz, et al. 1997):

- alterations in *affect or impulse regulation* (e.g., severe anger, suicidality, risk taking);

- alterations in *consciousness or attention* (e.g., pathological dissociation);

- alterations in *self-perception* (e.g., self viewed as damaged, shamed, or misunderstood);

- alterations in *perception of the perpetrator* (i.e., distorted view of an abuse perpetrator, if applicable);

- alterations in *relations with others* (e.g., distrust, revictimization, victimizing others);

- *somatization* (e.g., unexplained or exacerbated physical complaints); and,

- alterations in *systems of meaning* (e.g., hopelessness; distorted beliefs).

In brief, chronic relational trauma gives rise to an interaction of cognitive, emotional, somatic, and social symptoms (van der Kolk, 2003), which may be variously diagnosed under DSM-IV or ICD-10 criteria (van der Kolk, 2000). Efforts are under way to improve the diagnostic criteria and classification of complex trauma in DSM-V, planned for publication in 2007. Presently, the individual client can end up in many different parts of the social or healthcare system.

The interpersonal neurobiology approach offers a viable explanation (a) of how early neglect and trauma influences development by handicapping the growth of affect regulation and consequently of an integrated sense of self and functional social relationships, and (b) why multiple somatic, psychological, and social symptoms can result. The early deficits typically lead to cumulative effects throughout the life-span.

Given that early, traumatising relationships affect the maturation of the emotional and social brain, there are indications that it is possible to stimulate the brain at later stages, through appropriate conditions and activities, but clearly this is a field requiring a major research input. It is too early to say how much the emotional centres of the brain participate in neurogenesis, but there is much evidence that the brain is able to respond to appropriate motor stimulation. Klintsova (1998) showed the "therapeutic effects of complex motor training on motor performance deficits induced by neonatal binge-like alcohol exposure in rats."[4] Kramer and colleagues have shown how exercise improved problem-solving and other cognitive abilities of older people; they found effects on the frontal, temporal, and parietal cortex (*Science Daily*, 2003). These findings add to the discovery of "neurogenesis," the growth of nerve fibres and their linking in synapses.

More generally, the complexities of early stress, brain development, coping strategies, and social relationships imply the need for *complex treatment strategies,* that is, treatment modalities that involve body, emotion, social interaction, narrative, metaphor, etc. Ideally there should be both coherence and continuity over time because these clients generally suffer precisely from incoherent and discontinuous relationships, starting in early childhood and usually repeated later in life. Both of these requirements are a considerable challenge to public health services, which are under pressure to use simple rather than complex diagnoses, and "rapid responses" rather than long-term personal engagement with the patient.

Since the affective and relational problems addressed here start already in the first two years of life, it is not surprising that many of the symptoms are essentially *nonverbal*. Put in another way, many facets of self may be disturbed, wounded, or shattered

---

[4] This is one of a series of reports by the same team. For a brief summary of Anna Klintsova's work see http://psychology.binghamton.edu/faculty/klintsova.html

by early or later trauma. Many of these facets are non-verbal and they require non-verbal stimulation to develop and heal.

Van der Kolk's work gives some examples of such complex therapies. In a paper published in 2000 van der Kolk presented a "Phase oriented treatment of complex PTSD (DESNOS)". This programme included not only symptom management (through a variety of means) but creating narratives, making connections between internal states and actions, EMDR, body-oriented work, learning interpersonal connections, and so on. In his discussion he focused on the following topics (with the author's terminology added in brackets):

- Trauma and the body (= sense of an embodied self)
- Symptom management (= sense of an affective self)
- Resource identification and installation (= sense of agency)
- The use of language and the creation of narratives (= sense of verbal and narrative self)
- Trauma processing (can involve the creative self, using a variety of art media).

The first two of these are essentially "pre-verbal" and are particularly salient when working with problems arising from the first two years or so. *Dance movement therapy* seems particularly appropriate here. DMT works with the body (both activation and relaxation; sensory and motor; efferent and afferent pathways) and with the "embodied self." It also works directly with the affective self through expressing and experimenting with "vitality affects" (Stern) or "Efforts" (Laban). DMT can work with abstract movement (e.g., "strong and direct") and does not need to identify it with a particular purpose, narrative, or relationship, until the patient is able to cope with such associations. Like meditation, DMT also works with breathing, focusing, and relaxation. Like EMDR (Shapiro & Maxfield, 2003) it works with cross-linking right and left hemisphere of the brain.

Van der Kolk's items 3 to 5 seem to involve both language, narrative (dramatic plots), and structured social relationships, i.e. roles; that is they are close to the essential elements of *drama therapy and psychodrama*. Van der Kolk's "phases" may indeed be related to the need to progress through a developmental sequence, building up the "infantile" pre-verbal sensory and motor foundations and their neural substrates before proceeding to the "preschool" verbal and dramatic. DMT operates primarily at this "foundation" level but can also include elements of drama, such as role-playing, verbalizing the movement/dance experience, and shaping it into poetry or narrative.

We may reasonably assume that the dynamics of social interaction in the treatment situation are particularly relevant *where the problem has arisen as the result of interpersonal trauma,* resulting in "insecure", "ambivalent", or "disorganised" bonding, to use the language of attachment theory (Bowlby, 1971; Ainsworth, et al. 1978; Mains & Solomon, 1986). Not only does long-term physical, sexual, or emotional abuse influence the development of the brain, particularly with respect to affect-regulation, but it also often means that the patient is dubious, ambivalent, and demanding with respect to the therapist.

THE AFFECTIVE SELF IN DMT

DMT builds upon an extensive training in embodiment, movement skills, non-verbal expression, mirroring, and attunement which is invaluable in relating to the client (cf. Goldman, 2004). The interaction between therapist and client (or between clients in a group) provides opportunities for the client to experience and experiment with expressive movement and attunement in the "safe space" of the studio. The importance of this perspective has also been recognised by other approaches (e.g., Fosha, 2003).

Dance and improvisational movement offer scope for working with relational trauma at two necessary levels: the *poeitic* and the *cathartic*. The poietic level refers to a playful, creative exploration of new modes of being, enabling growth of the self (and probably neurogenesis, the generation of new brain cells and synaptic connections in the brain) in a safe physical and social space. The cathartic level enables the working through of emotional trauma, *once the self is developed enough* to cope with it without freezing up in defence or collapsing into psychosis.

These two aspects of therapy are particularly relevant to trauma. In many cases of PTSD the assumption is that the client is "normal" before the traumatic incident. The shock of the trauma is "frozen" and catharsis in such cases leads to constructive re-experiencing, releasing of the emotional reaction, and integration (cf. Levine, 1997). In reality, this is more complicated, and the client may experience re-traumatization. This is particularly the case in extreme cases of interpersonal trauma, including sexual abuse and torture. In such cases, it is important to build up all facets of the injured self (poeitic work), for example, by exploring a variety of pleasurable motor, sensory, and relational experiences. As the self heals, the person is more able to cope with and face up to the traumatic memories.

In the case of *complex* trauma, we are faced with the possibility that basic affect regulation mechanisms are deficient. Again, the poietic phase is essential. For here it is not so much a question of "restoring the self" (Kohut, 1977) but of *constructing* the self. The need is for a rich variety of growth-promoting experiences, alone and with others, over a substantial period of time: in brief, what has been termed a "second-chance childhood."[5]

Hubble, Duncan, & Miller (1999) concluded that it is *the people involved* in therapy (patient and therapist), and the nature of their *interaction,* that are more important than the techniques used: the *quality of the interaction may be the most important factor under the (partial) control of the therapist.* The success of dance movement therapy may in large part be due to the educational/training focus on non-verbal attunement with the client, a field in which DMT training has a unique emphasis via Laban movement analysis and its derivatives (Laban, 1948/1988; Laban, 1960/1998; Lamb & Watson, 1979; Kestenberg, 1985; Moore & Yamamoto, 1988/1992; Kestenberg-Amighi et al., 1999; Goldman, 2004).

In psychotherapy we are obliged to act according to what we think other people might do and what *we* think *they* think about *us*. We cannot rely on the systematic observations of natural science: we are forced into the hermeneutics of social science, more specifically, into the subtleties and complexities of *intersubjectivity* (e.g., Trewarthen, 1993; Crossley, 1996).

Dance therapists typically interact with their patients in ways, which are probably unique in the entire field of medicine, psychotherapy, and healing. *Both patient and*

---

[5] This term is from Marcia Leventhal, former head of the dance therapy programme at New York University.

therapist factors -- and thereby factors related to the quality of their *interaction* -- are relevant in DMT.

CONCLUSION

If it is true that many problems of pathology result from insufficient integration between the affect-regulation centres of the brain, then recent findings that movement can stimulate neural growth and change in the brain are particularly interesting.

DMT may work at a combination of physiological, cognitive, emotional, experiential, and social levels -- exactly the kind of complex intervention that the findings of interpersonal neurobiology would suggest are needed to compensate for early deficiencies and later trauma. The interpersonal neurobiology of emotion adds to the neurobiology of movement, cognition, and metaphor (cf. Lumsden, 2002) and contributes to the theoretical underpinnings of dance movement therapy. The beauty of dance movement therapy, like the *pas de deux* of the classical dance, lies in the meeting of affective selves, in their attunement, and kinesthetic resonance.

REFERENCES

Ainsworth, M., Blehar, M., Waters, E., & Wall, S. (1978). *Patterns of attachment.* Hillsdale, NJ: Erlbaum.

Bartenieff, I., & Lewis, D. (1980). *Body movement. Coping with the environment.* New York: Gordon & Breach.

Bowlby, J. (1971). *Attachment.* Attachment and Loss, Vol. 1. Harmondsworth: Penguin.

Bradley, S. J. (2000). *Affect regulation and the development of psychopathology.* New York/London: Guilford Press.

Cooley, C. H. (1902). *Human nature and the social order.* New York: Scribner's.

Cozolino, L. (2002). *The neuroscience of psychotherapy. Building and rebuilding the human brain.* New York & London: Norton.

Crossley, N. (1996). *Intersubjectivity. The fabric of social becoming.* London/Thousand Oaks/New Delhi: SAGE.

Fosha, D. (2003). Dyadic regulation and experiential work with emotion and relatedness in trauma and disorganized attachment. In M. F. Solomon & D. J. Siegel (Ed.). *Healing trauma. Attachment, mind, body, and brain* (pp. 221–281). New York & London: Norton.

Gallese, V., Keysers, C., & Rizzolati, G. (2004). A unifying view of the basis of social cognition. *TRENDS in Cognitive Sciences, 8*(9), 396–403.

Glass, J. M. (1993). *Shattered selves. Multiple personality in a postmodern world.* Ithaca, NY: Cornell University Press.

Goffman, E. (1959/1990). *The presentation of self in everyday life.* London: Penguin.

Goldman, E. (2004). *As others see us. Body movement and the art of successful communication.* New York & London: Routledge.

Herman, J. L. (1992). *Trauma and recovery.* New York: Basic Books.

Hodgson, J., & Preston-Dunlop, V. (1990). *Rudolf Laban. An introduction to his work and influence.* Plymouth: Northcote House.

Hubble, M. A., Duncan, B. L., & Miller, S. D. (1999). *The heart and soul of change: What works in therapy.* Washington, DC: American Psychological Association Press.

Humphrey, D. (1958). *The art of making dances.* New York: Rinehart.

Kestenberg-Amighi, J., Loman, S., Lewis, P., & Sossin, K. M. (1999). *The meaning of movement. Developmental and clincal perspectives of the Kestenberg Movement Profile.* Amsterdam: Gordon & Breach.

Kestenberg, J. S. (1975). *Children and parents. Psychoanalytic studies in development.* New York: Jason Aronson.

Klintsova, A. Y., Cowell, R. M., Swain, R. A., Napper, R. M., Goodlett, C. R., & Greenough, W.T. (1998). Therapeutic effects of complex motor training on motor performance deficits by neonatal binge-like alcohol exposure in rats. I. Behavioral results. *Brain Research, 800*(1), 48–61.

Kohut, H. (1971). *The analysis of the self.* New York: International Universities Press.

Kohut, H. (1977). *The restoration of the self.* New York: International Universities press.

Laban, R. (1948/1988). *Modern educational dance.* (Rev. Lisa Ullmann.) Plymouth: Northcote House.

Laban, R. (1960/1998). *The mastery of movement* (Rev. Lisa Ullmann). London: Macdonald & Evans.

Lamb, W., & Watson, E. (1979). *Body code. The meaning in movement.* London: Routledge & Kegan Paul.

Levine, P. A. (1997). *Walking the tiger. Healing trauma.* Berkeley, CA: North Atlantic Books.

Lumsden, M. (2002). *Psyche's dance -- movement, cognition and the self.* Paper presented at the NOFOD -- Nordic Forum for Dance Research. International Conference on Cognitive Aspects of Dance, NTNU, Trondheim, 11 January 2002.

Mains, M., & Solomon, J. (1986). Discovery of a new, insecure-disorganized/disoriented attachment pattern. In T. B. Brazelton & M. Yogman (Ed.). *Affective development in infancy.* (pp. 95–124). Norwood, NJ: Ablex.

McKenzie, C. D., & Wright, L. S. (1996). *Delayed posttraumatic stress disorders from infancy. The two trauma mechanism.* Amsterdam: American Health Association/Harwood.

Mead, G. H. (1934). *Mind, self, & society* (C. W. Morris, Ed.). Chicago & London: University of Chicago Press.

Moore, C.-L., & Yamamoto, K. (1988/1992). *Beyond words. Movement observation and analysis.* Philadelphia, PA: Gordon & Breach.

Niedenthal, P.M., Barsalou, L.W., Winkielman, P., Krauth-Gruber, S., & Ric, F. (2005). Embodiment in attitudes, social perception, and emotion. *Personality and Social Psychology Review, 9,* 184-211.

Pelcovitz, D., van der Kolk, B. A., Roth, S. H., Mandel. F. S., Kaplan, S. J., & Resick, P. (1997). Development of a criteria set and a structured interview for disorders of extreme stress (SIDES). *Journal of Traumatic Stress, 10*(1), 3–16.

Perry, B., D., Pollard, R. A., Blakely, T. L., Baker, W. L., & Vigilante, D. (1995). Childhood trauma, the neurobiology of adaptation and use-dependent development of the brain: How states become traits. *Infant Mental Health Journal, 16*(4), 271–291.

Preston-Dunlop, V. (1998). *Rudolf Laban. An extraordinary life.* London: Dance Books.

Reich, W. (1945/1972). *Character analysis.* Third ed. (V. R. Carfagno, Trans.). New York: Farrar, Stauss & Giroux/Noonday Press.

Roth, S. H., Newman, E., Pelcowitz, D., van der Kolk, B. A., & Mandel, F. S. (1997). Complex PTSD in victims exposed to sexual and physical abuse: Results from the DSM-IV field trial for posttraumatic stress disorder. *Journal of Traumatic Stress, 10*(4), 539–555.

Rowan, J., & Jacobs, M. (2002). *The therapist's use of self.* Philadelphia: Open University Press.

Schilder, P. (1950). *The image and appearance of the human body.* New York: International Universities Press.

Schore, A. N. (1994). *Affect regulation and the origin of the self. The neurobiology of emotional development.* Hillsdale, NJ: Erlbaum.

Schore, A. N. (2003a). *Affect dysregulation and disorders of the self.* New York & London: Norton.

Shapiro, F., & Maxfield, L. (2003). EMDR and information processing in psychotherapy: Personal development and global implications. In M. F. Solomon & D. J. Siegel (Ed.). *Healing trauma. Attachment, mind, body, and brain* (pp. 196–220). New York & London: Norton.

Sharaf, M. (1983). *Fury on earth. A biography of Wilhelm Reich.* New York: St. Martin's/Marek.

Sroufe, L. A., Duggal, S., Weinfield, N., & Carlson, E. (2000). Relationships, development, and psychpathology. In A. J. Sameroff, M. Lewis & S. M. Miller (Ed.). *Handbook of developmental psychopathology.* New York: Kluwer Academic/Plenum.

Stern, D. N. (1973). On kinesic analysis. A discussion with Daniel N. Stern. *The Drama Review, 17,* 114–126.

Stern, D. N. (1985). *The interpersonal world of the infant.* New York: Basic Books.

Stolorow, R., Atwood, G., & Brandchaft, B. (Ed.). (1994). *The intersubjective perspective.* New York & London: Jason Aronson.

Taylor, G. J., Bagby, R. M., & Parker, J. D. A. (1997). *Disorders of affect regulation. Alexythimia in medical and psychiatric illness.* Cambridge: Cambridge University Press.

Teicher, M. H. (2002). Scars that won't heal: The neurobiology of child abuse. *Scientific American,* March/02.

Trewarthen, C. (1993). The self born in intersubjectivity: The psychology of an infant communicating. In U. Neisser (Ed.). *The perceived self: Ecological and interpersonal sources of the self-knowledge.* New York: Cambridge University Press.

van der Kolk, B. A. (2000). The assessment and treatment of complex PTSD. In R. Yehuda. (Ed.). *Current treatment of PTSD.* Washington, DC: American Psychiatric Press.

van der Kolk, B. A. (2003). Posttraumatic stress disorder and the nature of trauma. In M. F. Solomon & D. J. Siegel (Ed.). *Healing trauma. Attachment, mind, body, and brain* (pp. 168–195). New York & London: Norton.

van der Kolk, B. A., McFarlane, A.C., & Weisæth, L. (Ed.). (1996). *Traumatic stress: The effects of overwhelming experience on mind, body, and society.* New York: Guilford Press.

Waters, E., Merrick, S., Treboux, D., Crowell, J., & Albersheim, L. (2000). Attachment security in infancy and early adulthood. A twenty-year longitudinal study. *Child Development, 71*(3), 684–689.

Winnicott, D. W. (1971). *Playing and reality.* London: Tavistock.

THE TRI-PARTITE MODEL OF BODY IMAGE AND ITS APPLICATION TO EXPERIENCES IN BUTOH

Päivi Pylvänäinen

The tri-partite model of body image organizes the contents of the psychological experience of the body into image-properties, body-self, and body-memory. Image-properties refer to one's perceived appearance of the body. Body-self is the body-based, interactive, experiencing, and emotional core-self. Body-memory stores the lived experiences and serves as a background for evaluating present experiences. The contents of body-memory and image-properties tune the action that the body-self carries out. These together are the body image and shape it continuously. The tri-partite model is based on pertinent literature from phenomenology, psychology, dance, and dance/movement therapy. The model offers theoretical grounding for dance/movement therapy. Its application and relevance is illustrated through a retrospective analysis of the author's movement experiences in butoh.

Keywords: body image; body-self; body-memory; butoh.

THE TRI-PARTITE MODEL OF BODY IMAGE AND ITS APPLICATION TO EXPERIENCES IN BUTOH

Body image is a central concept for dance/movement therapy (DMT) because it addresses the psychological experience of the lived body. This chapter aims to stay with the fundamental question of the structure of body image within the individual. In order to get a view of the research presently done on body image, the author made a search through the journals of the Taylor and Francis publishing company on their website (http://taylorandfrancis.metapress.com, February, 2005). Taylor and Francis publishes a wide selection of journals, among which there were approximately 20 journals that might discuss body image from various perspectives. These are journals related to philosophy, arts and humanities, education, health sciences, psychology, and psychotherapy. The author used these as a sample and included the journal issues since 2000. The word body image was used as the basic search criterion. 35 references to articles that discuss body image resulted.

The majority of the articles focused on body shape and weight control issues (11 references). This reflects the common understanding that body image is a person's perception of her physical appearance. When the research articles applied a wider understanding of body image and a psychological perspective was included, they focused on the question of self-esteem and satisfaction with the body (9 references). Several studies treated the body image issues in cancer, breast cancer specifically (7 references). There were only four articles that related the body image issues with perception, cognition, or consciousness. Three studies discussed the relationship between body image and mental health, and in two of these the focus was on pain problems. One article (Green, 2001) took into account the role of body image in active experiencing and functioning in the context of dance classes.

The word body-self as the search criterion rendered five articles that discussed body as an experiencing totality which responds to changes in life and plays a role in cognition, learning, and social interaction (Ellis-Hill, Payne, & Ward, 2000; Mullen & Cancienne, 2003; Shotter, 2004; Smith, 2002; Tsakiris & Haggard, 2005). None of these studies were from the field of DMT, yet they were written with an attitude that echoes DMT approach. The lived, experience-based description and understanding of body image is paramount to DMT. This functional, phenomenological sphere is the space where DMT essentially happens. This is also the perspective on body image to which DMT is excellently able to contribute. In doing so, DMT is building its own theory basis.

None of the research articles was specifically aiming at constructing the body image concept itself. This chapter aims at clarifying the concept of body image per se in the portrayal of the tri-partite model of body image. This model is based on pertinent literature from the fields of philosophy, psychology, and DMT. The body image is seen as a systemic structure consisting of image properties, body-self, and body-memory. To give an embodied and practical illustration of the application of the tri-partite model, the author complements the theoretical presentation with an analysis of her experiences in butoh.

UNDERSTANDING THE BODY IMAGE

The root of the body image is in the body. The body has been actively reflected on by philosophers Husserl, Heidegger, Merleau-Ponty and Foucault. Husserl brought into attention the difference between the lived-body and the body under a strict physical or physicalistic description. Heidegger continued with the phenomenological approach to the body and considered the question of embodiment. He stated we are embodied, and thus the relationship between embodiment and being should be studied. Merleau-Ponty illuminated the internal connection between the body, actions, and perception. At the start of the 1980's Foucault brought up the perspective of different nexuses of power and their role in the constitution of the body. Foucault observed the diciplinary power of social institutions such as the medical system, political regimes, and schools. The disciplinary power gains its dominance by inciting desire, attaching individuals to specific identities, and addressing real needs. Its emphasis is on normalization, to the point that it is the individual herself who will be doing the monitoring. The goal is to render the body more useful and effective, yet more docile. Husserl's, Heidegger's, and Merleau-Ponty's phenomenology offers a philosophical and theoretical basis for inquiries into body image (Welton, 1999; Price & Shildrick, 1999). Foucault's view is poignantly true -- today maybe even more than at the time when he initially presented it. It is important to keep it in mind as a reminder of the social reality we live in.

The classic definition of body image by Schilder (1950), stated that body image is the mental picture of one's own body. The word mental may easily lead to de-emphasis of the physical basis and emotional tones of body image. The word picture emphasizes the visual mode of perceiving the body image contents. However, Schilder's definition of the body image allows the perspective that body image is something multilayered, as the word mental also refers to the individual's total intellectual and emotional response to reality. Schilder took an important step on the way to bringing to attention the psychological significance of the physical body. Almost twenty years after Schilder, Fisher and Cleveland (1968) defined the body image as an individual's reference to the body as a psychological experience. In their definition the quality of body image as a phenomenological and lived phenomenon becomes apparent.

Gallagher (1995) proposed a more detailed description of the contents of this psychological experience of the body. According to him, the body image contains the subject's perceptual experience of her body; the subject's conceptual understanding of the body in general, including mythical and/or scientific knowledge; and the subject's emotional attitude toward her own body. This description takes into account the varied qualities of the contents, but it does not discuss the function of this information for the individual. The contents are centered on the individual. The link between the body image and the social reality around the body seems to be constituted of information, which is mediated through language.

Chace was one of the first dance/movement therapists to voice the DMT perspective of body image. She noted that body image is inseparably involved with emotion and action, and its formation is primarily a social creation (Chace in Sandel, Chaiklin, & Lohn, 1993). Her emphasis was functional. She attended to the lived body experience, which takes place in a social context.

After Chace, some new dance/movement therapists have tackled the task of detailing what the body image contents and its functions are. Gross (1992) organized the body image into four dimensions: the sensorimotor level of experience, which refers to the bodily perceptions through the sensory system; the boundary dimension, which refers to the differentiation by the skin between the inside and the outside of the body and thus constitutes a fundamental cognitive baseline; the space dimension, which refers to the bodily perception of personal and interpersonal space; and lastly, the dynamic dimension which refers to the energetic and expressive aspects of the body image. Gross saw the evolution of body image as the result of a developmental process in the context of object relations, containing conscious and unconscious qualities.

Becker (1993) offered another DMT definition of body image. She defined the body image as the individual's representation of conscious and unconscious aspects regarding the body. She filled this general statement with the notions that body image encompasses the individual's attitude to her body; personal space and boundary perception, sensorimotor qualities, and the relationship to the environment through groundedness.Groundedness means the energetic contact with the ground. The quality of grounding relates to balance, to the range of movement, and to coping. There is a pattern of perceptual organization that arises from body sensations. This pattern becomes the primary way the body works to interpret the surrounding environment.

There are many similarities in Beck's and Gross's perspectives on body image. They may to some extent reflect Beck's and Gross's background of DMT training at the Hahnemann University (Philadelphia, USA). Also, the similarities may be an expression of the general view of body image in the field of DMT.

THE TRI-PARTITE MODEL OF BODY IMAGE

This chapter proposes a tripartite model for the sake of organizing the information on body image in a systemic way. The intention is to increase the clarity of the concept and to give special emphasis to the lived body experience. The model reaches towards a profound understanding of the phenomenological and psychological contents of the body image. The tri-partite model offers a deeper grounding of the concept itself and of the statements, which refer to the concept of body image. In this chapter the focus is on a healthy body image. Thus the pathologies that may disturb the body image will not be addressed specifically.

Initially, the idea for organizing the body image concept into the three aspects of image-properties, body-self, and body-memory, arose from the reading of Schilder's (1950) text (Pylvänäinen, 2003). As Schilder described the contents of the body image, he was creating a potpourri of impressions, sensations, and experiences past and present. When organizing these phenomena with the macro-level concepts of image-properties, body-self, and body-memory, the meta-concept, i.e. body image, appeared in a clearer and systemic form.

The Image-Properties

The image-properties refer to a "looks" aspect of the body. They are a set of beliefs about the body, attitudes about its appearance, evaluations of good and bad regarding the outward view of the body, ideas about the treatment of the body and about transformation of the body appearance. These beliefs are often strongly influenced by cultural idealizations and attitudes (Dosamantes, 1992; Gallagher, 1995). The body is represented as something that is owned, as an object that can be expressed visually and articulated in words (Gallagher, 1995). Image-properties can incorporate objects that do not belong to the body itself, such as rings, eyeglasses, bags, and clothing items. The image-properties are part of the persona the individual creates for her social performance.

In the society and the media the body is primarily presented via the visual channel. The outside view of the body gains the greatest attention. Thus the image-properties of body image are emphasized. This bias makes the common understanding of body image concept external and superficial. An analogy would be to focus on studying the appearance of a book cover instead of studying the contents of the book. The focus on the external appearance of the body reduces the body image to a one-dimensional, superficial, judgmental, and manipulative construct. Idealizations and suggestions regarding the image-properties tend to lead into commercial and consummative behaviors, which may be alienating for the individual's relationship with her own body. It is through the image properties that the Foucaultian disciplinary power gets a hold on us. On the positive side, image-properties may allow the individual pleasure, self-nurturing behaviors, and accepting attention from others. Also, because the image-properties are so frequently referred to in the media, the image-properties may serve as a starting point in attending to one's body.

Dance/movement therapists' roles in the encounter with the image-properties are subtle. Even though the therapist's intention usually is to express some positive emancipation from the stereotypical image-properties requirements, the situation can turn more complex in the context of the therapeutic process: what does the therapist's own appearance express for the patient regarding the image-properties? If the therapist works as medical or educational staff member, how much will the patients project on her the Foucaultian disciplinary qualities? What will it do to the movement work, if the patient feels in herself a heavy load of dismissive and non-accepting associations to her own image-properties? How can one get started inspite of this barrier?

The Body-Self

In the field of DMT, the body-self concept has been discussed by Dosamantes-Alpersson (1981) and Pallaro (1996). They proposed that the lived sensations, when they form the core content of the lived body, are contained within the idea of body-self. According to Dosamantes-Alpersson (1981, p. 35), the body-self refers to "the totality of what is experienced kinesthetically, emotionally, and cognitively by individuals when they attend to the sense of their physical being." When in general the self-concept refers to the conscious, reflective personality of an individual and to the non-physical inner contents, the body-self refers to the acting and sensing body and the individual's consciousness of it in a lived, interactional moment. Pallaro discusses the concept in terms of object relations theory. She remarks that object relations theorists posit the primary experience of the body as the basis of the individual's sense of self.

Stern (1985) offers an interesting description of the development of the layers of self. Before language acquisition the development of the layers of self is fundamentally related to the body and to movement interaction. Stern's formulation can be taken as a description of the early stages of body-self. These layers of self, which are based on body experience and movement interaction, continue to function throughout the entire life-span.

The body-self is the experiencing and interacting core-self. It fundamentally creates the sense of self. It is the essence of the individual. The perception of one's own body-self and the body-selves of others are the primary data of experience. The actions and responses shape the body-self. It reaches out to connect with others. It is our basic medium for fulfilling the object relational desire to be in relation with the other. Everybody builds her own body-self in the interactional contact with others. The better one is grounded in her body-self, the better able she is to connect with the other's body-self. In the context of interaction, the body-self responds affectively. Schilder's (1950) description of the body image encompassed these qualities as well. The affectivity in the body-self appears and is experienced in body sensations, in body shape, and in the flow and dynamics of movement. By sensing, perceiving, and responding through the body-self, one appreciates her affective influence on others (see Campbell, 1995).

The body-self relates and responds to the physical environment as well. As Chace (1993, in Sandel, Chaiklin, & Lohn) said, a healthy body-self is in tune with and related to the reality of the world. The body-self does the experiencing and living in the present moment, it is at the core of the individual's actions and tendencies to emotions. Yet the body-self is also sensed, experienced, lived by the individual's attentiveness. Inward attention refers to the conscious effort by the individual to carefully perceive the sensations in the body-self. Consequently, the body-self holds a double role (Schilder, 1950; O'Shaughnessy, 1995). Tsakiris and Haggard (2005) identified these two roles as a sensing agent and an acting agent in their discussion of the concept of the embodied self. Both the awareness of one's own actions and awareness of one's own body are necessary conditions for the experience of selfhood. The body-self as the medium for the interaction is essentially engaged in DMT.

Body-Memory

Body-memory is the container of past experiences in the body. It is the way the body remembers and stores experiences within itself. Body memories are wordless and independent of conscious will (Casey, 1987). The body sensation in the background of an event may anchor the moment to the individual's autobiography, although the person may not have been paying intentional attention to storing the event into episodic or autobiographic memory. This is how body-memory contributes to the shaping of the totality of the self. The constantly present background that body-memory provides us with a basic factor in constructing the continuity of the experiencing self (Kinsbourne, 1995). Body-memory is interrelated with the body-self as body memories of past experiences can shape the responses the body-self carries out in the present.

Casey (1987) identified three spheres of body-memory: habitual body-memory, traumatic body-memory, and erotic body-memory. Habitual body-memory is defined as the active presence of the individual's past in the body. It holds experiences of everyday routine actions and situations. It is the container of the learned movement repertoire the person has. This constitutes the sense of body coherence, continuity, familiarity, and orientation, which are the foundations of mental health. Thus for example a neurological injury, which damages the movement repertoire, is not only a physical problem, but also a great challenge for the continuity of selfhood and mental health.

Traumatic body-memory (Casey, 1987) contains sensations in the body that are aroused in the moments of painful experiences. These sensations become stored whether the person experienced the trauma herself or whether she saw someone else in the traumatic situation. In traumatic body-memories, the body is fragmented, which disturbs the integrity of the body image and prohibits spontaneous and integrated action. The fragmentation is augmented by physical pain and fearful and anxiety-laden affects related to the situation. Patients suffering from trauma can be treated effectively by DMT.

Erotic body-memory is the container of the experiences of pleasure. Erotic body memories are essentially interpersonal because they are rooted in interactions with others (Casey, 1987). Not only the pleasurable and arousing adult sexual experiences are stored in erotic body-memory, but also the pleasurable and joyous body experiences in other developmental stages. Furthermore, the pleasure and excitement that the positive, non-sexual interaction and connectedness arise in the individual, are stored in erotic body-memory. It is the container of vitality affects and positive life energy, and thus is a very important element for mental health. Activating and enriching this part of body-memory can supply energy that spurs the therapeutic work and brings the feelings of optimism and vitalization.

The tri-partite model focuses on the systemic description of the psychological significance of the body and movement experiences. Keeping in mind the body image description by Gross (see p. 5), which emphasizes physical and sensory movement qualities contributing to the body image, it becomes apparent that it is possible to approach the body image on many levels. They all are equally needed when creating a good connection to one's body. At the crux of the connectedness to one's body image is the awareness of the body-self, which means consciousness of physical movement, body sensations, and emotions in the present moment. The consciousness of the moving and sensing body-self can develop in attentive moving. Dance can offer a unique possibility for attentive moving. Fraleigh (2004, p. 9) writes: "When we dance, we have access to a supple and unpredictable self in flowing cycles of descend-dance [...] connecting form with feeling in the ascendance back again." She views dance as a special kind of being-in-the-world and as knowledge, which is based on a non-dualist, dancing consciousness.

THE ENCOUNTER OF BODY IMAGE IN BUTOH EXPERIENCES
Why Butoh?

For the purpose of a practical illustration of the application of the tri-partite model and for searching whether the contents the model describes appear in movement experiences, movement material was taken from the author's butoh experiences. The author had been practicing butoh for five months at the time this writing project started and had journaled her experiences focusing on describing the movement work and reflecting on her own responses. Building on the idea of artistic inquiry as a research method, this chapter incorporates her notes.

Artistic methods in research are based on using art-making as a tool for collecting, anlyzing, and/or presenting the data (Hervey, 2000, 2004). The practice of butoh with a preeminent butoh artist can be seen as one kind of dance making. In this practice the goal was to learn butoh, which meant the focus was on indwelling in body expression and emotional communication. Emotion was central to knowing the art form and the knowledge that arises from the art. The instrument was the movers's body, which in the notes became the root of her self-reflection; the major instrument was the investigator herself. The journal notes were grounded on a systematic integration of sense-based and introspective methods. Also, they contained narrative, expressive language, and imagery, and the result was a distinctly individuated expression. These characteristics are in line with the artistic inquiry.

In empirical practice, the application of the tri-partite model focuses on inner experiences of the mover and their communication, which can be expected to be rich in emotional, intuitive, imaginative, and embodied content. This is another reason for using artistic inquiry as a method for collecting the data (Hervey, 2004). Because the author practiced butoh and journaled her experiences before she knew she was to use them in this chapter, her responses were free from specific intentions to handle body image issues through movement. This is important for the authenticity of the movement work and of the appearing results, because now the appearing body image related experiences will demonstrate the way the body and consciousness respond spontaneously.

There are some fundamental similarities in the attitudes with which butoh and DMT approach movement: allowing any kind of movement and emotion, ignoring the traditional requirements of beauty, gazing inside rather than focusing on the external movement performance. Fraleigh (1999, p. 34) writes: "Butoh is most of all a process of finding an expression, a primal body utterance. Its cathartic field is composed of gestural images rising to form out the subconscious in whatever sublime or awkward manner they take." This search for movement expression and communication is at the root of DMT as well. Butoh is wisdom of the body. Yoshito Ohno, a famous butoh teacher whose butoh workshops the author attends to, says: "Butoh is forte in pianissimo". When a dancer dances butoh, she is expressing herself, emotion, spirit, and spirituality. In butoh, the understanding is that the body becomes truly human, when the distinction between spirit, mind, and body disappears. Butoh body includes one's personal body, the body of others, and the world's body (Fraleigh, 2004).

Yoshito Ohno is the son of Kazuo Ohno. Kazuo Ohno is now 98-years old, and over his life long path of expressing himself in movement, he has tried to transcend the human and the animal, and to reach to the spirit. Kazuo Ohno's dance has roots in emotion (Ohno & Ohno, 2004). His direction is towards freeing "the innocent body". He teaches conscious awareness through movement by guiding into tuning an inner eye to the movement and oneself (Fraleigh, 1999). Yoshito Ohno is continuing his father's work, and also passing on some of the tradition of Tatsumi Hijikata, with whom the Ohnos collaborated a lot.

The Butoh Practice and Narrative

The workshops took place in the Kazuo Ohno Studio in Yokohama. The studio space was 7x14 meters large, with a wooden floor and windows on one wall.

Yoshito-san's (san-ending is a Japanese way for addressing a person respectfully) teaching was translated from Japanese into English by some of the Japanese students in the workshop. Yoshito-san offered movement suggestions, music, and some props, and then the participants moved. Often the movement was very basic movement like walking, standing, going down and up, exploring density (binding) or circular form in movement. Music was often classical. Flowers, tissue paper, parasols, and high heels were typical props.

The notes used here cover eight sessions from the very beginning of the author's participation in the workshops, June 2004 to November 2004. This was her first encounter with butoh, which she was interested in, because it was new to her and uniquely Japanese. The notes were written after each session based on her memory of the sequence of movement explorations during the 2-hour workshop. When writing these notes, she wanted to store Yoshito-san's teachings and to make notes of the different movement experiences, so she could remember them and maybe use them later in DMT work.

To analyze the journal in an organized way, the author identified movement episodes in it. A movement episode is a movement experience during a workshop, an experience with a theme that begins and ends. Usually, an episode was initiated by Yoshito-san's movement suggestion, e.g. "please walk through the studio", and it would end when he would turn the music off. Thus the timing and the suggestions were not under the participants' control. However, the author felt free in the workshops to respond spontaneously to the suggestions, music, and props with the movement impulses and emotions that they activated in her. 41 movement episodes were identified in the notes.

To overview the contents of these 41 movement episodes, the author checked whether they could be identified as relating to image-properties, the body-self, or body-memory. On the basis of the tri-partite model, the following criteria were set: 1) An episode would relate to image-properties, if it focused on the appearance and looks of the body. 2) In an episode related to body-self, the experience focused on movement action with an affect and with personal association to relationships and own being. 3) A body-memory related movement episode brought up past experiences, i.e. memories of body sensations, body based memories of past moments, and/or interactions.

Applying the criteria described above, out of the 41 movement episodes, 21 were related to the body-self, nine to body memory and two to image-properties. Some episodes related to two criteria, for example to the body-self and body-memory, or to image-properties and body-memory. Also, there were ten episodes where there was no specific body image related content, only plain movement experience and no personal association or emotion related to it. In five movement episodes, a more general thought or insight was related to the movement. In the following, examples of the movement episodes relating to body image will be presented.

One movement episode related to image-properties begun by us watching one of the students to move in vertical position while having a rope tightly around his whole body. Then the suggestion for the whole group was to step on the ground extremely quickly with strength, high muscle tension, and control. This movement was very strenuous and tiring to do. Afterwards the movement quality naturally turned into softness. Now Yoshito-san suggested the females would put high heels on and walk across the studio with a rose in hand. The continuum of these three movement themes constituted one movement episode. In the beginning, when watching the other student and then stepping myself, I felt confused and unsettled, wondering what I was doing in this workshop. When I got the high heels and a rose, they made me feel, with some bitterness, that now the confusion was gone and I had a direction given to me from the outside. I felt that the role of a woman is to be sexy and sexual, to balance with this quality, and to tolerate the pain it generates: the sexy shoes squeeze your feet, the sexuality generates children, which set limits and constrains on the woman. The image properties appeared in the moment of sensing the stereotypical female appearance in high heels and in a narrow body shape. It was about being bound, and the theme of being bound continued as the body-self related issues of womanhood, i.e. associations to what kind of actions womanhood puts into my body, became dominant in this movement episode. In retrospect I wondered, how much my confusion and the initial lack of connectedness to my own actions contributed to the emphasis of image-properties in this episode.

Once Yoshito-san said: "How do you walk across the space? Encounter the air around you!" As I walked I got a feeling I must walk on, no matter how terrifying it would be. Even though I felt I was walking slowly, others around me walked even more slowly. I noted that I and my sons escalate each other into speed. I thought I should try to find a more languid tempo into my action. This body-self related episode made me observe an issue related to my everyday interactions and to my motherhood. In my notes I did note explore in more detail the fleeting moment of anxiety. Yet that moment was a true hint at the struggles the body-self goes through in life.

Incidentally, in a workshop on my son's birthday, Yoshito-san played Japanese children's songs and asked: "How is the feel of a child and childhood in you?" As I moved to the music, I encountered a contained, safe joy. Then a bubbling, jumping excitement emerged. I did not express it in external movement, but held it inside my body, condensing the emotion and sensations related to it, thus feeling it stronger. Then I started to walk like my one-year old son, sensing the excitement and shakiness of the first steps. I realized, I carry memories of my child in my body, memories of his essence and of our being together. In this way I can be part of his memory, because I have the words now when he does not have them yet. I felt a strong, pleasant will and wish to be able to get thickly imprinted by memories. In this movement episode two qualities of body-memory appeared: affective body-memories related to my own past and body-memories related to a relationship and the other.

A movement episode, which carried a strong emotion and was related to body-memory was initiated by Yoshito-san's suggestion to explore aggression through a fist. As I squeezed my hand into a tight fist, I remembered my burst of anger towards my son a couple of days earlier. This memory of a moment of anger made it easy to find the aggression in my body: the immense tightness and binding in my hands and arms; a sharp, strong and direct gaze in my eyes; rapid, audible breath; grounded, wide posture. It was tiring to maintain this bodily aggression, and as I stayed with it quite a while, I eventually had to let it ease away because I simply did not have the stamina to keep it going any longer. In that moment I realized how often aggression arises from egocentric internal talk: I have been strained too much, I did not get what I thought I should have gotten. Yet the tiring aggression turns against the ego as well, strains it more. Right after this Yoshito-san divided the group in two, and as the one half observed the others moving, we continued the theme of aggression through a fist. This time my hands, both in a tight fist, started to tremble quickly in front of my chest with binding, as if trying to hit each other but never getting there. This was the physical expression of uproaring. My fists and elbows were horizontally aligned in front of my body, elbows tucked out, expressing blocking out of any contact. Uproaring, the deliberate withdrawal from and rejection of contact to others started to wear me out, my posture begun to sink, shrink, and weaken. I felt drained. This movement episode, through a body-memory and emotion, made me understand something about the nature of my aggression and what it does to me.

DISCUSSION

The author's narrative of movement experiences in butoh workshops demonstrated that her movement experiences did spontaneously reflect body image aspects as described by the tri-partite model. To fully use the informing potential of those movement experiences, it is important to analyze their context in detail in order to identify factors that may have contributed to the rich appearance of body image related movement experiences. Why did butoh workshops evoke so much? The movement frame was simple, such as walking, and even though the same movement is frequently done in everyday life, in butoh it was done with attention, awareness, and presence; with an inward gaze. The movement was so basic that the author could fully embody it and indwell in it. There was a group of people practicing an attentive approach to presence and movement together; it may have enhanced the experience compared to practicing it in solitude. Even though butoh was new to the author, this kind of approach to moving and movement experiencing was familiar to her. She was willing to move this way. While she was not actively thinking about the body image model when moving in butoh workshops, the knowledge of the model must have had some impact on her accepting and appreciative approach to movement. In her life situation she had nothing so anxiety causing going on that she would have felt a strong need to suppress or reject some of her reactions or emotions in the workshops. She was free to experience her movement as it was.

Presumably in an individual's life situation some factors promote experiencing movement with attentiveness, some withhold the person from movement experiencing. From her experiences in butoh, the author assumes that some of the factors influencing movement and consequently body image experience are:

- the nature of movement suggestions
- the level of experience in moving with attentiveness
- person's willingness to move
- the anxiety level in life and in the specific movement situation
- the tolerance of emotional response
- sensitivity for perceiving body sensations
- cognitive knowledge of the body image and body related theories

The assumption is, the more favorable these factors are toward movement experiencing, the better access the person has to her body image. These factors are not separate from the body image itself. Instead, many of them relate specifically to the body-self. In the future, it would be relevant to research in more detail how these factors co-influence the way a person experiences movement. This information would constitute a praxis-side of body image knowledge, to accompany the structure and content description the tri-partite model offers. This could be helpful for dance/movement therapists in foreseeing how a client may experience the movement work and what would be most supportive for the client in her body image exploration. It is only when a person can really allow herself to experience the movement that the change begins to take place.

The tri-partite model may serve as a tool for explaining and understanding movement experiences and processes. It can be applied in constructing treatment goals. It may be fruitful to consider the inclusion of the cognitive knowledge of the tri-partite model in the education of the general public about mental health and well-being because the knowledge of the tri-partite model may help people to recognize their body and movement responses in a more grounded and supportive way. The tri-partite model can be helpful in educating the colleagues of dance/movement therapists about the perspective DMT holds to body and movement communication. Also, with some populations, an education about the body image concept might be a helpful element in the treatment, paving the way for rich movement experiencing which may bring embodied connectedness to one-self and others.

The tri-partite model helps to recognize the interrelated interaction of body-self, the image-properties, and body-memory, which continuously shape the body image. The awareness of the experience and of the psychological significance of the body is developed through moving with attentiveness. Conscious movement experience brings embodied connectedness to the body-self. This supports mental health and the ability to connect with others. The continuing study of body image will enrich both the theoretical and practical body of knowledge in the field of DMT.

REFERENCES

Becker, M. G. (1993). *A discussion of metaphor as a vehicle for understanding body image in dance/movement therapy.* Unpublished Master's Thesis, Hahnemann University, Philadelphia.
Campbell, J. (1995). The body image and self consciousness. In J. L. Bermúdez, A. Marcel, & N. Eilan (Eds.). *The body and the self (pp. 27-42).* Cambridge, MA: MIT Press.
Casey, E. S. (1987). Remembering: A phenomenological study. Bloomington, IN: Indiana University Press.
Chace, M. (1993). Selected writings: Body image and physiology. In S. L. Sandel, S. Chaiklin, & A. Lohn (Eds.). *Foundations of dance/movement therapy: The life and work of Marian Chace (pp. 75-97).* Columbia, MD: The Marian Chace Memorial Fund of American Dance Therapy Association.
Dosamantes, I. (1992). Body-image: Repository for cultural idealizations and denigrations of the self. *The Arts in Psychotherapy, 19,* 257-267.
Dosamantes-Alpersson, E. (1981). Experiencing in movement psychotherapy. *American Journal of Dance Therapy, 4,* 33-44.
Ellis-Hill, C. S., Payne, S., & Ward, C. (2000). Self-body split: issues of identity in physical recovery following a stroke. *Disability & Rehabilitation, 22,* 725-733.
Fisher, S., & Cleveland, S. (1968). *Body image and personality.* New York: Van Nostrand.
Fraleigh, S. H. (1999). *Dancing into darkness: Butoh, Zen and Japan.* Pittsburgh, PA: University of Pittsburgh Press.
Fraleigh, S. H. (2004). *Dancing identity -- metaphysics in motion.* Pittsburgh, PA: University of Pittsburgh Press.
Gallagher, S. (1995). Body schema and intentionality. In J. L. Bermúdez, A. Marcel, & N. Eilan (Eds.). *The body and the self (pp. 225-244).* Cambridge, MA: MIT Press.
Green, J. (2001). Socially constructed bodies in American dance classrooms. *Research in Dance Education, 2,* 155-173.
Gross, C. (1992). *Body image concept in dance/movement therapy.* Unpublished Master's Thesis, Hahnemann University, Philadelphia.
Hervey, L. W. (2000). Artistic inquiry in dance/movement therapy. *Creative alternatives for research.* Springfield, IL: Charles C Thomas.
Hervey, L.W. (2004). Artistic inquiry in dance/movement therapy. In R.F. Cruz & C. F. Berrol (Eds.). Dance/movement therapists in action. *A working guide to research options (pp. 181-205).* Springfield, IL: Charles C Thomas.
Kinsbourne, M. (1995). Awareness of one's body. In J. L. Bermúdez, A. Marcel, & N. Eilan (Eds.). *The body and the self (pp. 205-223).* Cambridge, MA: MIT Press.

Mullen, C. A., & Cancienne, M. B. (2003). Re'sume' in motion: sensory self-awareness through movement. Sex Education: Sexuality, *Society and Learning, 3*, 157-170.

Ohno, K. & Ohno, Y. (2004). *Kazuo Ohno's world from without & within.* Middletown, CT: Wesleyan University Press.

O'Shaughnessy, B. (1995). Proprioception and the body image. In J. L. Bermúdez, A. Marcel, & N. Eilan (Eds.). *The body and the self (pp. 175-203).* Cambridge, MA: MIT Press.

Pallaro, P. (1996). Self and body-self: Dance/movement therapy and the development of object relations. The *Arts in Psychotherapy, 23,* 113-119.

Price, J., & Shildrick, M. (Eds.). (1999). *Feminist theory and the body -- A reader.* New York: Routledge.

Pylvänäinen, P. (2003). Body image: A tripartite model for use in dance/movement therapy. *American Journal of Dance Therapy, 25,* 39-55.

Schilder, P. (1950). *The image and appearance of the human body.* New York: International Universities Press.

Shotter, J. (2004). Responsive expression in living bodies: The power of invisible 'real presences' within our everyday lives together. *Cultural Studies, 18,* 443-460.

Smith, M. L. (2002). Moving Self: the thread which bridges dance and theatre. *Research in Dance Education, 3,* 123-141.

Stern, D. (1985). *The interpersonal world of the infant.* New York: Basic Books.

Tsakiris, M., & Haggard, P. (2005). Experimenting with the acting self. *Cognitive Neuropsychology, 22,* 387-407.

Welton, D. (ed.). (1999). *The body -- Classic and contemporary readings.* Malden, MA: Blackwell.

DANCE/MOVEMENT THERAPY FOR PEOPLE LIVING WITH MEDICAL ILLNESS

Sharon W. Goodill

This chapter proposes and describes five core foci for medical dance/movement therapy (DMT). Medical DMT is offered as a term to denote the application of DMT for people who are living with primary medical illnesses. In this context, DMT is a psychosocial support service for patients, their families and caregivers, and is part of the continuum of integrative health care. This discussion is oriented to the needs of adults with chronic medical illnesses, including cancer and diabetes. The five foci discussed are Vitality, Mood, Body Image of Illness, Relationship-focused Coping, and Self-efficacy.

Keywords: DMT, chronic illness, self-efficacy, mood.

INTRODUCTION

This chapter introduces theoretical concepts to support and inform the practice of dance/movement therapy (DMT) with medically ill people and their loved ones. For the purposes of this discussion, medical illness shall refer to conditions that present initially and primarily as physical (as opposed to psychiatric or behavioral) in nature. Dance/movement therapy is a mind/body approach to psychotherapy and increasingly offered in the conventional medical arena as a psychosocial service. The tenets and basic clinical methods of DMT, applied for decades in mental health areas, are intrinsically suited for adaptation to those with medical conditions, even if the capacity for physical movement is compromised. Dance/movement therapy interventions are directed to the places in human experience where psyche meets soma, where the kinaesthetic and the cognitive intersect, and where bodily-felt emotions can find motoric expression in the interactive context of a therapeutic relationship. It is logical to surmise that if phenomena and changes in the physical body are a source of pain, distress, anger, or isolation, then a somatically oriented method of psychosocial support and intervention will have meaningful impact.

The chapter is concerned mostly with the needs of adults with various chronic medical conditions. Chronic illness now is the leading cause of death in the world in both developed and developing countries, having recently eclipsed the threats of both infectious and acute diseases (Hyman, 2005). The comorbidity rates for medical conditions and psychiatric disorders demand our attention and are part of the rationale for integrating mental health services into standard medical care plans. Globally,

"one in four patients visiting a health service has at least one mental, neurological or behavioural disorder but most of these disorders are neither diagnosed nor treated....Mental illnesses affect and are affected by chronic conditions such as cancer, heart and cardiovascular diseases, diabetes and HIV/AIDS. Untreated, they bring about unhealthy behaviour, non-compliance with prescribed medical regimens, diminished immune functioning, and poor prognosis." (World Health Organization, n.d.)

In addition, people living with chronic illness are well aware of how the medical condition can impact every aspect of life. Vocational, spiritual, relational, sexual, emotional and psychological functioning are all affected to some degree. Thus, comprehensive health care should include services and professionals who can help patients and their families cope with the many attendant stressors and adjust to the inevitable changes and limitations.

Dance/movement therapists have professionalized as mental health specialists, and are also aligned worldwide with the complementary therapies and arts in healthcare movements. Inherently multidisciplinary in nature, dance/movement therapy (DMT) can play an integrative and humanizing role in the health care system. Dance/movement therapists who specialize with patients who are primarily medically ill have completed the requisite education and training for entry into the field of DMT, and have generally acquired additional knowledge and expertise particular to the conditions and issues faced by medical patients.

This application of DMT requires an integrated theoretical repertoire for the therapist, to include constructs developed in health psychology and in the neurosciences. Five core foci for medical DMT have been proposed: Vitality, Relationship-focused Coping, Self-efficacy, Body Image of Illness, and Mood (Goodill, 2005a). In this chapter, these foci are examined from biopsychosocial and holistic perspectives with linkages to and extensions of the existing theory and practice of DMT (see also, Melsom, 1999).

Vitality

In the dance/movement therapy literature, vitality has been described as "a positive quality of aliveness..." (M. Chace, 1975 cf. Schmais, 1985, p. 24), and vitalization as "an increase of energy which mobilizes the entire body" (Erhardt, Hearnes & Novak, 1989, p. 49) and "to be invigorated and enlivened" (Erhardt et al., p.59). In 1985, Schmais articulated the therapeutic factors, or healing processes in DMT, naming vitalization as one of eight such factors and describing it as, "investing people with the power to live" (Schmais, 1985, p. 25). She put the concept in movement terms, as follows:

> *"In the dance therapy session there is a synergistic effect resulting from the stimulation of being in a group situation and from the activation that is caused by moving.... freeing the impulse to act and the energy to do so. The flow of motion connects limbs to torso and feelings to actions."* (p.25)

Schmais further observed how "synchronous expressions of deep feelings to concordant rhythms vitalize the individual and the [dance/movement therapy] group, generating a reservoir of physical and psychic strength that can be used to further expression, communication and competence" (p. 26). Erhardt and colleagues (1989) conducted a three-part study of psychiatric patients who participated in DMT sessions using a modification of Yalom's Q-sort method (Yalom, 1995) that involved both structured interviews and participant responses to videotapes of DMT sessions. Sixty-six patients ranked the healing processes in both interviews and video review. Vitalization was ranked first and most frequently by this sample, regardless of age or gender. The researchers advised dance/movement therapists to "keep in mind that vitalization, an increase of energy that mobilizes the entire body, is the healing process clients value most" (p.59) and surmised that the clients in their study "valued Vitalization most because it affords an antidote to the sedentary patterns of their lives" (p.54).

For people whose illness results in a sedentary life, the sense of vitality offered in DMT can open the door to more invigorated ways of functioning and problem solving. Erhardt and colleagues noted the similarity between vitalization and the curative factor Instillation of Hope, described by Yalom (1995), and hope can be very important to the medically ill (Folkman & Moskowitz, 2000).

Two recent DMT studies focused on vitality (or closely related constructs) as a dependent variable. Over a 14-month period, Bojner-Horwitz, Theorell and Anderberg (2003) studied women with fibromyalgia who participated in a course of dance/movement therapy and viewed themselves moving on videotape. Based on the video viewings, the participants rated themselves on perceived life energy, mobility and pain. The researchers reported significant differences between the groups in ratings of perceived life energy, with the treatment group's perception of life energy increasing and that of the controls decreasing. The outcome variable, life energy, was defined in their study as how the patients' emotional and physical state is affected by the medical condition, in this case fibromyalgia. Coccari and Weiler (2003) reported a pilot study of wellness-seeking individuals who participated in an 8-week program of DMT. Outcomes were measured with self-report and showed statistically significant increases in energy and stamina as well as overall physical vitality.

Anecdotal data also suggest that medical patients find vitality in DMT. In a workshop I recently led for cancer survivors, one man shared, "I never feel so alive as when I am dancing". In her description of her own work leading DMT for people in cardiac rehabilitation, Seides (1986) observed how these patients need to "come to grips with the fact that renewed vitality may be slow in returning. Movement gives individuals opportunities to regain a sense of aliveness within the boundaries of their own limitations" (p.91).

Mood

Any psychosocial intervention of value to medically ill patients will give attention to the overlapping issues of mood, emotion and affect. Lazarus (2000) differentiates emotion from affect, saying "the former is a more inclusive concept that includes impulses to act and embodied emotional states" (p. 670), whereas mood has been defined as a "temporary disposition, and a state of the mind in regard to passion or feeling"(Thatcher & McQueen, 1977). Psychosocial interventions would do well to focus on the complementary goals of decreasing negative emotions (commonly including distress, sadness, fear, and anger) and supporting positive affect and emotions. The emotions often identified as positive: eagerness, excitement, confidence, happiness, pride, love, hope and relief, can occur even during stressful times or in the context of serious health problems (Folkman & Moskowitz, 2000; Lazarus, 2000). In addition, the positive emotions are linked to better coping, mastery, and even spiritual transformation in the face of stressful experiences (Folkman & Moskowitz).

Persistent negative emotions can both accompany and erode health status: "Patients with chronic medical illnesses have higher rates of depression and anxiety and these ...are associated with poor adherence to medical regimens and adverse medical outcomes." (Katon, Unützer, & Simon, 2004, p.1153). Having noted this, it is also important to give expression to the negative emotions. Pennebaker and colleagues have conducted numerous studies showing the health benefits of emotional expression through writing (Berry & Pennebaker, 1993). In a study of health status in college students Krantz (1994) demonstrated that psychophysical expression about troubling emotions (i.e., a DMT therapy method) decreased negative affect, and when combined with writing was associated with fewer visits to the health center.

Dibbel-Hope's controlled study (2000) of DMT to assist women in adaptation to breast cancer is an example of how DMT can enhance mood and emotion for people with chronic illness. The 22 women who participated in her 6-week course of group DMT (using the Authentic Movement method) showed statistically significant improvements in two components of mood. Mood was measured by the Profile of Mood States, a robust and commonly employed self-report instrument with six subscales: tension/anxiety, depression/dejection, anger/hostility, vigor, fatigue and confusion (McNair, Lorr & Broppleman, 1981). Dibbel-Hope's participants reported increased vigor and decreased fatigue. Serlin and colleagues (2000) reported similar benefits from 12-week programs of existentially based DMT groups for women with breast cancer. Their data showed significant decreases in fatigue and tension and increases in vigor, as measured also by the Profile of Mood States.

Body Image of Illness

Vamos (1993) developed a model for assessing and understanding body image in the context of chronic physical disability or medical condition. She suggests we "regard the body image as the portion of the self concept relating to the psychological representation of the body or the physical self" (p. 163) and notes that "the advent of physical illness increases its importance in overall self-representation and may therefore have considerable impact on overall self-esteem" (p. 163).

Vamos' model includes four major components:

- *Comfort:* pain, tiredness, dyspnea (difficulty with breathing), quality of sleep, parasthesias, nausea, enjoyment of food.

- *Competence:* cognitive ability, perceptual clarity, respiratory function, mobility, nutritional function, sexual function

- *Appearance:* self-evaluated, other-evaluated, visibility of disorder

- *Predictability:* degree of variability, suddenness of change, age appropriateness of disability.

Each medical condition creates its own constellation of these challenges to the body image. The body image is an appropriate focus for DMT, first because the heath of the body image has implications for other areas of functioning and health:

"Successful psychosocial adaptation to CID [chronic illness and disabilities] is said to reflect the integration of physical and sensory changes into a transformed body image and self-perception. Unsuccessful adaptation, in contrast, is evidenced by experiences of physical and psychiatric symptoms such as unmitigated feelings of anxiety and depression, psychogenic pain, chronic fatigue, social withdrawal, and cognitive distortions." (Livneh & Antonak, 2005, p. 13)

Secondly, as Kinsbourne (2002) suggests, the body image is essentially a "somatosensory background" that is formed through a coordination of "the somatic senses with intention and action, at times supplemented by vision" (p. 27). Kinsbourne purports the attentional view of the body image, that localizes it not to any part of the brain, but as providing a repository of information the body/brain has about itself. According to Kinsbourne, we attend to the body image when necessary, by slowing down, when in injury or pain, or when learning something new. Schilder (1950/1970) provided strong rationale for dance/movement based rehabilitation of the body image when he described its malleability this way: "Tension and relaxation of muscles, moving the body with and against gravity, with and against centrifugal impulses, may have an enormous influence on the body image. The phenomenon of the dance is therefore a loosening and changing in the body image" (p.207).

Seides (1986) described the way post-surgical cardiac patients feel as though they are "coming apart" (p. 90), as though the body's integrity has been disrupted, and that "movement can help to re-establish a sense of body integrity". Considering Vamos' model along with the methods and attributes of dance/movement therapy, one can hypothesize that movement interventions would impact body image in the areas of self-evaluation of Appearance, aspects of Comfort that relate to vitality (e.g. tiredness) and the mobility and perceptual clarity aspects of Competence. Seides' patients were dealing with the suddenness of change in the body (the Predictability component), as surgical patients must do when a body part has been removed or altered, whether of not this entails a change in outward appearance.

Relationship-Focused Coping

The concept of coping has been central to research on psychosocial aspects of medical illness. It seems that how patients and their loved one appraise the stressors associated with illness, how they respond to those stressors, and the resources they mobilize (or don't) in these responses have a clear and significant impact on quality of life, and sometimes on the medical course of the illness. This is particularly important in chronic conditions, because adherence to self-care regimens is essential for the maintenance of function and control of symptoms. Self-efficacy plays a role here, and is discussed in more detail below. Emotions play a role, and in paradoxical ways: Prolonged venting of emotions as the primary way of coping with stressors turns out not be effective, although (as seen in the work of Pennebaker, Krantz and colleagues) the expression of emotions is good for one's psychological and physical health. Emotional expression, problem-solving, and other forms of coping occur in a social and relational context (Coyne, 2000).

The concept of relationship-focused coping extends the process of coping with stressors from an individualistic model "to dyadic-level coping and also considers coping within the interpersonal context of the health care system" (Revenson, 1994, p. 126). Findings by Rohrbough and colleagues (2004) focus on relationship-focused coping and the importance of relationships in the adaptation to chronic illness. Their study of 191 congestive heart failure (CHF) patients and their spouses investigated both the patients' self-efficacy and the spouses' confidence in the patients and how each predicted patient survival over the ensuing four years. Both bode well for patient survival, but when compared, spousal confidence is a statistically stronger predictor than is the patient's own self-efficacy. The researchers concluded that spousal confidence in a CHF patient's ability to recover and survive constitutes a "fundamentally social protective factor" (Rohrbaugh, et al., p. 1).

In DMT, the therapeutic relationship is considered a mechanism for change whether in individual or group therapy formats (Fischer & Chaiklin, 1993) and dance/movement therapists work to help their clients generalize what is learned in sessions to their everyday and intimate relationships. We see that DMT supports the building of relationships through socialization, physical interaction, sharing in creative processes, movement rituals, and nonverbal communication (Serlin, 2000). Seides also emphasized the importance of the inclusion of spouses in the cardiac rehabilitation DMT work.

In dance/movement therapy assessment, elements of the dynamic and expressive movement repertoire are considered coping resources (Bartenieff, 1980). From a behavioral standpoint, these observable and patterned building blocks of movement comprise humans' habitual and unique ways of responding to events and experiences, including stressors. It is for this reason that dance/movement therapy treatment goals often include expansion the dynamic movement repertoire: increasing the range and mastery of Effort usage, the options for organizing movement in phrases, shaping in the kinesphere and ways of moving through space (Bartenieff, 1980). When the expressive movement capacity is enhanced in range, variation, intensity and mastery, the individual has more resources at his or her disposal for coping with stressors and challenges. Shaping in space with directional, planal and three-dimensional movement patterns is associated with how one relates to the physical and social environment, and relationships are built in the process of moving through shared space with attention to oneself and other movers (Kestenberg-Amighi, et al., 1999).

Using a single subject experimental design, Guthrie (1999) measured progress due to dance/movement therapy in a head injured man who struggled with both motoric/physical issues and psychosocial challenges. She documented clear improvements during the DMT intervention phase in the dynamic movement range and in self-reported movement confidence, and suggested a link between the psychomotor realm (movement qualities, spatial variables) and the psychosocial realm (confidence).

Self-Efficacy

Self-efficacy has been defined as "the belief that one can successfully perform behaviors to produce a desired outcome" (Berkman, 1995, p. 251) and "the belief that one can do what one has set out to do" (Endler, et al., 2001, p.618). The patient's perception of his or her own capacities is the key to assessing self-efficacy which, when strong, is associated with better self care and adherence to medically prescribed regimens (Farrell, Wicks & Martin, 2004). Even if self-efficacy is low at the point of diagnosis, it can be bolstered through interactive and social processes, particularly interventions that encourage independent activity on one's own behalf (Berkman, 1995).

DMT may be uniquely suited to the goal of increasing self-efficacy and internal health locus of control for medical patients who need intervention in these areas. Consider how in DMT it is the patient, not the therapist, who usually initiates expressive movement themes that are then shaped through improvisation into metaphors and for problem solving. Basic features of DMT, patient initiated physical activity, and responsive attention between the therapist and patient to the patient's own perceptions of bodily sensations, combine to replicate the conditions needed for encouraging self-efficacy. Bartenieff emphasized the connection between the patient's intent to act and his or her "independent participation" in recovery through movement (Bartenieff 1980, p.3).

A very few DMT studies to date have explored this notion. There is a substantial outcome study by Bräuninger (2006) that included self-efficacy as a moderator variable. Recently, Yang (2004) explored the fit between DMT methods and the components of self-efficacy as outlined by Bandura (1977). The components of Bandura's model of self-efficacy can be briefly summarized as, 1) Enactive Mastery Experience which is brought about through authentic experiences of success, 2) Vicarious Learning/Modeling, attained through observing others' behavior and success, 3) Allied Social Influences which occur through verbal persuasion or support, and 4) Judgment of Physiological and Affective States, meaning how people feel about their physical and emotional states (Bandura, 1986 and 1997, cf. Yang, 2004). Yang proposed that the following DMT techniques can facilitate an increase in self-efficacy: turn-taking in mirroring technique, the use of Shaping in the Vertical plane (Kestenberg-Amighi, et al., 1999), expanding movement repertoire, stress management methods. These techniques and their impact on self-efficacy and adherence were addressed in a case study of DMT with a diabetic woman who had co-morbid substance abuse problems. Statements made in her final session give qualitative evidence of some treatment success: "What I have achieved is that I've learned to take care of myself, exercise, and 'patience'.... Body and mind are both important for me and I didn't know it before.... I am confident. I can take care of my diabetes"(Yang, pp. 64-66).

In a randomized, controlled pilot study of mood and adherence in adults with cystic fibrosis, Goodill (2005b) found that participants who received a brief course of DMT (n=14) did report better adherence to nutritional self-care regimens one month after the completion of the therapy, when compared to the control group (n=10). Self-efficacy was not measured as a dependent variable, but the strong link between self-efficacy and adherence invites the possibility that a belief in ones' capacity for self-care was involved. Because the DMT intervention included body awareness methods, both active and in stillness, it is possible that learning to pay better attention to one's bodily cues may have led to an appreciation of the body's needs for self-care.

It is proposed herein that good adherence and self-care may be cultivated through both body awareness and self-efficacy, perhaps in a sequential process. In other words, one first must attend to the body's sensory and kinesthetic messages and then draw on a belief in oneself to engage in self-care behaviors. The fact that DMT supports and enhances body-self awareness is well-documented elsewhere (Cruz & Sabers, 1998). The integration of these attributes of DMT with concepts of self-efficacy and adherence constitutes a potent area for future research.

CONCLUSION

Two cautions are appropriate here. First, the five foci discussed herein are all constructs: abstractions of the lived experience that help us, as therapists, conceptualize our patients' plights and needs and inform clinical decision making. In practice, dance/movement therapy interventions could and generally do address all five foci in an integrated way.

As an example of how the five foci co-occur and overlap in clinical practice and research, consider the following excerpts and summaries from Dibbel Hope's (2000) report of her study of group DMT for survivors of breast cancer. Findings related to each of the five foci are italicized with references to the medical DMT focus in brackets.

Treatment groups "showed significant improvement over the control groups in Vigor, Fatigue [mood/vitality], and Somatization (p<.05), all of which related to sense of physical well-being." (p. 57) In self-report assessments of the DMT experience, 49% reported less depression and anxiety, less worry, more pleasure, and/or more hope [mood], 50% of the women reported an increased awareness and appreciation of their own strength and or knowledge [self-efficacy] and 75% of the participants reported increased appreciation of the body, more acceptance of the body "as is", and/or positive feelings about the body [body image]. At post-treatment, 63% of the participants reported receiving social support and in a 3-week follow-up survey using a 5-point Likert scale,"69% of the participants rated sharing and support as Extremely (5) or Moderately (4) helpful." (p.64) [relationship-focused coping].

Another example is the outcome study by Mannheim included in this volume. Findings showed that cancer patients who participated in the DMT sessions reported statistically significant reductions in anxiety, depression and fatigue as well as increases in emotional, social, physical and role-related aspects of quality of life. In these findings, the foci of mood, vitality and possibly relationship-focus are evident.

The second cautionary note is that this is by no means a complete list of themes and clinical concerns in DMT for adults with medical conditions. Pain relief, spirituality, grief, freedom, meaning, isolation, death and other issues (see Serlin et al., 2000) can be equally important to individual patients and their loved ones. The five foci described here provide a framework only, and can serve as a point of departure for therapists working with chronically medically ill adults. Holistic interventions such as DMT accept that any or all of these issues may seem pressing on a given day, and that an intervention directed to one problem may well bring some relief or clarity in another area. Numerous works in the psychology literature show the overlap of and relationships between these constructs (e.g. Endler, Kocovski & Macrodimitris, 2001; Spira, 1997). The enhanced body awareness achieved in DMT may manifest in better self-efficacy and adherence as proposed above, or may bolster the body image. Better mood state may be part of an increase in vitality and may also enable active engagement in supportive relationships. All this would suggest that good psychosocial support will not parse its focus, but rather approach the medically ill patient and his or her loved ones in a holistic way.

REFERENCES

Bandura, A. (1977). Self-efficacy: Towards a unifying theory of behavioral change. *Psychological Review, 84*, 191-215.

Bartenieff, I., & Dori Lewis (1980). *Body movement: Coping with the environment.* New York: Gordon and Breach Publishers.

Berkman, L. (1995). The role of social relations in health promotion. *Psychosomatic Medicine, 57*, 245-254.

Berry, D. S., & Pennebaker, J. W. (1993). Nonverbal and verbal emotional expression and health. *Psychother Psychosom, 59*, 11-19.

Bojner-Horwitz, E., Theorell, T., & Anderberg, U. M. (2003). Dance/movement therapy and changes in stress-related hormones: A study of fibromyalgia patients with video-interpretation. *The Arts in Psychotherapy, 30*(5), 255-264.

Bräuninger, I. (2006). *Tanztherapie. [Dance Therapy].* Weinheim, Germany: Beltz / PFA.

Coccari, G., & Weiler, M. (2003). *Exploring the impact of dance/movement therapy on personal vitality in well-ness-seeking individuals.* Poster presented at the American Dance Therapy Association 38th Annual Conference, Denver, Colorado.

Coyne, J. (2000, February). *Social Relationships, distress, and survival among CHF patients.* Paper presented at the Mind/Body Programs Symposium Series, MCP Hahnemann University, Philadelphia.

Cruz, R., & Sabers, D. (1998). Dance/Movement Therapy is more effective than previously reported. *The Arts in Psychotherapy: An International Journal, 25*, 101-104.

Dibbel-Hope, S. (2000). The use of dance/movement therapy in psychological adaptation to breast cancer. *The arts in psychotherapy, 27*, 51-68.

Endler, N. S., Kocovski, N. L., & Macrodimitris, S. D. (2001). Coping, efficacy, and perceived control in acute vs. chronic illnesses. *Personality and Individual Differences, 20*, 617-625.

Erhardt, B. T., Hearne, M. B., & Novak, C. (1989). Outpatient clients' attitudes towards healing processes in dance therapy. *American Journal of Dance Therapy, 11*, 39-60.

Farrell, K., Wicks, M., & Martin, J. (2004) Chronic disease management improved with enhanced self-efficacy. *Clinical Nursing Research, 13*, 289-308.

Fischer, J., & Chaiklin, S. (1993). Meeting in movement: The work of the therapist and the client. In S. Sandel, S. Chaiklin & A. Lohn (Eds.). *Foundations of Dance/Movement Therapy: The life and work of Marian Chace.* Columbia, MD: The Marian Chace Memorial Fund of the American Dance Therapy Association.

Folkman, S., & Moskowitz, J. T. (2000). Positive affect and the other side of coping. *American Psychologist, 55*(6), 647-654.

Goodill, S. (2005a). *An Introduction to Medical Dance/Movement Therapy: Health care in motion*. London: Jessica Kingsley Publishers.

Goodill, S. (2005b). Research Letter: Dance/Movement Therapy for Adults with Cystic Fibrosis: Pilot Data on Mood and Adherence. *Alternative Therapies in Health and Medicine, 11*, 76-77.

Guthrie, J. (1999). Movement and dance therapy in head injury: An evaluation. *Dance Therapy Collections, Dance Therapy Association of Australia, 2*, 24-30.

Hyman, M. (2005). Quality in healthcare: Asking the right questions: The next ten years: The role of CAM in the "quality cure". *Alternative Therapies in Health and Medicine, 11*(3), 18-20.

Katon, W. J., Unutzer, J., & Simon, G. (2004). Treatment of depression in primary care: where we are, where we can go. *Medical Care, 42*, 1153-1157.

Kinsbourne, M. (2002). The role of imitation in body ownership and mental growth In A. N. Meltzoff & W. Prinz (Eds.). The imitative mind: development, evolution,and brain bases (pp.311–330). Cambridge: University Press.

Kestenberg-Amighi, J., Loman, S., Lewis, P., & Sossin, K.M. (1999). *The Meaning of Movement: Development and clinical perspectives of the Kestenberg Movement Profile*. New York, NY: Gordon & Breach.

Krantz, A. (1994). *Dancing Out Trauma: the effects of psychophysical expression on health*. Unpublished Ph.D. Dissertation, California School of Professional Psychology, Berkeley, CA.

Lazarus, R. S. (2000). Toward better research on stress and coping. *American Psychologist, 55*(6), 665-673.

Livneh, H., & Antonak, R.F. (2005). Psychosocial adaptation to chronic illness: A primer for counselors. *Journal of Counseling and Development, 83*, 12-20.

McNair, D. M., Lorr, M., & Broppleman, L. R. (1981). *EITS Manual for the Profile of Mood States*. San Diego, CA: Educational and Industrial Testing Service.

Melsom, A. M. (1999). *Dance/movement therapy for psychosocial aspects of heart disease and cancer: An exploratory literature review*. Unpublished Master's thesis, MCP Hahnemann University, Philadelphia.

Revenson, T. A. (1994). Social support and marital coping with chronic illness. *Annals of Behavioral Medicine, 16*(2), 122-130.

Rohrbaugh, M. J., Shoham, V., Coyne, J., Cranford, J. A., Sonnega, J. S., & Nicklas, J. M. (2004). Beyond the "Self" in self-efficacy: spouse confidence predicts patient survival following heart failure. *Journal of Family Psychology, 18*, 184-193.

Seides, M. (1986). Dance/movement therapy as a modality in the treatment of the psychosocial complications of heart disease. *American Journal of Dance Therapy, 9*, 83-101.

Schilder, Paul (1950/1970) *The image and appearance of the human body*. NY: International Universities Press.

Schmais, C. (1985). Healing Processes in Group Dance Therapy. *American Journal of Dance Therapy, 8*, 17-36.Serlin, I. A., Classen, C., Frances, B., & Angell, K. (2000). Symposium: Support groups for women with breast cancer: Traditional and alternative expressive approaches. *The Arts in Psychotherapy, 27*, 123-138.

Spira, J. (1997). Understanding and developing psychotherapy groups for medically ill patients. In J. Spira (Eds.). *Group Therapy for Medically Ill Patients* (pp. 3-54). New York: The Guilford Press.

Thatcher, V., & McQueen, A. et al. (Eds.) (1977). *The new Webster encyclopedic dictionary of the English language*. Chicago: Consolidated Book Publishers.

Vamos, M. (1993). Body image in chronic illness -- A reconceptualization. *International Journal of Psychiatry in Medicine, 23*, 163-178.

WHO. (n.d.). *Mental Health: The bare facts*. Retrieved April 23, 2005, from http://www.who.int/mental_health/en/

Yalom, I. (1995). *Theory and Practice of Group Psychotherapy*. New York: Basic Books.

Yang, Hsiu-ling (2004). *The Impact of Dance/Movement Therapy on Self-Efficacy in Adults with Diabetes Mellitus: A Case Study*. Unpublished master's thesis, Drexel University, Philadelphia.

DANCE/MOVEMENT THERAPY WITH CANCER INPATIENTS: EVALUATION OF PROCESS AND OUTCOME PARAMETERS

Elana G. Mannheim & Joachim Weis

Dance/Movement Therapy, a psychotherapy using the body, helps cancer patients to cope emotionally and physically in the process of treatment. After medical therapies which can be invasive and aggressive, women, in particular, use Dance Therapy as part of a psycho-oncology rehabilitation program in order to come to terms with changes in the body, experience a new feeling of movement, express their emotions, and increase their self-confidence. Both quantitative and qualitative methods were used in a three-year research project at the Tumor Biology Center in Freiburg, Germany, to examine the effects of Dance Therapy: Standardized questionnaires for measuring quality of life, well-being, and self-image were employed in addition to using semi structured interviews that focused on patients' personal experiences in Dance Therapy. Additionally, external raters evaluated the movement patterns of selected patients using the Kestenberg Movement Profile (KMP). The results suggest significant improvements in quality of life, reduction of anxiety and depression, and increased self-esteem. The quality of movement progressed toward more healthy movement. The results may not be attributed to Dance Therapy alone, yet the qualitative assessments clearly show that Dance Therapy has a positive influence on the coping process. Methodological issues and future research needs are discussed.

Keywords: DMT, psycho-oncology, quality of life, coping;

INTRODUCTION

A wide variety of psychosocial pressures leading to emotional changes and loss of confidence can arise as a result of cancer. These may also manifest as psychological problems. For example, helplessness, inability to act, and severe existential anxiety are some of the feelings experienced by cancer patients (Weis, 1977). In view of this, modern cancer treatment increasingly takes account of psychosocial aspects and offers patients support in improving quality of life and coming to terms with the illness (Larbig & Tschuschke, 2000). Over the last 20 years, comprehensive psycho-oncology interventions have been developed in order to help patients adapt to the changes caused by the illness and maintain the best possible quality of life. In this process, the strengthening of appropriate coping strategies, reduction of anxiety and symptoms of depression such as negative thoughts or brooding phases, and the search for social support play a central role (Larbig & Tschuschke, 2000). This recognition has given rise to an important professional field involving creative arts therapies. Using artistic media, patients can express inner images of their current feeling states and these states can be transformed in the creative process (Luzzatto & Gabriel, 1998).

In recent years, German psycho-oncology treatment has begun to include dance therapy. Dance therapy offers an opportunity to convey experiences on a primarily nonverbal level, combining emotional processes and physical experience. Dance therapy can address the cancer patient as a whole person, both emotionally and physically, and to support the process of coming to terms with the illness. Our experience to date shows that it is mainly female cancer patients who are drawn to this form of therapy. Following medical therapies that may be invasive and aggressive, they wish to move freely and authentically, accept the changes in their bodies, and build new self-confidence. It is a fundamental principle of psychosocial therapy methods in oncology to work with healthy aspects of functioning as a starting point and tries to develop or strengthen personal resources.

In oncology rehabilitation integrated medical and psychosocial treatment measures are implemented with the aim of treating problems arising from the illness, promoting self-responsibility and initiative, and increasing patients' ability to cope with the illness. To this end, along with various relaxation therapies, individual and group psychological therapies, the psychosocial department of the Tumor Biology Center offers a wide-ranging selection of art therapies including painting, sculpture, poetry and bibliotherapy, music therapy, and dance therapy.

To date, there has been little research on dance therapy and oncology in Germany. Our working group carried out the first German pilot study on dance therapy with cancer inpatients (Mannheim, Liesenfeld, & Weis, 2000). Standardized instruments and semi-structured interviews were used to assess quality of life in terms of health. Individual case analyses showed significant improvements in quality of life. As the Tumor Biology Center uses a variety of treatment methods these improvements could not be solely attributed to dance therapy, but on a subjective level, patients perceived dance therapy to be an important support in the process of coming to terms with the illness.

While no further studies on dance therapy in psycho-oncology were available in German, we found a small number of publications in English. Dibbell-Hope (2000) conducted a study of 33 female breast cancer patients in an outpatient setting. The study involved a randomized control group, and standardized tests, and interviews. Evaluation of the tests showed a slight improvement in mood, perceived stress, body image, and self-esteem. The interview evaluations showed a marked improvement in emotional well-being, self-esteem, and acceptance of body image. The participants felt generally more hopeful, more optimistic, and extremely supported by the group on a social level.

In their study of cancer patients, Serlin, Classen, Frances and Angell (2000) found significant improvements with respect to fatigue, vitality, and reduction of fear and depression. The women had taken part in supportive-expressive group therapy with integrated dance therapy over a 12-week period. Sandel and Judge (2004) investigated 35 women with breast cancer who took part in outpatient dance therapy over a 12-week period. Significant improvements in quality of life were detected in comparison with the waiting group, and shoulder symptoms and body image also improved over the course of the intervention.

In sum, there has been little research on dance therapy in cancer patients and further systematic evaluation is needed. Initial results show that dance therapy can lead to emotional changes and improvements in body image and self-esteem. In view of this, it was the aim of a three-year study to evaluate dance therapy within a psycho-oncology rehabilitation facility and to investigate to what extent this type of therapy can improve physical and emotional well-being and promote self-esteem. The study aimed to describe how dance therapy affects this target group. The following results relate to the pilot phase carried out in 2002 at the Tumor Biology Center, Freiburg, Germany.

METHODS

Design

The pilot phase employed a one-group, pre-post design with quantitative and qualitative processes to examine quality of life with respect to health, anxiety and depression, self-esteem, and the influence of dance therapy on physical and emotional changes and on movement. This phase of the research project served to obtain information on which patients took advantage of the therapy and to test the suitability of the measuring instruments.

Description of the Sample

Dance therapy was offered to all inpatient rehabilitation clinic patients who showed interest in this group therapy. There were no exclusion criteria. Ninety patients were recruited for participation in the study from Mai to November 2002. Owing to acute illness whilst at the center, time conflicts with other therapies, general weakness or premature discontinuation of the therapy for other reasons, the sample decreased to N=81. In order to ensure greater homogeneity, only female patients were included into the pre-post comparison. The data of N=77 patients were evaluated.

The average age of the female participants was 52 years. The youngest was 25 and the oldest 83 years old. Two thirds of these female patients were married, divorced, or widowed. Just under a third had had no children. Approximately half of them were employed (either full or part-time). Most of the 77 female patients had been diagnosed with a tumor between two and ten months previously. For two thirds of these female participants, the dance therapy was the first experience of psychotherapy.

The patient group was heterogeneous in terms of diagnosis, tumor and treatment status. The largest group was the 51 female breast cancer patients, of whom 40 had had tumors removed without mastectomy and 11 had undergone mastectomy. Almost all had undergone radiotherapy and/or chemotherapy, 6 were continuing to receive chemotherapy during their stay, and 15 were there due to a new tumor or a relapse.

Instruments

The study employed both standardized and qualitative instruments for data collection (questionnaires, interviews, and movement analysis). The dance therapy participants' expectations were recorded using a self-constructed assessment inventory using questions based on the Dortmund Questionnaire on Movement Therapy (DFBT -- Dortmunder Fragebogen zur Bewegungstherapie, Hölter, 2001). Factor analysis of the new inventory on one of our clinical samples identified four scales: relaxation, self-esteem, emotional expression, and social/interaction skills.

The dimensions of quality of life relating to cancer were obtained using the Quality of Life Questionnaire -- EORTC QLQ-C-30 (Aaronson et al., 1993). The 30 items encompass five functional scales (physical, role, emotional, social, and cognitive functions) as well as various symptom scales such as fatigue, pain, nausea and sickness, sleeplessness, shortness of breath, etc. Patients were also asked for a general assessment of their physical condition and quality of life.

The German version of the Hospital Anxiety and Depression Scale HADS-D (Herrmann, Buss, & Sneith, 1995), which was developed specifically for use with the physically ill, was used for self-assessment of anxiety and depression. Each scale for anxiety and depression consists of 14 items.

To assess participants' self-image, four scales from the Frankfurt Self-Image Concept scales (Frankfurter Selbstkonzeptskalen -- FSKN, Deusinger, 1986) were selected: evaluation of self-esteem, ability to deal with problems, sensitivity and mood, and ability to interact socially. Evaluation of the success of the dance therapy was carried out using the Dortmund Questionnaire on Movement Therapy (DFBT, Hölter, 2001), which contains 60 statements on how the movement therapy worked. The 7 DFBT subscales relate to an assessment of therapeutically helpful elements in the dance/movement therapy including awareness, catharsis, re-experience, insight and learning, as well as well-being and group cohesion.

Additionally, feedback from the patients written in response to an open-ended question ("What did you personally gain from the dance therapy?") was evaluated. Observation and analysis of movement was used as a therapy-specific assessment instrument. The purpose of the movement assessment was to judge the success of the therapy using defined therapy goals relating to movement, and to record changes in movement behavior and emotional features. The movement of 3 patients was recorded on video while they were taking part in the dance therapy sessions. Two trained and qualified movement analysts rated their movement on 15 minute video clips using the Laban/Bartenieff Movement System (Laban/Bartenieff-Bewegungssystems LBBS), in order to record qualitatively complex movements. The movement data was used to discover how physical changes showing improved movement were reflected both within dance therapy session and in the course of dance therapy treatment.

Clinical Procedures

Dance therapy was offered as a group intervention. Guided dance improvisation was used with the aim of stimulating awareness of the remaining healthy parts of the body, re-creating confidence in the patient's own body, and awakening joy of life. The aim of non-verbal access to emotions is to give patients the opportunity to experience the so-called "negative" feelings of fear, sorrow, and anger and express them through dance. The human contact through the dance therapy group offered an escape from potential isolation and encouraged new social relationships with other cancer patients. Each group session was divided into four phases:

Phase 1 consisted of an exercise phase designed to create a trusting atmosphere, to stimulate breathing and movement, and improve the contact to the floor (grounding). The exercises were repeated in a similar way in each group lesson, so that the patients could learn them and continue with them at home.

Phase 2 was a phase of experiencing. It involved either strong movements (such as stamping), associated with willpower, assertiveness, and self-assertion, or gentle movements leading to lightness, carefreeness, and exhilaration. The qualities of the movements were designed to awaken intense feelings of enjoyment and zest for life.

Phase 3 centered on themes. The themes were introduced by the therapist and served as motifs for exercises and improvisation activities. The main themes were: awareness of one's own needs, finding space/refuge, coping with one's own limitations, coping with difficult emotions.

Phase 4 consisted of a discussion at the end of each dance therapy session. The discussions allowed patients to reflect on the experiences of the lesson and share them with the group. The aim was to integrate the experiences into everyday life and open up new perspectives for shaping life in the future.

This relatively high-structured approach was chosen because patients usually participated in only about 7 therapy sessions, due to their brief average stay at the center. Two dance therapy groups, with a maximum of eight participants each, were offered at varying intervals. Group I took place three times a week, Group II twice a week. Both were ninety minutes long. Because of the varying dates of the patients' arrival at and departure from the Tumorbiology Center the structure of the group was flexible and membership changed relatively frequently. The participants took part between 3 and 14 times. Most of them (81%) took part between 5 and 9 times.

RESULTS

Concerning the patients' expectations of dance therapy (see Figure 1), the most important issue was to seek active relaxation, the desire for inner peace and equilibrium. Similarly, improvement in self-esteem and emotional expression were high on the list of expectations. It seems striking that the need for contact with other patients was of minor importance at the start of the dance therapy treatment.

Figure 1: Expectations
Means of n = 77 patients (T1)

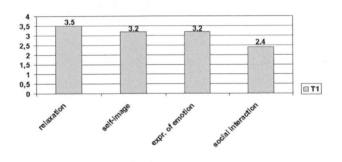

Scale values: 1=disagree entirely - 4= strongly agree

In the subjective assessment of the dance therapy, participants particularly confirmed the improvement in well-being. This was followed by similarly high values concerning learning, awareness, catharsis, and insight. At this point, group cohesion was valued relatively highly, with a mean of 4.69, which may show that, contrary to the original expectations of the participants, social interaction in the dance therapy was seen as helpful.

The resulting mean of the DFBT (M=4.90) was significantly higher than that of a study on movement therapy with psychosomatic patients (Hölter, 2001; M=4.20), and may indicate high success of dance therapy in this sample test (see Figure 2).

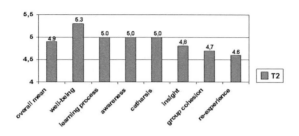

Figure 2: Effects of Dance Therapy (DFBT)
Means of n = 67 patients (T2)

Scale values: 1 = disagree entirely – 6 = strongly agree

We received answers to the open question: *"What did dance therapy do for you personally?"* from 59 patients. Using content analysis, it was possible to form categories, which confirmed the effectiveness parameters of the dance therapy (see Figure 3; left side: categories; right side: examples for patients' quotes).

Ability to express emotions	"expressing negative feelings, too, through dance"
	"knowing one's own limitations"
Expressive movement	"to dance as lightly as a butterfly"
Vitality	"joy in movement"
Relationship to own body	"I feel more in touch with my own body"
Self esteem	"feeling good about myself"
Group cohesion	"feeling trust towards other group members"

Figure 3: „How effective was Dance Therapy for you personally?"
Multiple Nomination n = 59

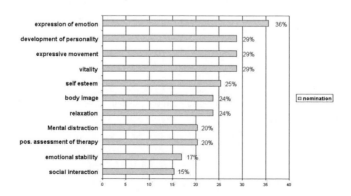

With respect to quality of life, the illustration of the results concentrates on the scales, which were relevant to the group under investigation (see Figure 4). The data at the outset of the investigation showed marked impairment on the function and symptom scales compared with the normal population. During the intervention period (T1 to T2) there was a statistically significant improvement in the mean values of the role function, emotionality, fatigue, and physical function scales (p<.01), and mean values of social function also improved moderately (p<.05; see Table I). Although the patients' values during the relatively short intervention period became more similar to the reference data of the normal population, they remained far below the average values of the normal German female population (Schwarz & Hinz, 2001).

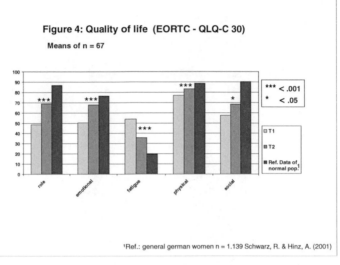

Figure 4: Quality of life (EORTC - QLQ-C 30)

Means of n = 67

¹Ref.: general german women n = 1.139 Schwarz, R. & Hinz, A. (2001)

TABLE I: STATISTICS OF THE QUALITY OF LIFE SCALES (EORTC-QLQ-C30)

Scales	Means (SD) T1 (n=77)	Means (SD) T2 (n=67)	Means (SD) Ref. Data (n=373)	F (67,66)	p	Eta²
Role functioning	48,5 (30,5)	68,9 (26,9)	86,6 (23,7)	26,4	P<.001	.29
Emotional functioning	50,3 (25,1)	67,8 (26,2)	76,3 (22,2)	29,6	P<.001	.31
Fatigue	53,8 (26,3)	35,8 (21,9)	19,5 (23,1)	36,8	P<.001	.36
Physical functioning	76,8 (17,2)	83,3 (13,9)	88,7 (17,5)	16,4	P<.001	.20
Social functioning	57,4 (28,4)	68,2 (30,1)	90,3 (20,1)	6,8	P<.05	.09

The value of the anxiety scale prior to the intervention lay significantly higher than the reference values of German women aged 40 to 59 years (see Table II; and Figure 5). Within the treatment period this value decreased significantly and became more similar to the reference values. Similar positive changes were shown for depression.

TABLE II: STATISTICS OF THE ANXIETY AND DEPRESSION SCALES (HADS)

Scales	Means (SD) T1 (n=77)	Means (SD) T2 (n=67)	Means (SD) Ref. data (n=1142)	F (67, 66)	p	Eta²
Anxiety	7,0 (3,5)	5,2 (3,5)	5,2 (3,4)	26,2	p<.001	.28
Depression	4,8 (3,4)	3,3 (3,1)	4,8 (3,7)	18,9	p<.001	.22

Figure 5: Anxiety and Depression (HADS)
Means of n = 67

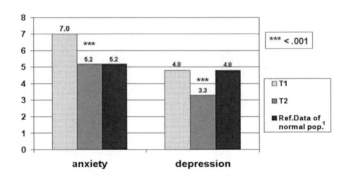

¹Ref.: General German women, (40 - 59 years), n = 373/1142; Schwarz, R. & Hinz, A. (2001)

Figure 6: Self image (FSKN)
Means of n = 67

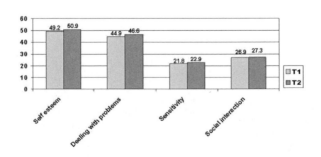

The self-image scales showed initially high values, which changed only slightly during the course of the treatment (see Figure 6). However, there was a significant improvement of values for self-esteem, and general ability to deal with problems. "Social contact and ability to interact socially" was the factor, which showed the smallest change (see Table III).

TABLE III: STATISTICS OF THE SELF IMAGE SCALES (FSKN)

Scales	Means (SD) T1 (n=77)	Means (SD) T2 (n=67)	F (67, 66)	P	Eta^2
Self esteem	49,2 (7,8)	50,9 (6,4)	16,8	p<.001	.20
Dealing with problems	44,9 (5,2)	46,6 (5,4)	13,2	p<.01	.17
Sensitivity	21,8 (3,7)	22,9 (4,4)	8,7	p<.01	.12
Social interaction	26,9 (3,6)	27,3 (3,8)	2,4	p=n.s.	.04

In the movement analysis, the movement characteristics of three patients videotaped during the sessions were rated by external raters on scales from 0 to 3. The higher the point score, the higher the relevant movement characteristics of the patient.

The results of dance therapy session 1 were compared to those of dance therapy session 5 (see Figure 7). In the course of the treatment period the movement behavior of the three patients improved and became more similar to healthy movement behavior.

The raters who were blind to actual sequence of sessions agreed in 90 of 141 possible cases (63.8% agreement). The total scores of the mean values of the two raters are illustrated in Figure 7. Because of the small sample of 3 patients and the low rater agreement, the results are not further interpreted here.

Figure 7: Movement Analysis

Summary Score

Means of Rater A + B

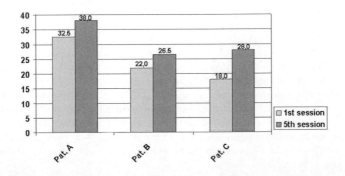

The participants in the study took part in other therapies besides dance therapy during their rehabilitation. Almost all took part in sport therapy, Qi-Gong, and a relaxation process. Three quarters of the participants took advantage of individual psychological support and a quarter received another creative arts therapy. This level of participation in psychosocial support services provides evidence of a heavy psychological burden, and the search for support in coming to terms with the illness.

DISCUSSION

During rehabilitation many inpatients are still in a shock following their cancer diagnosis and subsequent treatment. They are under considerable physical and psychological tension. Emotional reactions of depression and fear of relapse are common amongst them. Physical weakness, limitation of physical functions and pain hinder them to a varying extend.

In addition to dealing with symptoms of the illness and symptoms caused by treatment or subsequent problems, the main focus in psycho-oncology rehabilitation is generally the promotion of resources and remaining health. Promoting self responsibility and self control, and reduction of anxiety and depression are important therapeutic goals. The few studies that investigated the influence of dance therapy interventions on various goal parameters in cancer patients report positive effects with respect to the emotional well-being, and body and self image of female cancer patients. This pilot study suggests that at the beginning of the rehabilitation the patients generally suffered from poor physical well-being, and were strongly psycho-socially burdened. Participation in dance therapy provided them with access to positive body-related experiences, and to emotional processes that helped them to cope with the illness. In this way, dance therapy actively supported their process of coming to terms with the illness and strengthened their self confidence. There is thus initial evidence that dance therapy can play an important role in oncology rehabilitation for the specific subgroup of women.

The pilot phase showed that the majority of the instruments used are appropriate for the main study. An exception is the Questionnaire on Movement Therapy (DFBT), which is still being developed. Here, the test theoretical analyses and factor-analytical calculations showed that this procedure is clearly not yet sufficiently standardized and requires further development. The investigation instrument we developed with reference to the DFBT on the expectations of dance therapy can continue to be used on the basis of the good factor-analytical results (see appendix). The movement analysis showed unsatisfying results, in particular with respect to inter-rater reliability. It is assumed that the low inter-rater agreement in the pilot phase is attributable on the one hand to the procedure used, and on the other hand to the different levels of training of the raters. Consequently, for the main phase, the Kestenberg Movement Profile (KMP) will be selected, for which trained raters are available. In addition, the movement observation will take place using a standardized setting.

In this pilot study, it was not the primary aim to evaluate the effects of dance therapy. Especially since, because of the multi-modal treatment concept in inpatient treatment, the changes can not be attributed solely to the dance therapy. Rather, the pilot study provides important information on the central mechanisms of dance therapy, which must be investigated more systematically in further studies. With respect to the methodology, future studies should employ qualitative as well as quantitative procedures, on the basis of our experience because of the nature of dance therapy. The main phase of our project may show to what extent the selected, and in some cases modified, instruments can lead to further results. A follow up after three months is planned for the main phase in order to investigate to what extent positive effects are maintained in this period. In addition, it must be controlled whether the patients are continuing a comparable intervention at home, and to what extent transfer of that intervention's influence on emotional well-being takes place in everyday life.

REFERENCES

Aaronson, N.K., Ahmedzai, S., Bergmann, B., Bullinger, M., Cull, A., Duez, N.Z., Filiberti, A., Flechtner, H., Fleishman, S.B., & de Haes, J.C. (1993). The European Organization for Research and Treatment of Cancer QLQ-C30: a quality-of-life instrument for use in international clinical trials in oncology. *Journal of National Cancer Institute, 85,* 365-376.

Deusinger, I. (1986). *Frankfurter Selbstkonzeptskalen, FSKN.* Göttingen: Hogrefe.

Dibbell-Hope, S. (2000). The use of Dance/Movement Therapy in Psychological Adaptation to Breast Cancer. *The Arts in Psychotherapy, 27 (1),* 51-68.

Hinz, A., & Schwarz, R. (2001). Angst und Depression in der Allgemeinbevölkerung. *PPmP Psychotherapy, Psychosomatic, medical Psychology, 51,* 193-200.

Herrmann, C., Buss, U., & Sneith, R.P. (1995). *Hospital Anxiety and Depression Scale, HADS – German Version.* Bern: Huber.

Hölter, G. (2001). Bewegung, Spiel und Sport mit psychisch kranken Menschen, Ziele, Akzeptanz und Evaluation [Movement, play and sports with the psychic ill. Goals, acceptance, and evaluation.]. In Fischer, K. & Holland-Moritz, H. (Eds.). *Mosaiksteine der Motologie* (pp. 233-253). Schorndorf: Hofmann.

Larbig, W. & Tschuschke, V. (2000). Psychologische Interventionseffekte bei Krebs – eine Einführung. [Effects of psychological interventions with cancer patients. An Introduction.] In W. Larbig, & V. Tschuschke (Eds.). *Psychoonkologische Interventionen* (pp. 12-20). München: Ernst Reinhard Verlag.

Luzzatto, P., & Gabriel, B. (1998). Art-Psychotherapy. In Holland, J.C. (Ed.). *Psycho-Oncology* (pp. 743-757). New York: Oxford-University Press.

Mannheim, E.G., Liesenfeld, M., & Weis, J. (2000). Tanztherapie in der onkologischen Rehabilitation: Konzepte und empirische Ergebnisse zu Auswirkungen auf die Lebensqualität. [DMT in oncology rehabilitation. Concepts and empirical results on improvement of quality of life.] *Zeitschrift für Musik-, Tanz- und Kunsttherapie, 11(2),* 80-86.

Sandel, S.L., & Judge, J.O. (2004). Dance and movement program improves quality of life measure in breast cancer survivors. In American Dance Therapy Association (Eds.). *Choreographing health: Dance/Movement Therapy 2004. Proceedings from the 39th Annual Conference* (pp. 105-108). New Orleans: Hampton Inn & Suites.

Schwarz, R., & Hinz, A. (2001). Reference data for the quality of life questionnaire EORTC QLQ-C30 in the general German population. *European Journal of Cancer, 37,* 1345-1351.

Serlin, I.A., Classen, C., Frances, B., & Angell, K. (2000). Symposium: Support groups for women with breast cancer: traditional and alternative expressive approaches. *The Arts in Psychotherapy, 27 (2),* 123-138.

Weis, J. (1997). Das Konzept der Salutogenese in der Psychoonkologie. [The concept of salutogenesis in psychooncology] In Bartsch, H. & Bengel, J. (Eds.). *Salutogenese in der Onkologie* (pp. 164-184). Basel: Karger.

APPENDIX

Erwartungen an die Tanztherapie

Welche der folgenden Erwartungen haben Sie? Bitte kreuzen Sie an, welche Aussage für Sie stimmt....
Durch die Teilnahme an der Tanztherapie erwarte ich:

	stimmt gar nicht	stimmt wenig	stimmt ziemlich	stimmt sehr	
1. körperliche Entspannung	1	2	3	4	verw_1
2. seelische Ausgeglichenheit	1	2	3	4	verw_2
3. wieder Spaß an der Bewegung zu finden	1	2	3	4	verw_3
4. mich ohne Leistungsdruck bewegen zu können	1	2	3	4	verw_4
5. belastende Gedanken eine Zeit lang abzuschalten	1	2	3	4	verw_5
6. Schmerzen zu mindern	1	2	3	4	verw_6
7. wieder Zugang zu meinem Körper zu bekommen	1	2	3	4	verw_7
8. meinen Körper annehmen zu können	1	2	3	4	verw_8
9. im Tanzen auch mal „Dampf ablassen" zu können	1	2	3	4	verw_9
10. die momentane Stimmung oder Gefühle zum Ausdruck bringen zu können	1	2	3	4	verw_10
11. mich selbst besser kennen zu lernen	1	2	3	4	verw_11
12. Kontakt zu Mitpatientinnen zu finden	1	2	3	4	verw_12

EVALUATING DMT IN FIBROMYALGIA PATIENTS -- CONSEQUENCES OF VERBAL, VISUAL AND HORMONAL ANALYSES

Eva Bojner Horwitz

This randomized control trial presents hormonal, emotional, physical and visual status changes in thirty-six female fibromyalgia patients (FMS) after six months of dance/movement therapy (DMT). FMS is a stress related chronic pain syndrome involving musculoskeletal aches, stiffness and pain with perturbations in the stress-axis. Serum concentrations of different stress hormones, different verbal self-ratings scales, a video interpretation technique (VIT) and self-figure drawings were analyzed. The results show that six month of DMT improved the psychological and physiological function. The VIT and self-figure drawings captured treatment effects that were not evident from verbal scales or reflected in hormone levels. The use of different assessment techniques has affected the treatment outcome. Difficulties perceiving information through verbal/cognitive modalities as well as alexithymia are factors discussed. This study indicates that both DMT and the VIT have great influence on the FMS patients' well-being, life energy, perception of pain and self-perception.

Keywords: DMT, Fibromyalgia, RCT, Self-figure drawing, Stress hormones, Video interpretation.

INTRODUCTION

This chapter describes a study with the principal aim to determine whether and how the hormonal, emotional, physical, and visual status changed in female FMS patients, following treatment with dance/movement therapy (DMT), comparing this to a randomly assigned control group of female fibromyalgia (FMS) patients. The study used different assessment methods: hormone analyses, video interpretation technique, self-figure drawing and questionnaires. The video interpretation technique (VIT) has been analyzed using both a quantitative and a qualitative method. The study also aimed to detect possible differences between verbal, visual, and hormonal analyses, which will be the main focus of this chapter.

Specific questions were:

I. Is it possible to find corresponding changes in stress-related hormones and movement patterns (measured by video interpretation) in female FMS patients after DMT?

II. Is it possible to detect differences between verbal, visual and hormonal assessments after treatment with DMT in FMS patients?

III. Is it possible to identify changes in self-figure drawings after DMT compared to a control group?

IV. How do female FMS patients think about themselves when they see themselves on videotape? The phenomenon under scrutiny was self-perception after video viewing.

V. Whether and how do visual stimuli, as detected from patient's own movement patterns on videotape, affect female FMS patients' assessments of their own condition?

MATERIAL AND METHODS
Subjects

Thirty-six female FMS patients participated. FMS is a stress related chronic pain syndrome involving musculoskeletal aches, stiffness and pain where perturbations in the stress-axis and high scores on somatic anxiety and muscular tension have been found. Mean age was 57 years (SD 7.2 years) and the mean duration of the disease was 7 years in the treatment group and 8.7 years among controls. Pain duration was much longer in both groups (>12 years on average). The patients were randomized into either a DMT treatment group (20 patients) or a control group (16 patients). 20 patients were randomized to the treatment group to secure sufficient evaluated numbers of patients.

The treatment (experimental) group (20 patients) was randomly divided into two groups (of 10 patients each). Patients participated in weekly one-hour DMT sessions for 6 months. The subjects in the control group did not participate in the treatment but were invited to use DMT after the study was completed. A detailed description of the randomization procedure of each DMT session can be found in Bojner Horwitz (2004a).

In the interview, eight female FMS patients participated (Bojner Horwitz et al., 2003a). Description of the randomization procedure, see Bojner Horwitz (2004a).

Treatment Method

The DMT model is constructed on a bio-psycho-social basis. All therapy sessions involve both verbal and non-verbal processes (Bojner Horwitz 2004a).

Music was used in all DMT sessions and the patients voted on desired music genres, with the majority deciding the choice. Five genres of music were presented: pop, instrumental, classical, folk music and rhythmic world music.

Hormone Analysis

Blood samples were obtained in order to assess serum concentrations of the hormones prolactin, dehydroepiandrosterone sulphate, cortisol, neuropeptide Y and saliva samples of cortisol at baseline, after 4, 6 and 14 months (Bojner Horwitz et al., 2003b).

Video Interpretation Technique

Video interpretation is a method adapted by the author (Bojner Horwitz et al., 2003a) for FMS patients to measure changes in their self-perception as well as changes in movement patterns over time after DMT. Do motor functions change in chronic pain patients after DMT? Over the years, the method has come to play a quantitative, qualitative, and therapeutic role. Patients were videotaped individually before and after treatment periods. The patients were told to perform standardized movement sequences in video recordings (Bojner Horwitz et al., 2003a, Bojner Horwitz et al., 2004b). The patient interpreted herself as she appeared in the videotapes and used a five-point scale to indicate whether and how her mobility, movement pain, and life energy had changed over time. The video interpretation gave patients a retrospective view of their movement patterns prior to treatment, as well as after treatment and follow-up.

Self-Figure Drawing

The self-figure drawing data used was collected individually both in the treatment and control group at baseline, after 6 and 14 months. A sample of 48 drawings from the study population was taken in order to evaluate the responsiveness to this non-verbal method. 24 drawings from eight patients in the treatment group and 24 drawings from eight patients from the control group were randomly selected for the derived measurements and the corresponding analyses. Patients were given a blank sheet of paper (A4) and crayons of the following colors: red, orange, yellow, green, blue, violet, black, brown and white. The study leader (the author) instructed the patients to draw a picture of themselves on the theme of self-image. All patients were given a total of two minutes to complete the drawing. The prominence of the following variables was calculated: the amount of body details, the number of colors used in the drawing, percentage of the paper used, and the number of kilobytes used for scanning the drawing (Bojner Horwitz, 2004a, Bojner Horwitz et al., 2005b).

Questionnaires

The different questionnaires used were: MADRS: Montgomery Åsberg Depression Rating Scale (MADRS; Montgomery et al., 1979), CPRS: Comprehensive Psychopathological Rating Scale (Svanborg et al., 1994), SOC: Sense of Coherence (Langius, 1995), SSP: Swedish Universities Scale of Personality (Gustavsson et al., 2000), Life Events (Anderberg et al., 2000), VAS: Visual Analogue Scale (Anderberg, 1999), Global assessment of well-being and pain, and ranking of dance, music, and drawing (Bojner Horwitz, 2004a, Bojner Horwitz et al., 2005b).

Qualitative Aanalyses

A phenomenological hermeneutic method was used to obtain a deeper perspective on the "viewing oneself on video". The method was inspired by the French philosopher Paul Ricoeur (Ricoeur, 1976; Bojner Horwitz et al., 2003a).

RESULTS

Concerning the hormone analyses, the result showed a tendency to increased levels of cortisol in plasma and saliva in the treatment group at 14 months. This may indicate a revitalization of the HPA (hypothalamic-pituitary-adrenal)-axis. No significant differences appeared between treated -- and none treated patients (Table I).

TABLE I: RESULTS FROM EVALUATION: HORMONE DATA WITH ANOVA REPEATED MEASURES DESIGN

Effect	df	MS	Df Error	MS Error	F	p-value	Effect size Baseline: month 14	
DHEA-S							Control	Treatment
Between groups	1	16.65	31	12.54	1.33	0.26		
Within groups (time)	3	0.42	93	0.40	1.06	0.37	2.8-3.0	3.4-3.5
Interaction (groups*time)	3	0.28	93	0.40	0.70	0.56		

Plasma cortisol

Between groups	1	5408.68	31	20737.80	0.26	0.61		
Within groups (time)	3	8273.03	93	6137.59	1.35	0.26	74.9-289.2	77.2-339.2
Interaction (groups*time)	3	5890.00	93	6137.59	0.96	0.42		
Saliva cortisol								
Between groups	1	65.94	22	28.64	2.30	0.14		
Within groups (time)	3	66.15	66	35.77	1.85	0.15	6.2-8.4	7.9-11.9
Interaction (groups*time)	3	18.75	66	35.77	0.52	0.67		
Prolactin (log (prol+1))								
Between groups	1	0.04	31	0.69	0.05	0.82		
Within groups (time)	3	0.35	93	0.05	7.54	<0.001*	5.2-6.9	5.3-7.8
Interaction (groups*time)	3	0.01	93	0.05	0.22	0.88		
NPY								
Between groups	1	6.45	30	36.81	0.18	0.68		
Within groups (time)	3	278.83	90	18.42	15.14	<0.001*	14.6-17.0	13.2-18.1
Interaction (groups*time)	3	16.03	90	18.42	0.87	0.46		

*Note: Dependent variable time (4 levels) and group (treatment and controls); * indicates statistical significant results.*

The results also showed significant functional improvement, as reported by the patient's interpretation of the videos at 14 months. This improvement was observed in the treatment group as increased mobility and life energy and as decreased movement pain assessed by video interpretation (Table II).

*TABLE II: CHANGES IN MOVEMENT PATTERN SCORES BEFORE AND AFTER VIDEO
INTERPRETATION (BASELINE TO MONTH 14)*

Parameter	Assessments before video		Assessments after video		Change within groups (effect size)			
	Control	Treatment	Control	Treatment	Control	Treatment	p-value	
	median (min-max)		median (min-max)		median change from Baseline to Month 14			
Movement pain	3 (1-4)	4 (3-5)	3 (1-4)	4 (4-5)	0	-1	p<0.001	
Mobility	3 (2-5)	2 (1-3)	3 (2-5)	1 (1-2)	0	-1	p<0.001	
Life energy	3 (2-4)	2 (1-4)	3 (2-5)	1 (1-2)	0	-1	p<0.001	

Note: Significant p-values demonstrate difference between treatment and control group with respect to changes in scores before and after video interpretation after 14 months.

The difference scores derive from a five-point-scale and represent the following:
1 = significant increase, 2 = increase, 3 = unchanged, 4 = decrease, and 5 = significant decrease regarding the three items movement pain, mobility, and life energy Assessment before video represents change from baseline to rating before video viewing. Assessment after video represents change from baseline to rating after video viewing.

In the self figure drawings, significant differences were seen in the variables "amount of body details" and "amount of paper use" between the treatment group and controls. The treatment group showed a significant increase in the "amount of body details" and "amount of paper use" compared to controls (Table III). Specific parts of the verbally oriented ratings in CPRS, "bodily discomfort" and "compulsive act", were positively correlated to "number of different colors" in the self figure drawing. The variable "pain and ache" in the CPRS correlated negatively to the "amount of paper use", i.e. the more pain, the less paper used.

TABLE III: RESULTS OF ANOVA REPEATED MEASURES DESIGN FOR THE DIFFERENT VARIABLES IN THE SELF-FIGURE DRAWINGS

Variable	ANOVA factor	df	MS	df	MS			Effect size (Baseline: month 14)	
		Effect	Effect	Err.	Err.	F	p-level	Control	Treatment
Amount of body details									
	Between groups	1	217	14	68.2	3.2	0.10		
	Within groups (time)	2	20	28	11.3	1.8	0.18	11.9-8.9	11.1-16.1
	Interaction (group*time)	2	11	28	11.3	6.7	0.004		
Amount of paper use in %									
	Between groups	1	2002	14	969	2.1	0.17		
	Within groups (time)	2	175	28	111	1.6	0.22	50.0-40.0	48.8-68.8
	Interaction (group*time)	2	908	28	111	8.2	0.001		
Amount of Kb when scanning									
	Between groups	1	3675	14	1642	2.24	0.16		
	Within groups (time)	2	133	28	287	0.46	0.63	136-135	148-156
	Interaction (group*time)	2	104	28	287	0.36	0.70		
Amount of colours									
	Between groups	1	3.5	14	6.6	0.5	0.48		
	Within groups (time)	2	2.1	28	1.0	2.1	0.14	3.5-3.3	3.3-3.8
	Interaction (group*time)	2	2.6	28	1.0	2.6	0.09		

The patient's global rating of the items "well-being" and "pain" after 14 months showed significant differences between the treatments and controls. The median value for "well-being" was "increased" in the treatments and "unchanged" in controls and median value of "global pain" assessment was "decreased" in the treatments and "unchanged" in controls.

Concerning the evaluation of the patient's perception of which of the modalities -- dance, music or drawing that had the strongest influence; most FMS patients (74%) evaluated dance as having the strongest, music (21%) second strongest and the drawing process of the DMT process as having the third strongest (5%) influence. There were no other treatment effects seen in the verbal questionnaires.

The qualitative part of the study showed that the video interpretation in combination with interviews facilitated a communication and understanding between the therapist and the patient. The patient's awareness of body and self was improved and the patient's body- and self image was better integrated. The "paradoxical integration process", which was the result of the complete interpretation of the VIT, laid the groundwork for the patients new body conception with the result that the video interpretation technique evidently had therapeutic qualities.

DISCUSSION

DMT is a treatment form suitable for patients with FMS, as seen in the results. However, the different hormonal, visual, and verbal instruments presented in this study may affect the outcome of this treatment. The visual instruments of video interpretation and self-figure drawings showed significant improvements both in physical and psychological function and in emotional and psychological variables. On the other hand, the verbally based instruments showed no physical, psychological, or emotional improvements in the treatment group compared to controls. The assessment methods consequently influence the treatment outcome. The FMS patients appear to find it easier to understand and relate to changes in their bodies when visual modalities are involved in the questionnaires.

The focus is on the cognitive function of the FMS patient when discussing assessment of treatment effects. Stress and alexithymia may be factors that could decrease the patient's perceptiveness that, in turn, may trigger difficulties in focusing on the issue at hand. Symbols and less intellectualized processes may therefore be prioritized and easier to deal with when discussing assessment techniques in FMS patients after DMT. That can explain why the verbal questionnaires did not show any differences between the groups.

When measuring treatment effects, some processes in our body may be slower to signal change than others. Changes in the hormonal system may take longer to emerge than changes in body movements and self-figure drawings. It would therefore have been interesting to follow up further changes in the biological markers. Verbal assessments of the patient's personality and emotions may also have been affected differently with longer follow-up. It may be that we underestimate the body's capacity as a modulator of treatment effects since certain levels of our consciousness, such as verbal/cognitive, visual, emotional, sensational and motor levels appear to be more responsive to treatment than others in different phases of a treatment process. Different stages of the disorder may also be reflected in the varying results of these studies.

Which results are critical for the patient to achieve after treatment? Video assessment showed significant improvement in the treatment group in terms of functional variables (pain, life energy, and mobility) and of well-being. These factors signal improved capacity both physically and mentally. It is open to speculation whether results would have been different if the mean age had been lower. More patients in the treatment group would probably have returned to work as a result of improved functionality. One patient in the study actually did so.

What aspects of DMT had the greatest effect on the patients? Was it the dance, the art, or the music, or the combined effect of these elements? Or was it a social and psychological effect resulting from patients with the same problems being together in a group: the sense of coherence? Or was it a combination of all these aspects? When patients were asked, they rated the dance element as the strongest influence, the musical element as the second strongest, and the art as the third strongest influence. Earlier studies have shown that music and dance are inseparable, which in this study may be interpreted as the dance having stimulated and activated the patients' ability to perceive the music, and vice versa (Bojner Horwitz, 2002).

Decrease in "Alexithymic" Movement Patterns

Researchers have lately shown that endocrine stress responsiveness probably has a large genetic component, which is of interest in the discussion of personality and responses to treatment (Hellhammer et al., 1993). As seen in the sample group of FMS patients in this study, different aspects of life events and alexithymic characteristics may have played a role in the treatment outcome. As an example, the fact that 25% of patients in the treatment group reported sexual abuse in their life history may have led to perceptive difficulties during treatment analyses.

Alexithymic characteristics in FMS and the patients' rigid movement patterns suggest that dance/movement therapy is appropriate for this clientele due to the primary focus on sensorimotor communication rather than verbal communication. Movement patterns as well as well-being and life energy increased among the FMS patients. It would have been interesting to ascertain whether the decrease in "alexithymic" movement patterns corresponds to a decrease in alexithymic personality, with reference to Schilder's work on body image where he explains that changes in body movements also change inner psychological factors (Schilder, 1970).

A hypothetical explanation of the increase in movement patterns after DMT may also be found in a decrease in the activity of the vegetative system as a result of symbolic movement expression. The autonomic system does not have to trigger vegetative reactions as seen in an alexithymic state (Ursin, 1995). Instead, the patient's limbic system starts to communicate feelings through dance movements where symbols arise from movements and words in order to bring unconscious ideas to awareness for them to lose their hold on the personality.

From Cortical to Limbic Behavior

If we hypothetically may explain the rigid and awkward movement patterns, seen at the outset of this study as "cortical behavior", the symbolic and emotional exploration through DMT upgrades the movements to so-called "limbic behavior". The sympathetic activity is triggered by emotional exploration through dance and music and the patient's gestures become more filled with emotional content. ACTH (adrenocorticotropic hormone), which is secreted by the pituitary, triggers the cortisol response. In the treatment group, cortisol levels at 14 months showed a slight tendency to increase compared to controls, which may be interpreted as a result of this behavioral transformation; from "cortical" to "limbic" behavior.

Hormones Linking Bodily Expression with Emotions

Hormones are said to aid communication between the central and autonomous nervous systems on the one hand, and behavioral and emotional bodily expression on the other. On this premise we may interpret the video interpretation technique (VIT) results as a mediator of triggered hormones. However, changes in the patient's movement patterns may be a result of changes in inner biological systems (hormones) and it is unclear whether or not hormones always link bodily behavior and emotions. Had our results shown significant changes in hormone levels between groups, how should that have been interpreted? Are changes in hormone levels more important than the visual effects observed between the groups? The current study suggests that the patient's own visual perception of increase in functionality appears to be a more valuable result of the DMT treatment seen in this perspective.

Hormone Levels -- Reflecting Syndrome Stages

Research into variables that affect hormone levels is in its infancy and it is therefore critical to be able to use the results of hormone measurements as an indicator of the patient's condition. Hormone measurements may for instance depend on when the patient first sought medical help and when the blood samples were drawn. Hormone levels may also vary depending on how long the patient has suffered from pain and other symptoms, and may fluctuate with different stages of the disorder. Patients in this study had a mean pain duration of over 12 years, which could be interpreted as most of them being in a late stage of the disorder. However, a complicating factor is that many of these patients had unfortunately received insufficient help and therefore could be regarded as having earlier-stage disease. Are the patients at a stage where their HPA axis still reacts normally to internal and environmental demands? Or has the patient developed a state where the HPA axis no longer reacts at all and could be identified as "exhausted"? These factors are significant for the analysis of hormone levels since the results of hormone measurements may appear to be contradictory at different stages of the disorder for stress-related reasons. It seems highly plausible that these varying results reflect different stages of the syndrome. It is therefore important to determine which stage of the disorder the patient is in. A further complication is that hormone levels may not correlate uniformly with a specific stage of the disorder. As an example, NPY (neuropeptide Y) may be involved in the sympathetic nervous system and could therefore be regarded as a marker of stress (Anderberg et al. 1999). Elevated plasma levels of NPY have been found in female FMS patients (Anderberg 1999b). However, low levels have also been found in this patient group (Crofford et al. 1994, Clauw 1995). The contradictory results may be due to the HPA axis and sympathetic nervous system responding differently depending on the stage of the patient's disorder. While the unchanged levels of NPY seen in this study are difficult to interpret, the changed cortisol levels may be the result of a revitalization of the HPA axis. Cortisol, which increases with mental and physical activation, decreases with prolonged stress and distress. Low levels have been found in patients with post-traumatic stress disorder and in patients suffering from chronic stress (Gunnar et al. 2001, Oquendo et al. 2003, Rosmund et al. 2000).

DHEA-S is an adrenal hormone, which reflects well-being and good psychosocial circumstances (Theorell et al. 1998a). However, low levels have been found in patients who have recovered from depression (Fabian et al. 2001) and an increase in DHEA-S has been found in patients with PTSD (Söndergaard et al. 2002) as well as in patients treated with cognitive behavioral therapy (Cruess et al. 1999). In the current study the levels of DHEA-S did not differ between patients and controls.

In this study there were no changes in prolactin after treatment with DMT. Prolactin, which is said to increase in situations of loss of power and crisis, (Theorell 1992) does show inter-individual variations in FMS patients (Griep et al. 1993). Other researchers have later found decreased prolactin levels in FMS patients (Landis et al. 2001). Decreased levels of prolactin have also been found in refugees under increased strain and in dependency situations (Söndergaard et al. 2003). Other personality factors such as empathy and hypersensitivity also appear to affect prolactin levels (Sivik 2004).

As seen in a report on patients with different psychosomatic conditions who received treatment with art psychotherapy, serum uric acid concentration was measured and a significant increase was seen between a period of seven to eighteen months after treatment. After two years of treatment the levels decreased (Theorell et al. 1995, 1998). Serum uric acid concentration maybe more sensitive than hormones in mirroring increasing energy levels after art psychotherapy.

Video Interpretation Technique -- a Critical Therapeutic Tool

When treating stress-related disorders, video interpretation may be used to help patients perceive "healthy" body signals such as muscle tension and early onset of pain. This could be important as the onset of pain in FMS patients often occurs in connection with emotionally stressful life events (Anderberg et al. 2000). If it is true that the body can mirror more than words can express, the video interpretation technique may benefit patients who have difficulty verbalizing their feelings. It therefore appears more relevant to use somatically directed methods when measuring body movements and body language. Viewing and interpreting herself on videotape may also help the patient to reflect and deepen her sense of self-perception and give the therapist and patient a common understanding of the status of the patient's self-perception after treatment. Seen in this broader perspective, treatment tools that comprise self-perception may be very important due to their apparent ability to enhance treatment effects in FMS patients.

In another perspective, reading body signals may also help prevent stress disorders. The body has much knowledge and speaks its own language and is probably more alert in signaling changes before they become evident in inner biological systems. Using the language of the body may help therapists and patients gain insights that can prevent maladaptive movements and further progression of stress-related disorders.

Self-Figure Drawing -- a Mirror of Inner Senses

A picture appears to reflect non-verbal issues that are linked to the patient's inner senses. When comparing changes in the self-figure drawings of FMS patients after DMT to controls, it is interesting to note that the factors "amount of body details" and "amount of paper use in percent" differed significantly. Interestingly, the factor "number of different colors" in the self-figure drawing correlated positively to "bodily discomfort" and "compulsive act" in CPRS. The greater the physical discomfort and the more compulsive the actions, the more colors were featured in the patient's drawing. "Pain and ache" in the CPRS correlated negatively to the "amount of paper use in percent", i.e. patients appeared to "shrink" on the paper when in pain. Color appears to reflect comfort and compulsive thoughts, while picture size appears to represent degree of pain, and amount of body details may be related to well-being. This concurs with previous research which has shown that psychological and emotional problems can be mirrored in human figure drawings and in self-portraits (Offman et al. 1992, Morin et al. 1998).

Context Affects Musical Perception

Is it possible to separate dance from music? Music and dance have always been considered inseparable (Bojner Horwitz 2005). In some African countries music and dance even share the same word. The initiation of a movement depends on music to some extent. As part of one session, the patients in this study were invited to dance without music. The movement patterns and energy decreased directly. It would be interesting to know whether our results would have been the same if no music had been used in the dancing sessions.

The context in which music is presented affects our perception of the music. Biological, cognitive, social, cultural, and psychological aspects are always involved when we perceive music, and this must be taken into account in the choice of music for therapy (Bojner-Horwitz 2002, Bojner-Horwitz et al. 2005). In these studies we therefore allowed the patients to choose their desired music genres by voting, with the majority determining the decision.

Future Assessments

From research we know that negative behavioral and psychological factors are related to the risk of developing a chronic pain syndrome such as FMS. Techniques that help the patient gain increased awareness of her body, or help the therapist initiate dialogue with the patient are therefore highly relevant in the rehabilitation of both physiological and psychological injuries. Behaviors can be interpreted and analyzed in order to bring patients "back on track" and reduce the risk of developing chronic pain disorders.

In clinical work it is important to develop and increase our understanding of how psychotherapy, both verbal and non-verbal, works on a psychobiological level. Moreover, we need to better understand the potential role of specific biological markers (such as saliva tests) in the diagnosis of disorders. Research should be focused on developing assessment techniques, including objective markers, to monitor treatments over time and measure their effects.

More cost-effective tools are needed because of the increase in patients with stress-related disorders, one being FMS. These may include self-figure drawings and films in combination with other supportive verbal scales and standardized verbal ratings as well as visually orientated methods.

Matching Perception Level with Assessment Technique

Different levels or aspects of consciousness are discussed in the literature in terms of body-related psychotherapy and other self-development theories (Downing 1996). According to Downing, these levels are:

- The *verbal-cognitive* level, including thinking processes, which could be verbalized.
- The *visual* level, including visual fantasies or thoughts, which include visual gestalts or visual impressions of the environment. Images from audio stimuli are also included at this level.
- The *emotional* level, which represents the perception of a feeling, e.g. happy or sad.
- The *sensational* level, which focuses on bodily sensations, e.g. warm or stiff.
- The *motor* level, which includes the body's position and movement in a room.

Downing notes that no hierarchies exist among these levels. An important outcome from this study concerns the conscious levels at which our patients are receptive to therapy, and the levels we as therapists assign to our assessment tools. Ideally, treatment and assessment methods should match each other to provide a fair picture of the patient and of the potential effects of treatment on each individual. Figure 1 below describes the various techniques used in this study, classified according to Downing's definitions.

FIGURE 1: TECHNIQUES ACOORDING TO DOWNINGS DEFINITIONS

Dance/Movement Therapy	Perception Levels	Assessment Methods	
Verbal/Cognitive	Verbal/Cognitive	Video Interpretation	visual motor emotional
Visual	Visual	Self figure Drawing	visual emotional sensational
Emotional	Emotional	Hormones	indirect affected by and/or affect all levels
Sensational Motor	Sensational Motor	Questionaires	verbal cognitive

A hypothetical model of the different modalities involved in DMT and the patient's different conscious levels for receiving treatment effects are presented in Figure 1. The figure also identifies the different assessment methods used in this study and the referenced conscious modalities, according to Downing, presented in each assessment technique. We see that the conscious level, which is present in the questionnaires, is primarily the verbal/cognitive level where no significant differences were found between groups. The perception levels in the hormone analyses are not comparable with the self-rating scales, but may indirectly be affected by and/or affect all conscious levels. Both the video interpretation technique and the self-figure drawing covers perception levels where visual modalities are present. The perception of viewing seems to capture more information compared to the other perception modalities in this patient group. When words alone are used to evaluate symptoms and treatment effects, valuable information may be lost. Visual modalities may be a good starting point for capturing information that may be missing from verbal questionnaires.

It is important to know which assessment technique is most suitable at the patient's stage of the disorder. By using the video interpretation technique, patients can raise their awareness of these different modalities by discussing the options with the therapist. Another aspect of this is that the patients´ state of the disorder may involve activity of hyper arousal, depending of earlier life events and post traumas. If this is the case, the patients will not easily be taught complex cognitive information. The patient will instead focus on non-verbal cues as for example body movements, facial expressions, tone of voice; not the words which accompany this. In a state of fear or arousal, we can expect our patients to have access to their non-verbal memories and language (Perry 1997). This is important to have in mind when discussing therapeutic interventions and different assessment techniques.

Another aspect of the results of this study may be that treatment with DMT has not affected the patients at the verbal/cognitive level. That could indicate that the DMT method only has visual, sensational, emotional and motor effects in this cohort. The verbal/cognitive levels may take longer to trigger and affect.

With regard to the results of this study, where video analyses and self-figure drawings were better able to signal changes over time than verbal questionnaires, our findings are comparable with other research reports. Interestingly, another study has shown that video analyses were more nuanced in delivering information on certain variables compared to verbal questionnaires and other direct methods when measuring risk factors associated with tree seedling (Spielholtz et al. 2001). It is important to report such errors in order to avoid misclassification in e.g. epidemiological studies.

CONCLUSION

As indicated by the visual instruments in this study, six months of DMT appears sufficient to improve both physical and psychological function in FMS patients. The video interpretation technique and self-figure drawing captured treatment effects that were not evident from verbal scales or reflected in hormone levels. The body speaks its own language and is probably more alert in signaling changes before they become evident in inner biological systems. The biological markers probably need a longer treatment period to show significant differences between the groups and the verbal instrumentation may not be the most appropriate assessment technique in this patient group because of alexithymic factors. Video interpretation and self-figure drawing may offer a new way of assessing symptom changes after DMT. The video interpretation technique may also be useful for early identification of maladaptive movement patterns and as a mirror of bodily and facial expressions of emotions. The visual assessment tools can also be used therapeutically.

REFERENCES

Anderberg, U.M. (1999). *Fibromyalgia syndrome in women -- a stress disorder? Neurobiological and hormonal aspects.* Doctoral dissertation from the faculty of Medicine, Dept. of Neuroscience, Psychiatry, University Hospital, Uppsala, Sweden.

Anderberg, U.M., Liu, Z., Berglund, L., & Nyberg F. (1999b). Elevated plasma levels of neuropeptide Y in female fibromyalgia syndrom patients. *European Journal of Pain, 3,* 19-30.

Anderberg, U.M., Marteinsdottir, I., Theorell, T., & von Knorring, L. (2000). The impact of life events in female patients with fibromyalgia and in female healthy controls. *European Psychiatry, 15,* 295-301.

Bojner Horwitz, E. (2002). *Music in dance/movement therapy.* C-Uppsats University College of Dance, Stockholm, Sweden.

Bojner Horwitz, E., Theorell, T. & Anderberg, U. M. (2003a). Fibromyalgia patients own experiences of video self-interpretation: a phenomenological-hermeneutic study. *Scandinav. Journal of Caring Science, 17,* 1-8.

Bojner Horwitz, E., Theorell, T., & Anderberg, U.M. (2003b). Dance/movement therapy and changes in stress-related hormones: a study of fibromyalgia patients with video-interpretation. *The Arts in Psychotherapy, 30,* 255-264.

Bojner Horwitz, E. (2004a). *Dance/movement Therapy in Fibromyalgia Patients -- Aspects and Consequences of Verbal, Visual and Hormonal Analyses.* Doctoral dissertation from the faculty of Medicine. Dept. of Public Health and Caring Sciences, Uppsala Science Park, Uppsala University, Uppsala, Sweden.

Bojner Horwitz, E., Theorell, T., & Anderberg, U.M. (2004b). New technique for assessment of clinical condition in fibromyalgia -- a pilot study by video-interpretation. *The Arts in Psychotherapy, 31,* 153-164.

Bojner Horwitz, E., & Bojner G. (2005a). *Må bättre med musik.* [Improve your health with music.] ICA förlag, Västerås, Sweden.

Bojner Horwitz, E., Kowalski J., Theorell T., & Anderberg U.M. (2005b). Dance/movement therapy in fibromyalgia patients: Changes in self-figure drawings and their relation to verbal self-rating scales. *The Arts in Psychotherapy* (accepted May 2005).

Clauw, D. (1995). Fibromyalgia: More than just a musculoskeletal disease. *American Family Physician, 52,* 843-851.

Crofford, L.J., Pillemer, S.R., Kalogeras, K.T., Cash, J.M., Michelson, D., Kling, M.A., Sternberg, E.M., Gold, P.W., Chrousos, G.P., & Wilder RL. (1994). Hypothalamic-Pituitary-Adrenal axis perturbations in patients with fibromyalgia. *Arthritis Rheumathology, 37,* 1583-1592.

Cruess, D.G., Antoni, M.H., & Kumar, M. (1999). Cognitive-behavioral stress management buffers decreases in dehydroepiandrosterone sulphate (DHEA-S) and increases in the cortisol/DHEA-S ratio and reduces mood disturbance and perceived stress among HIV-seropositive men. *Psychoneuroendocrinology; 24,* 537-549.

Downing, G. (1996). *Kroppen och Ordet. Kroppsorienterad psykoterapi -- teoretisk bakgrund och klinisk tillämpning* [The Body and the Word. Bodily oriented psychotherapy -- theoretical background and clinical use]. Natur och Kultur. Centraltryckeriet Borås 1997.

Fabian, T.J., Dew, M.A., & Pollock, B.G. (2001). Endogenous concentrations of DHEA-S and DHEA-S decrease with remission of depression in older adults. *Biological Psychiatry, 15,* 767-774.

Griep, E.N., Boersma, J.W., & de Kloet, E.R. (1993). Pituitary release of growth hormone and prolactin in the primary fibromyalgia syndrome. *Journal of Rhematology, 21,* 2125-2130.

Gunnar, M.R., & Vasquez, D.M. (2001). Low cortisol and a flattening of expected daytime rhythm: potential indices of risk in human development. *Developmental Psychopathology, 13,* 515-538.

Gustavsson, J.P., Bergman, H., Edman, G., Ekselius, L., von Knorring, L., & Linder J. (2000). Swedish universities Scales of Personality (SSP): construction, internal consistency and normative data. *Acta Psychiatrica Scandinavia, 102,* 217-225.

Hellhammer, DH., & Wade, S. (1993). Endocrine correlates of stress vulnerability. *Psychotherapy and Psychosomatics, 60,* 8-17.

Landis, CA., Lentz, M., Rothermel, J., Riffle, S., Chapman, D., Buchwald, D., & Shaver, J. (2001). Decreased nocturnal levels of Prolactin and growth hormone in women with fibromyalgia. *The Journal of Clinical Endocrinology & Metabolism, 86,* 1672-1678.

Langius, A. (1995). *Quality of Life in a group of patients with Oral and Pharyngeal Cancer. Sense of Coherence, Functional Status and Well-being.* Dissertation from the Dep. of Medicine, the Center of Caring Sciences North. Karolinska Institute, Karolinska Hospital. Stockholm. Sweden.

Merleau Ponty, M. (1996). *Phenomenology of Perception.* NewYork: Routledge & Kegan Paul.

Montgomery, S., & Åsberg, M. (1979). A new depression scale designed to be sensitive to change. *British Journal of Psychiatry, 134,* 382-389.

Morin, C., & Bensalah, Y. (1998). The self portrait in adulthood and aging. *International Journal of Aging and Human Development, 46,* 45-70.

Offman, H., & Bradley, S. (1992). Body image of children and adolescents and its measurement: an overview. *Canadian Journal of Psychiatry, 37,* 417-422.

Oquendo, MA., Echavarria, G., Galfalvy, HC., & Grunebaum, MF. (2003). Lower cortisol levels in depressed patients with comorbid post-traumatic stress disorder. *Neuropsychopharm, 28,* 591-598.

Perry, BD. (1997). Incubated in Terror: Neurodevelopmental factors in the "cycle of violence". In J. Osofsky (Ed), *Children, Youth and Violence: The search for solutions* (pp. 124-148). Guilford Press: New York.

Ricoeur, P. (1976). *Interpretation theory: Discourse and the surplus of meaning.* Fort Worth. Texas Christian University Press.

Rosmond, R., & Bjorntorp, P. (2000). Low cortisol production in chronic stress. The connection stress-somatic disease challenge for future research. *Lakartidningen 20, 97,* 4120-4124.

Schilder, P. (1970). *The image and appearance of the human body.* New York: International Universities Press.

Sivik, T. (2004). Ur rapport om Psykosomatologi och psykosomatisk integrativ behandling och rehabilitering [Psychosomatology and psychosomatic integrative treatment and rehabilitation]. Medlemsblad Svensk Förening för Psykosomatisk Medicin, 1.

Spielholz, P., Silverstein, B., Morgan, M., Checkoway, H., & Kaufman, J. (2001). Comparison of self-report, video observation and direct measurement methods for upper extremity musculoskeletal disorder physical risk factors. *Ergonomics, 44,* 588-613.

Svanborg, P, & Åsberg, M. (1994). A new self-rating scale for depression and anxiety states based on the Comprehensive Psychopathological Rating Scale. *Acta Psychiatr Scand, 89,* 21-28.

Söndergaard, HP., Hansson, LO., & Theorell, T. (2002). Elevated blood levels of dehydroepiandrosterone sulphate vary with symptom load in posttraumatic stress disorder: findings from a longitudinal study of refugees in Sweden. *Psychotherapy and Psychosomatics, 71,* 298-303.

Söndergaard, H.P., & Theorell, T. (2003). A longitudinal Study of Hormonal Reactions Accompanying Life Events in Recently Resettled Refugees. *Psychotherapy and Psychosomatics, 72,* 49-58.

Theorell, T. (1992). Prolactin -- a hormone that mirrors passiveness in crises situations. *Integr Physiol Behav Science, 27,* 32-38.

Theorell, T., Konarski, K., Burell, A., Engström, R., Lagercrantz, A., Teszary, J., Thulin, K., & de la Torre, B. (1995). *Konstpsykoterapi vid långvariga psykosomatiska sjukdomstillstånd.* Statens Institut för Psykosocial Miljömedicin. Sektionen för Stressforskning. Karolinska Institutet, Stress Research Reports Nr 259. Stockholm, Sweden.

Theorell, T., Konarski, K., Westerlund, H. et al. (1998). Treatment of Patients with Chronic Somatic Symptoms by means of Art Psychotherapy: A Process Description. *Psychotherapy and Psychosomatics, 67,* 50-56.

Ursin, H. (1995). Psykosomatikk: Ett psykobiologiskat perspektiv [Psychosomatics: A psychobiological perspective]. In T. Sivik & T. Theorell (Eds.). *Psykosomatisk Medicin.* Lund: Studentlitteratur.

DANCE MOVEMENT THERAPY GROUP PROCESS: A CONTENT ANALYSIS OF SHORT TERM DMT PROGRAMS

Iris Bräuninger

This chapter investigates dance movement therapy (DMT) group process in short-term treatment programs. It examines and identifies common themes that evolve in twelve different DMT groups. The programs have been closely monitored through the writer as part of a major research project. The focus presented in this chapter rests upon the results gained from the qualitative method as part of a multi-centered randomized control trial: Ten sessions of short-term group DMT are compared to a wait-listed control condition regarding the improvement of quality of life and the reduction of stress (Bräuninger, 2006). Qualitative data on the group processes are gained from the Intervention-Checklist 2 (ICL2). Results are based on the subjective records of the dance movement therapists and have been objectified with some limitations: The use of Laban- and KMP-terminology simplified the process of analyzing the meaning of therapist's explanations. Across all twelve DMT treatment groups, parallels regarding themes and group process emerged, and different phases in the group process matched the group-phase-model introduced by Bender (2001).

Keywords: DMT, group process, short term treatment, intervention checklist / ICL, qualitative research

INTRODUCTION

The idea behind this inquiry is to improve the understanding of group theme formation and according group processes in short-term treatment programs in DMT. Is it likely that parallels emerge in different DMT groups that have been set up with the purpose to reduce stress and improve quality of life? Will the emerging themes and issues in these short-term treatment groups show some kind of commonality despite the fact that different DMT approaches have been applied in twelve DMT groups led by eleven dance movement (dm) therapists.

OUTLINE OF THE STUDY

The focus of this study is on the meaning and interpretation of the collected data derived from narrative descriptions of eleven dm therapists' perceptions of the group processes development. The nature of the study is qualitative. The research project combines quantitative and qualitative methods: The randomized control trial (RCT) included 162 participants with n=97 in short term DMT groups and n=65 in wait-listed control groups and a pre-, post-, and 6 months follow-up test including standardized measurements. The overall project is described in greater depth in the book "Tanztherapie: Verbesserung der Lebensqualität und Stressbewältigung" [Dance movement therapy: Improvement of quality of life and stress management] (Bräuninger, 2006).[6] Table I gives an overview of the RCT:

[6] The author gratefully acknowledges the Marian Chace Foundation of the American Dance Therapy Association for supporting this research project through a grant.

TABLE I: RCT (QUESTIONAIRE PRESENTED TO THE PARTICIPANTS)

Groups	Test Phases		
	t1: Pretest	*t2: Posttest*	*t3: 6-months Follow-up test*
	(1-2 weeks prior to onset of short term treatment programs)	*(ca. 10-12 weeks after t1)*	*(ca. 9 months after t1)*
Treatment group	Standardized questionnaires Written consent form	Standardized questionnaires	Standardized questionnaires
Wait-listed control group	Standardized questionnaires Written consent form	Standardized questionnaires	Standardized questionnaires

Eleven dm therapists conducted twelve groups and ten DMT sessions per group. After each session, every therapist filled out Intervention Checklist 1: One table column per participant and per DMT session that collects interventions per individual. Intervention Checklist 2, which was also completed, collects all group interventions per DMT sessions. It consists of quantitative and qualitative items. ICL1 and ICL2 were developed by the author as a "personal memorandum" for the therapists of each of the ten group sessions. A total of 103 ICL1s and 128 ICL2s were received and analyzed. The procedure how data were collected by the therapists is demonstrated in Figure 1.

FIGURE 1: DATA COLLECTION FROM DM THERAPISTS

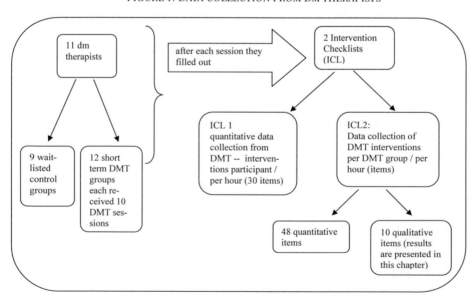

THEORIE

As the purpose of this chapter is on evaluating short term DMT programs, the focus of the overall research study on DMT's efficacy on improvement of quality of life and stress-management will be disregarded here.

The classical set-up of group process in DMT appears to be tripartite: The aim of the first phase, the Warm-up phase, is the physical and psychological warming up of participants the awakening and, at best letting go of tension, and the preparation of the body oriented process phase. In the second phase, the process phase, participants develop their individual (movement) themes or they are immersed in the group process. The aim is to foster communication by means of body action and nonverbal empathy, and to enhance the relief of bodily and emotional blockages through self-expression and symbolic communication. Being united through a common rhythm serves as a base from which trust can develop, personal isolation can be overcome, and community can be experienced as healing. During this phase communication can become symbolic, and movement images and metaphors can emerge on all sensory levels (Bräuninger 2000a, 2000b; Bräuninger & Blumer, 2004; Ellis, 2001; Meekums, 2002; Rose, 1995; Schmais, 1985; Stanton, 1992). The third phase, the closure, often includes a verbal ending serving intrapsychic, interpersonal, and cognitive processing. In the Chace approach the tripartite division is known as 1. Warm-Up, 2. Theme Development, and 3. Closure (Berrol et al., 1997; Levy, 1992; Penfield, 1994; Schmais, 1981).

The group-phase-model from Bender (2001) presents four phases that influence the group process regarding various questions and behaviors. Table II presents the Phase Model of Group Development (S. Bender, personal communication May 9, 2005) where the four phases are presented on the first row and the corresponding themes are on the left vertical column:

TABLE II: GROUP-PHASE-MODEL OF GROUP DEVELOPMENT (BENDER, 2005)

	Inclusion	*Responsibility*	*Openness*	*Termination*
question	in or out	top or bottom	open or closed	holding on or letting go
behavior of the team leader	integrating	confronting	respecting	terminating
interaction	one with many	one against one or many	one with/against one	one with one/many
feeling	I am significant/ insignificant	I am competent/ incompetent	I am likeable/ unpopular	I am autonomous/ dependent
fears	not being significant not being seen	having too much or too little influence	not being liked, to be too close, not close enough	not being able to manage it alone
need	Harmony	confrontation	differentiation	completion
boundaries	the team	in the team	the individual	the team

SHORT TERM TREATMENT PROGRAMS IN GROUP DANCE MOVEMENT THERAPY

Even though short-term treatment programs in DMT have not systematically been researched, some studies explore the efficacy of DMT in this context. The expression "short-term", as used in this chapter, describes the application of DMT from one session minimum up to twelve sessions.

In their pilot study, a randomized control trial, Erwin-Grabner Goodill, Schelly Hill and von Neida (1999) demonstrated that test anxiety is reduced through a four-sessions' DMT intervention.

A pilot study on a randomly assigned one-session DMT intervention by Brooks and Stark (1989) showed that people's affect improved significantly regarding depression, anxiety, and hostility in both the psychiatric group and the healthy group, compared to two control groups. In the intervention-study within a multi-treatment context, Mannheim (2004) explored the effect of DMT in an oncology rehabilitation program (average of 7 sessions). Results showed significant improvements in quality of life, reduction of anxiety and depression, and increase of self-esteem, although effects may not be attributed to DMT exclusively (Mannheim and Weiss, this volume). The qualitative assessments of interviews clearly demonstrated the positive influence of DMT on the coping process.

Further, an eight-week multidisciplinary intervention program by McComb and Clopton (2003) with participants randomly assigned to an intervention and a control group, verified the effects of movement, relaxation, and education on the stress levels of women with sub-clinical levels of bulimia. The intervention group showed significant reduction in anxiety compared to the control group but no significant improvement in self-esteem, attitudes or behaviors associated with bulimia nervosa. The randomized control trial by Astin and colleagues (2003) examined the short and long term efficacy of an 8-weeks training in mindfulness meditation plus Qi-Gong movement therapy in the treatment of fibromyalgia. Results revealed that both interventions register statistically significant improvements across time for the Fibromyalgia Impact Questionnaire, Total Myalgic Score, Pain, and Depression, and no improvement in the number of feet traversed in a 6-minute walk.

METHOD

Participants

Table III gives an overview of the average age and gender of the participants.

TABLE III: AGE AND GENDER OF PARTICIPANTS

Participants	N=162	Treatment Group n=97	Waitlisted-Control Group n=65
Means (M) Standard Deviation (SD)	M=44 yrs. SD=9 yrs.	M=44 yrs. SD=9 yrs.	M=44 yrs. SD=8 yrs.
Gender (%) Women	147 (90.7)	88 (90.7)	59 (90.8)
Men	15 (9.3)	9 (9.3)	6 (9.2)

RECRUITMENT

Dance Movement Therapists

The author invited qualified dm therapists from all over Germany who, if possible, already had received their certificate for "alternative practitioner in psychotherapy"[7]. Additionally, they had to be qualified as dm therapists approved by the BTD or accordingly. They already worked in private practice and were experienced in leading DMT groups. For the purpose of recruiting participants, they were provided with a PR text (supplied by the writer) that could be published in the local newspaper.

Participants

Non-hospitalized men and women who suffered from stress and who aimed to improve their quality of life were invited to participate in a ten session short term DMT group. They completed standardized questionnaires at three different times, had to tolerate the randomized assignment into either the treatment group or the wait-listed control group, and they gave their written consent for participation. Exclusion criteria were current psychological, psychotherapeutic and/or medical treatment on an out-patient, day-care, or in-patient basis, the existence of a psychiatric illness or a severe physical disability, psychotherapeutic treatment within the last twelve months, the missing of the consent form, or the prolongation of the ten session treatment.

Data Aquisitation Method

After each one of the ten DMT session the Intervention Checklist 2 (ICL2) on group process was completed by each dm therapist. The results of the quantitative ICLs will be presented in Bräuninger (in preparation). The ten qualitative items of the ICL2 enabled the therapists to briefly document and acquire the evolving group process through the following categorization: group process with four subcategories (verbal themes, verbal images, movement themes, movement images), other imaginative techniques, other relaxation techniques, other meditative (dance) therapeutic techniques, other DMT approaches, structure of the session, and content focus of the session (see Appendix).

Data Analysis

The process-oriented analysis of the DMT groups was gained through content analysis and description of the qualitative items through the ICL2: Data from all twelve DMT groups were collected per subcategories and per session (Mayring (2003) calls this procedure "induzierte Kategorienbidlung" [inductive category building]. They were presented according to verbal and movement themes from first to tenth session ("zusammenfassende Inhaltanalyse" [summarized content analysis] according to Mayring). Results are presented for each one of the ten sessions and combined in a concluding summary.

---

[7] In Germany, this certificate is required from the public health departments of the Bundesländer [States] in order to establish a private practice as a dance movement therapist or as any other psychotherapeutically oriented therapist.

RESULTS

The eleven participating dm therapists are abbreviated with the letters a, b, c, d, e, i, k, l, n, r, u. The letter b2 describes the wait-listed control group of therapist b that became treatment group after one year (therapist b filled out the ICLs for this group). Therapist c had two treatment groups at t1. For the purpose of better readability, quotes from the dm therapists are italicized.

1. Session Group Process

Verbal Themes

Organizational (i^8) and psycho-educational themes including the introduction of a stress-reaction-model (a) were mentioned. Additional verbal themes were introducing one-self and getting to know the group (c1, c2, l, u), clarifying members' motivation to participate (c1, c2) and questioning one's belonging (n). Participants apparently showed more abstract stress management strategies during the first session, for example they wished to evaluate one's own achievement or to express the appetite for freedom (e, u) and movement (d) and letting go of one-self, sensing the body, being light without effort (b). Themes emerged and already pointed to stress producing factors in participants' lives: a wailing mother (e), illness (d), one's own dissatisfaction and inadequacy (c2), or in relation to the concrete therapy situation a person mentioned his or her difficulty to get in contact with other group members (d).

Movement Themes

Different focal points became apparent in different groups: Two groups worked on the kinesphere (a, b) and the body image (c1, c2). In the latter, the purpose was to influence the self-image and self-reliance (c2). Images of persons were expressed through movement, for example to scoop water and take a cold shower as refreshment (i). Laban work was mentioned three times (a, b, c2): Shifting of weight and the work with two efforts namely weight and its two effort elements light and strong and flow and its two effort elements free and bound flow (b). Other movement qualities that appear were stamping, shaking, cutting, gathering (e) and jumping (b). A moved association (a), a body journey (l), a duette improvisation and relaxation (a) were other movement themes. Dance therapists described autonomy in movement, the awareness of own needs (c1) and to establish first contact (l) as goals for the first session.

Summary and Conclusion

A gentle start on a verbal and movement base seemed to be common. Group members strived to sense some equilibrium in their groups. Using flow and weight efforts seemed appropriate, as they fostered learning styles and coping strategies.

---

[8] The eleven different dance movement therapists are abbreviated with the letters a, b (b2 describes the wait-listed control group of therapist b that became a treatment group after the waiting period), c (c1 and c2 refers to the two intervention groups of therapist c), d, e, i, k, l, n, r, u. For the purpose of better readability, quotes from the dance movement therapists are italicized.

2. Session Group Process

Verbal Themes

Participants of one group expressed what they hope to achieve through therapy, they wanted to improve their body consciousness (c1). Body awareness and how participants experience hecticness (l) were themes in one group, one person wanted to know how a lump in the stomach might feel (an attritional talk with the employer prior to the DMT session had taken place) (c1). In some groups, strong emotions were already present such as letting go of anger (i), sense of delight towards the DMT session (c1), bothering feelings preceding the talk with the employer (c1), anxiety (d), enviousness (others get more) and resignation (b2). Two groups dealt with the issue: what would be the group norm (i) and do I belong (n)? Intrapsychic or interpersonal themes of stress were outlined: Depression (e), illness, decision, feeling of being externally directed (d), self-image (I am mean to others) (e) were introduced as well as subjects on partner conflicts (e), stress at the working place (c1) and violation of boundaries (b2). Two kinds of stress management strategies could be distinguished: One was applied within the DMT session; it helped to gain and to find the right energy for oneself (i). The other was adopted outside the therapeutic setting: Based on the experiences during the session, one participant has started to dance again in her home, another one was able to obtain ideas for the talk with her employer (c1).

Movement Themes

The Chace approach was mentioned once (r), and movement themes were analyzed through the Kestenberg Movement Profile (KMP): One group apparently worked mainly with tension flow rhythms (the first diagram of the KMP) such as twisting and on the floor and in standing position with strain and release (i). Another group used basic flow elements such as opening and closing (e). Two other groups concentrated on exploring the kinesphere (b, c2) and the personal and general space (c2). One group tried to convert their theme into movement with the assistance of expressive work and the use of Laban elements, introduced by the therapist (a). Laban work was also used in another group (c2), especially weight and time/tempo and the action flattering alternating with calmness (l). The door plane (r), person-centered movement composition (a), horizontal turning, strong loosening, strong and rhythmic punching (b) and gathering movements (i) were more movement qualities apparent. Sporadically, therapeutic objectives were specified, to sense and nourish one's own needs through moving singular body parts (c1) or to get grounded (r). The clients of one group expressed through movement, what was translated into verbal language through one person: Swim oneself free, detach and loosen, gain space, -- I am enough on the ground -- I want to search for lightness (i).

Summary and Conclusion

Through movement themes, the inner world was explored and the inner space is sensed. The personal expression was fostered by means of personal dance composition. The unifying process across the groups was the participants opening up, their sharing of stress related issues. At the same time, the movement process turned more towards intrapsychic work, opening and closing, and becoming aware of the boundaries between inner and outer world.

3. Session Group Process

Verbal Themes

Participants recalled having taken home a good feeling after the last session and having maintained a positive image and enjoyment (c2). In the third session, regressive wishes became significant in two groups: One of them expressed the strong need for a safe and conserved space to relax and to de-energize where no pressure exists. They also named familiar stressors (i). The other group stated their big desire for harmony: Individuals articulate the wish for symbiosis, which would procure a sense of security, as group conformity would develop. On the other hand, differing behaviour would be experienced as distancing (b2). Two other groups dealt with similar issues: Do I still belong to the group even if I say no once? (l) and what about group belonging and responsibility? (n). Painful early separation situations and the experience of death came up as themes in two groups (b2, d). One group discussed issues on power and powerlessness (e), another group focused on more abstract concepts such as space and one's personal experience in space (e).

Movement Themes

Two groups worked with the concept of kinesphere (a, l). Three groups put the theme leading and following into action (b, c1, c2) in trying to let body parts lead, they strike the note and dominate, while one participant decided, what should be done while the other follows (c2). Mirroring (c2) and the Chace circle (c1) were some more DMT techniques, respectively approaches used. One dance therapist integrated intervention that she had used in the previous session in order to deepen the personal movement motives of the second session (a). Other movement qualities were pushing, propelling, cutting (e), as well as experimenting with moving, pausing, using strength (b2). A joyful quality emerged in group b where participants played hide-and-seek. In another group, however, one person recalled unhappy early childhood experiences when she has been screamed at as an infant and her movement radius has been constrained. Other movement images that were activated were to sunbath, to stock up on some sunshine, but also seek shelter under the blanket in an embryo-like posture (e).

Summary and Conclusion

The main theme seemed to be the preoccupation with physical and mental adjustment: Adjusting to somebody and letting oneself be guided, adapting to somebody, letting go of and taking on responsibility. The "debate" was deepened through working on one's individual movement repertoire. The awareness grew for the interacting processes between one's current needs and past experiences.

4. Session Group Process

Verbal Themes

Verbal themes of the forth session demonstrated a different focus compared to the previous sessions: Indeed participants in several groups attributed the reason for their stress to external factors such as the approaching Christmas time (n), the forthcoming change of job (e). They also declared their own ambivalence as the cause of their stressful situations: the ambivalence between the external pressure to complete something and the internal claim to becoming contemplative (c2). One group focused on the own person: being under pressure or having too many things going on in the mind (d) or being in an inner conflict (b2), melancholy and no movement (i), anger (c2) and anxiety (d). However, throughout many groups a tendency towards resource orientation was recognizable: Strength was one of the terms which were mentioned, to feel courage (i, c1), to better confine oneself (c1, e, u) and to explore one's space and get grounded (l, u). Additional psycho-education explained what happens on a hormone base during stress (a), in another group members express that they sense their emotions stronger and that their awareness would be improved compared to the beginning of DMT (c1).

Movement Themes

In most groups the work with polarities was striking: On one side, the work with indulging qualities such as picking, gathering became obvious, on the other hand, punching, pushing, stamping movement qualities appeared as well (i). Fighting movement, strength was mentioned at the same time as letting go and calmness as antipole (a). This duality also became apparent in other groups: Dance therapists listed calmness and movement, equilibrium and pauses (c2), plenty of weight, little weight (c1), narrow and wide kinesphere (l), opening -- closing (k), and heaviness -- lightness (d). Parallels could also be found in the following movement descriptions: Use of weight (c2), the work with ground and stance (b) and strength (b2) and the focus on work including the kinesphere (b2), the space (lower, middle, superior) (e) and horizontal widening (r). Group specific themes were the concentration on body image, improvisation, exploration, composition (c1), the integration of voice, breath, body awareness (b2) or the incorporation of the Bartenieff Fundamentals (b). Emerging movement images are grain of seed → plant/tree (l) and karate (i).

Summary and Conclusion

Many groups concentrated on working with polarities during the movement process as well as identifying and naming one's own resources.

5. Session Group Process

Verbal Themes

To combine family, children and a 50% job is hard to balance and ends up in having no energy and feeling exhausted and being swamped, that is the tenor in group i. Other participants mention stressors like feeling the strain between the inner world (need for contemplativeness) and outer world (hectic, turbulences, work) around Christmas time (c2). Sporadically, emotions in the vein of aggression (b) and loneliness (b2) were described, someone mentioned killing (e), another one the handling of separations such as farewell and pause (c2). The debate with one's own role especially one's role as a woman seemed to become more important: the role of providing / being emotional, social, and barely egoistic (i). Relaxation, body awareness (a) and quietness obtained a greater significance (b). The verbal themes got easier and more playful in some groups: To experience strength and the improvement of somatic symptoms, to experience joy at the rediscovery of female movements and fighting impulses and improvement of self-worth (c1). Others enjoyed that they could easier engage with the group /with a theme / in the process (l), they discover lust (b2), try out, sense, and play (u).

Movement Themes

Several groups focused on body awareness work (i, k, l, a, b2): One group worked with the lower part of the back which was experienced as being very tactile and sensitive / vulnerable / painful (i), in another group it was the spine (k). The focal point on body part dominance (l) and the integration of shaking movement, activation of the meridian Qui Gong: 10 movements, partner massage (a) fostered the improvement of body awareness. Additionally, interactive movement with voice (b), deepening of the theme use of weight, partner modalities (in twos) and movement composition (c1) were listed as movement themes, in which nonverbal interaction was mentioned explicitly. Laban's action drives whipping, pushing, pressing were applied as fighting qualities (e). Occurring themes were the work with space / kinesphere (l), space, direct and indirect (b2) or pauses in movement: stoppage, quietness, transitions, phrasing (c2).

Summary and Conclusion

Verbal themes circled around strong emotions such as hate, sadness, isolation as well as joy. Personal vitality or the lack of vitality seemed to be strongly felt, also on a body level: On the one hand, the nonverbal process focused on quietness and relaxation; on the other hand, the growing awareness of internal and external strength and vital female resources was fostered.

6. Session Group Process

Verbal Themes

By comparing the documentation, it stands out that all the dm therapists made little notes on the process of the sixth session. Also, there were hardly any common themes to detect. In one group aggression, grounding and quietness played an important role (b), in another the theme on sexuality and partnership (b2) was dominant, respectively in two other groups farewell and transition (into the new year) were picked out as the central theme (c1, c2). Group d dealt with issues around anger, pressure, irritation and neglect, group u discussed if an individual or a collective is attached.

Movement Themes

Repetition, working with body part modalities (c1), body awareness, kinesphere (b2) and movement work with stick and chiffon cloths (a) and focusing on space, weight, time, and flow were movement themes of the sixth session. Movement processes revolve around the personal space (kinesphere) (c1), the experience of the space, and indulging qualities (e), sensing and filling one's own space (l). Apart from that, the focus was on weight (b), use of weight (c1) strength (r), time sudden transitions → as in the theme of time (c2), and on movement qualities such as bound flow (r) and authentic movement from the internal to the external (n).

Summary and Conclusion

The use of Laban's effort qualities *space, weight, time, and flow* and the work on the kinesphere unified the groups.

7. Session Group Process

Verbal Themes

In two groups, the issue of *separation* came up on the seventh session (i, c2), other groups centered on subjects such as *leading and following* (a) and the transference of positive experiences into daily life (a, c1). One group debated how to find *balance and halt* (c2) or how to *be better and to be familiar with* (e). Furthermore, the attention was also problem- and emotion-oriented, themes were *sadness, anger, disappointment, being at the end of one's robe,* partnership (b2, d) and one's own achievement *(where am I standing?)* (l).

Movement Themes

Movement themes were tensing up, grapping, stretching, bound flow (i) goal-orientation, grounding, fluttering, opening, closing, sensing (e) and tenderness, tranquility (b) or swing, strength, lightness (d), space, verticality, kinesphere, ground (l). A dance therapist mentions a plant (k), another one rolling and lolling (r), another one flow, directness and weight (b2). Leading and following (a), the work with strength (b), time, sustainess, suddenness, interruption of time (c1) and the structure of dance with quick and slow parts (c1) are recurrent issues of other sessions.

Summary and Conclusion

All the descriptions of the seventh session give the impression of a playful and flowing process with and against the force of gravity and the attempt, to rise, to stretch in the vertical plane and to take one's standpoint. This gives a light and delicate appearance, all the same the atmosphere is not anxious but goal-oriented and at the same time strong.

8. Session Group Process

Verbal Themes

The eighth session offered the possibility to address actual personal stress factors such as problems in the partnership (b2, c2) and sexuality (b2). Interim results were drawn in many groups as members recall resources which I had and which I learned and re-experienced in the DMT group (a), developments, keeping boundaries, self-worth, changes in lifestyle, planning: to quit the job, to start a new training course (c1). In other words: I listen to my inner voice (b) and I follow my inner impulses (u). Other themes were walking through life, rising, landing, being criticized, being afraid of critics, letting go (e) and standing up, strength, minimizing / maximizing (l) and last-not least farewell/past/future (d).

Movement Themes

The movement themes were very clear: One group discussed stress sequences and the desired move, working in the here and now: what remains, what has changed? (a) One group expresses their actual state and the target state (e), how it was being in the center. Time, respectively sustained / sudden, a lot of time, interruptions in time, change (c1) or weight sensing → the ground and the air (theme of space) (c2) were additional movement themes. Repeatedly, the occupation with polarities (c1, d, r) and with space and boundaries appeared, to capture the space and the boundaries around the space as well as seeing the limits of others and of oneself, defending one's boundaries and taking the space (n). Some were moving with one and another through free dancing -- bonding to each other (u), others focused more inside and listen to inner impulses (b). Some groups mentioned little efforts, strength, stamina, flow (b2) or concentrated themselves on different themes such as leg work, connection between trunk and ground, and lightness (e).

Summary and Conclusion

Verbal and movement themes centered around one's personal core and inner space, individual resources, and the ground and supporting factors which kept oneself ashore. The viewpoint also went outwards to the others, to the past, the present, and the future.

9. Session Group Process

Verbal Themes

The most important theme was the farewell. Issues from previous sessions were addressed again such as problems in the partnership and with sexuality (b2), separation, resumée (n), dosing the use of strength and devotion/protection (l), and space and ego grounding (u).

Movement Themes

Several groups danced the "journey through time": It was a journey where they crossed and came back to the stages of the individual sessions thereby including the used music (e, n, l) or creating a stress management path: movement and composition with media (a). The defined goal was the integration of all themes (l). The work with the wheel plane (r) or with the pathway round / square (c2) was mentioned. Other groups experimented with force, tension, relaxation, flow, rest (b), pushing, pulling, shifting (e), body contact with hands, stretching, widening (narrowing), away from the body, towards the body (b2), round, angular, and own movement (c2) and track on the ground/track in the air/connection/image paint (c1).

Summary and Conclusion

Applying a journey through time was a characteristic of several groups. On the same alley, though more indirectly, the work on the sagittal plane, the wheel plane and the focus on pathways fostered the contention with and integration of the presence, the past, and the future.

10. Session Group Process

Verbal Themes

Participants used the tenth session to feedback to the dm therapist and to recall different stages in the group process (i, a, c1, c2, b2). One group made a journey through the ten sessions (e). Future prospective (c1, c2) and how one deals with one-self was discussed (b2). The attention was directed to centre, light -- shadow, treasure, strength (e), and to encounter, awareness, courage, and ego-identity (r). Nearly in all groups, the central issue was the farewell and good-bye from one and another (i, a, b, c1, c2, e, n, k, l, u, b2).

Movement Themes

Spatial group formations, the extended group, groups in two's or three's, an energy circle at the end where symbolic gesture are integrated (i) were described. Free movements and twisting, stamping and clapping movements (i) as well as free dancing to reduce stress, composition with props and symbols (u) terminate the last session of two groups. Three other groups end their last session by integrating all themes (l) with the aid of a time journey in movement and good-bye: expressing the experienced trough movement (n) and repeating stations on the way, >reminiscence of special individual movements, compositions (c1, c2). At the end tension and relaxation (b, i), strength (b), jumping and flattering (e) as well as the work on the kinesphere (e, r) were mentioned.

Summary and Conclusion

In the last DMT session, the main emphasis is on integrating all the experiences, insights, and perceptions as an individual and as a group member, to bring the shared process to a good end, to say good-bye, and to separate from one and another.

DISCUSSION

The aim of this research was to examine twelve short-term treatment programs in DMT and their group processes, thereby identifying common evolving themes. For this purpose, the 10 qualitative items of the ICL2 have been analyzed. To a certain degree, the investigation has approved that parallels in the group process exist. Nevertheless, these results should not be over-interpreted, as dm therapists' subjective documentation of the group process can only be objectified to a certain degree. Some descriptions could have been plurivalent and might have biased the analysis. Terms from Laban and KMP terminology simplified the communication of meaning. All dm therapists were trained in Laban and/or KMP terminology. As their amount of training had varied according to their training institution, the use of the terminology might have differed slightly. The ICL2 is not yet a standardized tool therefore the eleven therapists may have interpreted the items in different ways, despite the instructions on the meaning of the different items through the researcher. In general, using movement analysis can clarify the process. However further studies on the validity and interrater-reliability regarding the usage of common DMT terms as well as introducing standardized procedures into training programs are needed. Additionally, the researcher may have misinterpreted the descriptive material of her colleagues. The focus of the inquiry has been limited to analyzing the development of themes in the groups.

Subsequently, the results are compared with the group phase model of Bender (2001) who assumes that DMT groups pass through four different phases. Bender does not specify if the traverse of all four phases need a minimum of DMT sessions. Therefore, it is assumed that her model can also be applied to short-term treatment programs as described in this study. Affiliation occurs during the first phase of Benders group phase model. That is true in the first two hours of the DMT groups: They struggle with issues of how to find the equilibrium within the group. The use of flow and weight in the DMT groups overlap with flow, mentioned by Bender as relevant for that phase, it does not overlap with space which Bender described as another important effort quality used in the first phase. Responsibility enhanced by confrontation and autonomy during the second phase is a typical characteristic according to Bender. Comparing the DMT group process of the third and forth session with Bender's group phase model reveals that the responsibility phase seems to be present, because the main emphasis lay on attunement, being guided, accommodating, and letting go of and taking over responsibility. Confrontation and autonomy, as mentioned by Bender, deepens in the treatment groups through working on individuals' movement repertoires (during the third session), focusing on polarities in the movement process (forth session) as well as recognizing and labelling one's own resources. Openness is the core of the third phase in Bender's phase model, characterized by questions of being close or far, emotions of being amiable / not amiable, anxiety of being rejected or being to close or to far away, and the need for differentiation. In evaluating these characteristics in the DMT groups' verbal processes, it becomes obvious that openness is important while strong emotions are being expressed. In concordance with Bender, the dm therapists mention the predominance of the efforts space and weigh; additionally, they also list the time and flow efforts. Relating to themes of internal and external strength, female and vital resources, and kinesphere (sixth session), the DMT groups' processes are not concordant with Bender's third phase. Nevertheless, their goal-orientation during the seventh session can be interpreted as a need for differentiation in accordance with the phase model. The last phase described by Bender is the separation phase. The focus is on holding on and letting go, terminating interactions, feeling autonomy or dependency, and using the effort quality time. Several analogies exist in the treatment groups, especially in sessions eight to ten: The DMT themes seem to become centered, the effort time plays a very important role, and the main emphasis is on integrating experiences and insights, closing the collective process, and separation.

Concordance could not be found regarding the usage of planes: As far as the dm therapists reported usage of planes, their descriptions differed from those in the phase model. Concordance seems to exist with regard to the general schedule line of the ten sessions, and the four phases affiliation, responsibility, openness, and separation outlined by Bender (2001).

As a result, the phase model seems to offer a helpful reference frame to the group process development in short-term treatment programs. The present study validates the phase model of Bender in all but one point. Additionally, it facilitates assignment and categorization of emerging themes in the DMT process to the four phases of Bender. Even though the group processes of the twelve groups are not totally identical with the phase model, it is possible to confirm that parallels in the group process exist across all twelve DMT groups. This is an interesting result, keeping in mind that the DMT approaches applied varied extensively (Bräuninger, 2006, Bräuninger in press). It would be fascinating to examine in future research, whether these findings can be replicated in other DMT groups, for example, in groups for clients with a psychopathological or (psycho-)somatic diagnosis, groups for the elderly, or for adolescents.

Using the standardized ICL2 in this study was the first step in checking its usability for research purposes, with a positive result. Its application in future DMT studies will support and accelerate the process to validate the ICL2 as a reliable DMT research tool. The multi-centered RCT of which this study is part, has offered an invaluable resource of possibilities to combine qualitative with quantitative information on the same sample. This study offers a valid insight into group process development and emerging contents within short-term DMT group programs.

FINAL THOUGHTS

Across all twelve short-term DMT treatment groups, parallels have been detected regarding themes and group process that were in accordance with the four phases of Bender (2001), namely the phases: affiliation, responsibility, openness, and separation. Movement observation language from Laban Movement Analysis and Kestenberg Movement Profile simplified the evaluation of the qualitative group process data. Further research could evaluate the validity and interrater-reliability of common used language in DMT. The usage and further evaluation of the ICL2 can support to establish a standardized DMT research tool.

To conclude, parallels in groups themes presented in this chapter can sensitize dm therapists for leading short term DMT groups, choosing appropriate intervention options and setting specific treatment goals in short term DMT programs.

REFERENCES

Astin, J.A., Berman, B.M., Bausell, B., Lee, W.-L., Hochberg, M., & Forys, K.L. (2003). The efficacy of mindfulness meditation plus Qi Gong movement therapy in the treatment of fibromyalgia: a randomized controlled trial. *Journal of Rheumatology, 30*(10), 2257-2262.

Bender, S. (2001). Lasst die Gruppe tanzen, Teil 2[Let the group dance, Part 2]. *Zeitschrift für Tanztherapie, 8*(13), 3-11.

Berrol, C., Ooi, W. L., & Katz, S. (1997). Dance/movement therapy with older adults who have sustained neurological insult: A demonstration project. *American Journal of Dance Therapy, 19*(2), 135-160.

Bräuninger, I. (2000a). Tanztherapie mit Menschen in der zweiten Lebenshälfte: Möglichkeiten der Angst- und Suchtbewältigung [Dance movement therapy for people in their second half of life: Possibilities for treating anxiety disorder and substance abuse]. In P. Bäuerle, H. Radebold, R.D. Hirsch, K. Studer, U. Schmid-Furstoss & B. Struwe (Eds.). *Klinische Psychotherapie mit älteren Menschen. Grundlagen und Praxis* [Clinical Psychology with elderly people. Theory and practice] (pp. 136-141). Bern: Hans Huber.

Bräuninger, I. (2000b). Tanztherapie in der Gerontopsychiatrischen Tagesklinik bei Patienten mit Angststörungen [Dance movement therapy in a day clinic with patients with anxiety disorder]. In C. Kretschmar, R.D. Hirsch, M. Haupt, R. Ihl, R. Kortus, G. Stoppe & C. Wächter (Eds.), *Angst-Sucht-Anpassungsstörungen im Alter. Schriftenreihe der Deutschen Gesellschaft für Gerontopsychiatrie und -psychotherapie, DGGPP, Band 1* (pp. 202-206). Düsseldorf: Die Deutsche Bibliothek-CIP Einheitsaufnahme.

Bräuninger, I. (2006). *Tanztherapie. [Dance Therapy].* Weinheim, Germany: Beltz / PVU.

Bräuninger, I. (in preparation). What are successful dance movement therapy interventions?

Bräuninger, I. (in press). Treatment modalities and self-expectancy of therapists -- modes, self-efficacy and imagination of clients. *Body Movement and Dance in Psychotherapy, International Journal for Theory, Research and Practice (1)*.

Bräuninger, I., & Blumer, E. (2004). 7.4. Tanz- und Bewegungstherapie [Dance and movement therapy]. In W. Rössler (Eds.). *Lehrbuch Psychiatrische Rehabilitation [Psychiatric rehabilitation]* (pp. 380-387). Heidelberg: Springer Verlag, Fachbuch Medizin/Psychologie.

Brooks, D., & Stark, A. (1989). The effects of dance/movement therapy on affect: A pilot study. *American Journal of Dance Therapy, 11*(2), 101-112.

Ellis, R. (2001). Movement metaphors as mediator. A model for the dance/movement therapy process. *The Arts in Psychotherapy, 28*(3), 181-190.

Erwin-Grabner, T., Goodill, S.W., Schelly Hill, E., & von Neida, K. (1999). Effectiveness on Reducing Test Anxiety, *American Journal of Dance Therapy, 21*(1), 19-34.

Levy, F.J. (1992). *Dance Movement Therapy: A Healing Art* (rev. Ed.). Reston, VA: American Alliance for Health, Physical Education, Recreation and Dance.

Mannheim, E. (2004). Dance/Movement Therapy as a clinical intervention method in oncological rehabilitation. Evaluation of treatment effects -- results of Phase I. Paper presented at the *First International Research Colloquium in Dance/Movement Therapy, BTD, February, 13-14, 2004, in Hannover, Germany, preceeding the 10th annual BTD membership assembly.*

Mayring, P. (2003). Qualitative Inhaltsanalyse. Grundlagen und Techniken [Qualitative content-analysis and techniques] (8th ed.). Weinheim: Beltz.

McComb, J.J.R., & Clopton, J.R. (2003).The effects of movement, relaxation, and education on the stress levels of women with subclinical levels of bulimia. *Eating Behaviors, 4*(1), 79-88.

Meekums, B. (2002). Dance Movement Therapy. A creative psychotherapeutiv approach. London: Sage.

Penfield, K. (1994). Laban Movement Analysis and group process in dance movement therapy. Conference Proceedings of the First International Clinical Conference on Dance/Movement Therapy in Berlin, Germany >Language of Movement< from September 1-4, 1994 (pp. 162-165).

Rose, S. (1995). Movement as Metaphor: Treating Clinical Addiction. In F.J. Levy (Ed.). *Dance and other expressive art therapies. When words are not enough* (pp. 101-108). New York: Routledge.

Schmais, C. (1981). Group development and group formation in dance therapy. *The Arts in Psychotherapy, 8,* 103-107.

Schmais, C. (1985). Healing process in group and dance therapy. *American Journal of Dance Therapy, 8,* 17-36.

Stanton, K. (1992). Imagery and metaphor in group dance movement therapy. A psychiatric out-patient setting. In H. Payne (Eds.). *Dance movement therapy: theory and practice* (pp. 123-140). London: Routledge.

APPENDIX (Translation of ICL2 by the author)

INTERVENTION-CHECKLIST /ICL2 (group process related) Therapist-Code: Session Nr.:

LEADERSHIP STYLE:

Today, my predominant style was (please tick):	…direct ... combination ... non-direct
	…verbal ... combination ... non-verbal
	... assertive ... confrontative ... provocative
	... sensitive ... empathetic ... supportive
	... accepting ... explorative ... emotion-focussed

GROUP PROCESS: ... verbal themes:
(please fill in)   ... verbal images:
                            ... movement themes:
                            ... movement images (identified through the therapist):

IMAGINATIVE TECHNIQUES   ... Active Imagination
                                ... Visualization
                                ... others (which?):

RELAXATION TECHNIQUES: ... guided relaxation
                                        ... body awareness
                                        ... breathing exercises
                                        ... guided imagination
                                        ... elements from progressive muscle relaxation / Jacobsen
                                        ... others (which?):
                        ... open relaxation (minimum input, f. ex..music)

MEDITATIVE DANCE (THERAPY)   ... Elements of Authentic Movement (which?)
METHODS (which?):   ... Meditative / Ritual Dances
                                    ... others

DANCE THERAPY APPROACHES: ... Chace Approach (Chacian circle, mirroring, changing leadership, etc)
(which intervention?)   ... In-depth psychological oriented dmt
                                    ... Integrative Dance Therapy
                                    ... Authentic Movement (mover-witness, etc.)
                                    ... others:

MODUS
  Clients:
    Receptive Mode (relaxed, but consciously awake): ca. _____ % of session
    Active Mode (clients move actively)   ca. _____ % of session

  Therapists:
    Activly participating
    (accompanies the group in an active mode):   ca. _____ % of session
    Observing / witnessing   ca. _____ % of session
    (accompanies the group with words, looking, breathing,...)

STRUCTURE OF THE SESSION:
  ... Warm-up - process - closure (as in Chace Approach):
    Warm-up (please tick):   ... verbal   ... body-oriented   ... others
    Transition
    Process (please fill in):
    Transition:
    Closure (please tick):   ... intrapsychic   ... combination   ... interpersonal
                                      ... verbal   ... combination   ... body-oriented
  ... different structure (which?):

THE FOCUS on content of the session was   ... prepared   ...intuitively develpoed ... post worked
Which focus? (catchwords)

	No, not at all	0 - 1 - 2 - 3 - 4 - 5 - 6 - 7 - 8 - 9 yes completely
In this session, I felt at ease and free		0 - 1 - 2 - 3 - 4 - 5 - 6 - 7 - 8 - 9
In this session, I could achieve my therapeutic aims		0 - 1 - 2 - 3 - 4 - 5 - 6 - 7 - 8 - 9

DANCE MOVEMENT THERAPY IN THE LIGHT OF TRAUMA: RESEARCH FINDINGS OF A MULTIDISCIPLINARY PROJECT

Claire A. Moore

Over a period of two years, a university research project focused on four alternative methods of how to treat domestic violence. Besides investigating the specific effects of an interdisciplinary network, of public work on violence and of counselling, the main interest was to examine Dance Movement Therapy and its psychotherapeutic efficacy with traumatized clients. Of the 44 clients that were referred to therapy, 27 started therapy and 16 clients ended therapy. All the clients, that ended therapy, showed considerable changes in their symptoms, such as stress and pain reduction, less depression and less medication. Furthermore, they developed a better body image, more self-awareness and self-confidence. The small-scale results were gained by analysing questionnaires and documentation, and by comparing movement analysis, session notes and psychological tests (BDI & BSI) before and after therapy. The main conclusion is that Dance Movement Therapy with its body-mind approach can positively influence the specific symptoms of abuse because the body is the central factor in the memorizing of traumatic incidents.

Keywords: domestic violence, trauma, DMT, interdisciplinary work, clinical social work

INTRODUCTION

In the past 30 years, there has been an increasing social and political concern about domestic violence. Generally referred to as violence within a current or former, close relationship, awareness has grown of its deleterious consequences, both for the victim as well as for the wider social context in which the abuse takes place. Domestic violence is not restricted to physical violence. It may include physical, sexual, psychological[9], economic and social abuse, and these may occur together or separately. Furthermore, it is independent of ethnicity, socio-economic class, religion and age, and can be found in almost all cultures throughout the world (CWASU, 2005; Sullivan, 2000).

Most definitions of the term 'domestic violence' reflect a feministic understanding of domestic violence, viewing the occurrence of abuse within the gender dichotomy of a male perpetrator and a female victim. It is for this reason that research literature across disciplines mainly focuses on 'Violence against Women' (VAW) (Saltzman, 2004), and that published figures on prevalence and incidence rates are usually much higher for women than for men. Domestic violence, which accounts for 23% of all violent crime in the UK, is the only category of violence where the risks for women are deemed higher (1%) than for men (0.5%), with men being victims in 26% of domestic violence incidents.

In October 2004, the 'Ministry of Families, The Elderly, Women and Youth' (translated by the author) published the first German study on domestic violence (BMFSFJ, 2004a). Of the 10,000 women (aged 16-85) that were interviewed to their experiences, 37% reported one-time incidents of physical assaults and 40% reported to have experienced physical and/or sexual abuse. These figures concur with other international data (see CWASU, 2005). In the German BMFSFJ study, various forms of sexual abuse had been experienced by 58% of the women, and 42% said that they had been subjected to psychological violence at least once in their lifetime. Approximately 25% of these women reported physical and/or sexual abuse in their current or previous heterosexual

---

[9] 'psychological violence' refers to the harm of a person's psyche, i.e. the development and structure of the *psychological self* and the *body self* (Damasio, 1997)

or homosexual relationships. An evaluation of the Beratungs- und InterventionSStellen (BISS)[10] in Niedersachsen (Löbmann et al., 2004) shows that the majority of violent incidents occur between couples (80.7%; n=1917). The study also shows that in 63.8% of the cases children were witnesses of domestic violence (with 53.9% under the age of five). Similar figures can be found in a survey distributed via NCH Family Centres in the UK (Abrahams, 1994), in which 75% of mothers reported that their children had directly witnessed domestic violence, 33% had seen their mothers beaten up and 10% had witnessed sexual violence. Kavemann (2002) has pointed out that witnessing and experiencing violence are frequently connected, thus making children to dual victims. The incident will always be harmful to the child, regardless of whether violence is witnessed or experienced.

Recently, research shows that boys and men suffer from domestic violence, too, and that domestic violence is best viewed as 'gendered violence' (Hagemann-White, 1998). The findings of an albeit small-scale German pilot study 'Violence against Men' (translated by the author) (BMFSFJ, 2004b) reflect an increasing number of male victims that admit to the experience of physical and/or sexual abuse within closer relationships (6%-9%). As Mirrlees-Black (1999) and the British Crime Survey (BCS, 2000) point out, women are far more likely to say they had experienced domestic assault at some time in their lives and to admit that they were upset by the experience than men. One of the reasons for not reporting domestic violence is the view that the incident is a private matter and can be dealt with by the victim (BCS, ibid.). Feelings of shame and guilt, fear of the assailant and fear of not being taken seriously by the police or other helping agencies are also reasons for not reporting (BMFSFJ, 2004a). Furthermore, it appears that victims' perceptions of their experiences are closely linked to gender issues and gender identity, and the subjective construction of 'normality' and what constitutes a crime. Findings from the 1996 British Crime Survey self-completion questionnaire reveal that virtually no male victim defined their experience as a crime as opposed to 40% of the women (Mirrlees-Black, 1999), even though the questions asked about the incident would meet the legal definition of an assault.

On the basis of this gradual unfolding of the magnitude of domestic violence, the research outcomes and figures on prevalence rates must be viewed as the tip of an iceberg. It can be expected that an improved standardization of terminology and measurement within national and international research as well as a change in personal beliefs on abuse will reveal a far greater account on the nature of domestic violence.

For the purpose of the research project presented in this paper, it was important to understand the wider effects of violence, and to follow the questions of prevention and treatment. The most important traumatic effects of abuse include somatic and psychosomatic health problems, such as multiple injuries, gynecological problems, miscarriages, stress-related ailments, chronic pain or eating disorders (Taket, 2004), psychological difficulties, such as depression, extreme anxieties, self-harm, severe lack of self-esteem and self-confidence and/or dissociative states (Sachsse, 2004), and social problems, such as isolation from family and friends, difficulties in relating with others, change of home, or separation/divorce (Stephens & McDonald, 2000). In the above mentioned German study on violence (BMFSFJ, 2004a), two-thirds of the women reported physical injuries such as bruises, broken bones, or head injuries following vio-

---

[10] 16 counseling projects that act as a link between the criminal justice system and practical social work in a crisis

lent incidents. Every third to seventh woman needed therapy to cope with the somato-psycho-social effects.

Only gradually, domestic violence is seen as a major health issue for the victim (Taket, 2004). Still today, according to Williamson (2000), only every tenth case of domestic violence is recognized by the health system, and the effects are frequently not diagnosed as a result of the incident(s). Due to inappropriate diagnoses, women suffering from somato-psycho-social symptoms are very often treated with neuroleptic drugs, tranquilizers and pain-killers. As a result, the victim experiences dampened affects and an inability to willfully change stressful and destructive life circumstances, either on his or her own or with the support of others.

In addition to the effects on a personal level, domestic violence has an immense impact on the wider health-care and socio-economic system, too. The cost of male violence in Germany is estimated as high as 14.8 billion € per year (Niedersächsisches Ministerium für Soziales, Frauen, Familie und Gesundheit, 2002). The estimated cost of domestic violence in England and Wales in 2001 was £23 billion (Walby, 2004). These figures highlight an urgent need for early prevention and intervention programs.

Since 1990, there are a growing number of domestic violence projects in Germany that focus on the establishment of an interdisciplinary and inter-institutional support system for the victims of domestic violence as well as on intervention programs for perpetrators. The research findings of these projects identify interdisciplinary cooperation as crucial to the tackling of domestic violence (BMFSFJ, 2004b), as it improves the availability of information on domestic violence and on services for those who experience it. However, although the services of legal advocacy and social work have greatly improved, little has changed in the therapeutic services.

A relatively new approach within the psychotherapy schools is traumatherapy, viewing the phenomenon of trauma from a somato-psycho-social angle (Sachsse, 2004; van der Kolk et al., 1996). Instead of interpreting a person's behaviour purely as a reaction to unconscious, unresolved, intrapsychic conflicts, or as false conditioning, traumatherapy makes an attempt to understand and treat the body and mind as reacting to the effects and influences of real, existentially life-threatening situations. For exploring the experience of violence, intrapsychic and interpersonal coping strategies play as much a part in the therapeutic process as do the knowledge of biochemical and neurophysiological reactions to the stressful incident. For about 20 years, findings from stress and brain research are increasingly linked to psychoanalytic discussions on the dynamics of violence, and gradually to other therapies, such as Cognitive-Behaviour Therapy (CBT) or Gestalt Therapy, thus forming a new thinking model for the treatment of traumatized clients (see Sachsse, 2004, for an overview). However, inspite of the awareness that 'the body keeps the score' (van der Kolk, 1994), most psychotherapeutic approaches limit their interventions to talk and do not actively integrate the body in the treatment process. As van der Kolk says, "words can't integrate the disorganized sensations and action patterns that form the core imprint of the trauma" (in Sykes Wylie, 2004). The sensations and actions that have become stuck in and after the traumatic event need to be integrated in the treatment process, so that the person can regain a sense of familiarity and efficacy in his/her body. Following the quest for more effective treatments, it appears that body psychotherapies could have more to offer. In Germany, however, this awareness is only slowly setting off discussions on treatment models (Sachsse, 2004). Body psychotherapies are still viewed as adjunctive therapies, and are laden with the prejudices and fears of orthodox psychotherapies. Research is necessary to validate somatic approaches.

A well researched trauma-body-psychotherapy model is Sensorimotor Psychotherapy (Ogden & Minton, 2000). The treatment method aims at helping people view their bodies as separate from their (trauma-conditioned) emotions and to cultivate clients' self-awareness of inner body sensations. According to Ogden and Minton, this method is especially beneficial for clinicians working with dissociation, emotional reactivity or flat affect, frozen states or hyperarousal and other PTSD symptoms.

On the basis of the so far presented knowledge about the dynamics of violence, the traumatizing effects, and the effectiveness of interventions and approaches, it seems a reasonable assumption that victims of violence would most profit from a support centre that offers legal advocacy, counselling, publicity work, an interdisciplinary network and psychotherapy with a trauma-centred, body-oriented focus. Funded primarily by the Arbeitsgruppe für Innovative Projekte (AGIP) at the Niedersächsisches Ministerium für Wissenschaft und Kultur (MWK; Lower Saxon Ministry of Science and Culture, translated by the author), the Fachhochschule (University of Applied Sciences, translated by the author) Oldenburg/Ostfriesland/Wilhelmshaven put all these ideas into a doctoral research project for two years (September 2002-September 2004). Due to the inherent magnitude of the ideas, the focus was narrowed down to women, children and adolescents who had experienced or were still experiencing domestic violence, i.e. male adults were not included. The innovative aspects of this project, at least in Germany, were *for one* the uniqueness of merely one centre to offer such extensive, inter- and multidisciplinary support, *for two* the possibility for victims of violence to profit from Dance Movement Therapy in a non-clinical setting. The concept was to offer its services without bureaucracy, to be easily accessible, to be cost-free and to offer multidisciplinary support immediately.

For the purpose of this paper, the focus shall be on the psychotherapeutic services offered in this project. The approach was trauma-centred and insight-oriented, i.e. the interpersonal and intrapersonal management of trauma were viewed from a functional, neurobiological perspective as well as from a psychodynamic understanding of human behaviour. The treatment method included functional exercises to sensitize the client's body awareness, and diverse verbal and nonverbal interventions that served the client's stabilization, the growth of inner resources and self-acceptance. The aim of the research on Dance Movement Therapy was to investigate the effectiveness of this model for traumatized clients.

METHODS

Participants

Women, children and adolescents who had experienced or were still experiencing domestic violence were able to use the services of the centre. There were no restrictions regarding age, ethnicity, religion, or the number and severity of incidents. However, male adolescents were only able to participate up to the age of 19. As it was an outpatient centre, people with an acute psychosis were not included in the project.

The participants were either referred to the centre by local General Practitioners (GP), by other support agencies, such as shelters or the welfare office, by schools, by therapists, or they came on their own accord. Flyers of the project, regular newspaper articles on the work at the centre, bi-monthly public seminars on domestic violence issues, and bi-monthly interdisciplinary network meetings helped to make the project known to the region.

Materials[11]

The centre was based in a newly renovated house, with two rooms for the sole use of Dance Movement Therapy. A small room with a table and six chairs served for interviews, a large room with a wooden floor was used for the sessions. This room was equipped with audio equipment, cushions, balls, fabrics, puppets and other typical DMT props. Originally, video equipment was installed but had to be removed as the participants unanimously rejected it.

Session notes were made after each session, which included the prevailing themes, movement analysis, transference and countertransference issues, and afterthoughts.

The anamnesis and personal data of a client were recorded on standardized sheets, after the client had signed the required consent forms for the participation in the project. All data were anonymously locked away in a filing cabinet.

Two standardized tests, the Beck Depression Inventory (BDI) (Beck, 1995), and the Brief Symptom Inventory (BSI) (Franke, 1995), were used for all adult and adolescent clients. The tests were handed out at the beginning and at the end of therapy (t1 & t2). Due to individual differences in the length of therapy, the time between t1 and t2 varied from one client to the other. The BDI is a 21-item test presented in multiple choice format designed to measure the presence of depression in adolescents and adults. The statements are rank-ordered and weighted to reflect the range of severity of the symptom. Scores under 11 points can be viewed as negligible, points ranging from 11 to 17 indicate a mild to moderate depression, and scores over 18 points are considered to be clinically relevant. The BSI is a 53-item self-report scale used to measure nine primary symptom dimensions (somatization, obsessive-compulsive behavior, interpersonal sensitivity, depression, anxiety, hostility, phobic anxiety, paranoid ideation, and psychoticism), and three global indices [Global Severity Index (GSI), Positive Symptom Distress Index (PSDI), and Positive Symptom Total (PST)]. The BSI measures the experience of current psychological status and distress in the past seven days including the day the BSI was completed. Answers are on a 5-point scale, from 0 = "not at all", to 4 = "extremely". Raw scores were converted to T-scores using age and sex appropriate nonpatient norms. A client's status of psychological distress is considered high if at least two T-scores of the nine primary symptom dimensions or the T-score of the Global Severity Index (TGSI) are 63 points or above[12].

Movement analysis of the client's movements in the sessions was based on Laban Movement Analysis (LMA), and, in particular, on the two furthered systems BESS (Body, Effort, Shape, Space) (Bartenieff & Lewis, 1980) and KMP (Kestenberg Movement Profile) (Kestenberg-Amighi et al., 1999). As the clients rejected video recordings of their sessions, it was only possible to record by memory. Therefore, the only categories taken from the KMP were Bipolar Shaping and Tension Flow Rhythms.

---

[11] For space reasons, no data sheets are included in this paper. However, they can be sent out on request.
[12] The raw scores are converted to standardized T-scores (31 – 80 points; TGSI, TPST, TPSDI) which can be found in two norm-tables (adults, students) in the appendix of the test handbook. According to the handbook, gender is the only criteria for conversion, as the group of adults is ranked by the level of education and the students have a constant level of education.

At the end of therapy, i.e. after the whole treatment, the clients were asked to fill out a questionnaire on their subjective view of Dance Movement Therapy. The questionnaire contained six open questions that had been designed particularly for this project. These questions range from the more general of what had been particularly respective less helpful to more insight-oriented questions about somato-psycho-social changes. The questions are as follows:

- Which aspects of therapy were particularly helpful?
- Which aspects of therapy were less helpful?
- What has changed since you started therapy?
- Were you able to develop a better understanding for yourself and your life situation during this time?
- How do you perceive yourself and your body at the end of therapy?
- What are your wishes for your personal future?

Procedure

The client and the therapist had three initial sessions to clarify goals and to record the somato-psycho-social anamnesis. A contract for twelve sessions was only drawn up if the goals were jointly agreed upon. After the three initial sessions, i.e. at the beginning of therapy, t1 was filled out. A joint evaluation of the therapeutic process, and a possible renewal of the contract for an individually negotiable period, followed at the end of the twelve sessions. At the end of therapy, i.e. after the whole treatment, t2 was filled out.

RESULTS

Clients

From February 2003 to May 2004, 44 clients asked for Dance Movement Therapy. They were all German citizens. The age distribution was as follows (Table I):

TABLE I: AGE DISTRIBUTION OF REFERRALS (n=44)

	0-12	13-17	18-24	25-34	35-44	45-54	55-64	Over 65
Female	2	6	15	2	10	5	2	0
Male	0	0	1	0	0	1	0	0
Total	2	6	16	2	10	6	2	0

Note: Noticeable are three peaks: one at 18-24 years, another at 35-44 years and a third small peak from 45-54 years.

As mentioned in the methods section, clients came for three initial sessions first to clarify their aims and goals in therapy. From the 44 clients that had been referred, 26 female and one male client decided to start therapy. The following Table II gives a general overview of these clients.

TABLE II: GENERAL OVERVIEW OF CLIENTS (n=44)

	Clients	Average number of sessions (incl. interviews)	Reasons for drop-out
That ended therapy	16	28 sessions	--
That dropped out	- 6 individuals - 1 family (mother, 3 daughters -- 13/15/17 years, 1 son 19 years)	1 woman (48 years): 15 sessions 5 women (18-24 years): 4 sessions family: 13 sessions	serious somatic illness (hospitalization) not ready for therapy: returned to abusive relationships needed social worker to support them with current legal, social and financial difficulties

The educational standard of the 16 female clients was diverse, ranging from still being pupils (n=3), minimal schooling (Hauptschulabschluss) (n=5), secondary school qualifications (Realschulabschluss) (n=6) to higher academic degrees (n=2).

Types and Effects of Violence

The somato-psycho-social anamnesis of the 16 female clients revealed the following distribution of types of violence:

- As an adolescent: one-time incident of sexual violence by a male stranger (n=2)
- During childhood: chronic experience of sexual and psychological abuse by father (n=1)
- During childhood: chronic experience of sexual, psychological, physical, social and economic violence by parents (n=10)
- In marriage: chronic experience of sexual, psychological, physical, social and economic violence by partner (n=3)

In the three initial interviews, all clients reported psychosomatic symptoms, such as fear, reduced body sensations, eating and breathing disorders, as well as psychological syndromes such as lack of concentration, disturbed sleep, depressive symptoms, difficulties relating, and inappropriate feelings of humiliation, worthlessness and self-depreciation. Two women had developed severe chronic syndromes over the years in form of fibromyalgia and chronic back-pain, which limited their motility immensely.

The themes that all women and adolescents explored in therapy (11 in individual therapy, 5 in group therapy) were low self-esteem, fragmented body image and body sensations, fears, anger and grief, partnership conflicts as well as the construction of positive life visions.

Tests: BDI & BSI

Of the 16 clients that ended therapy, all except for the child filled out the BDI and the BSI. The two adolescents were 17 years old and therefore considered old enough to participate. The scores for both tests are given in Table III.

TABLE III: RESULTS OF BDI AND BSI

Nr.	BDI		Nr.	BSI					
	t1	t2		TGSI		TPST		TPSDI	
				T1	t2	t1	t2	t1	t2
1	20	5	1	74	50	80	52	63	45
2	23	3	2	80	56	80	53	80	59
3	13	5	3	74	40	80	63	66	56
4	46	13	4	80	74	80	80	80	63
5	14	1	5	60	44	59	45	59	45
6	38	24	6	80	74	80	80	74	62
7	25	20	7	74	68	67	63	74	67
8	23	8	8	80	80	80	80	80	74
9	53	20	9	80	80	80	80	80	68
10	4	3	10	68	48	52	49	76	45
11	4	3	11	68	48	52	49	76	45
12	33	4	12	80	49	80	51	74	45
13	16	3	13	71	40	74	40	62	45
14	45	12	14	80	43	80	44	80	45
15	24	1	15	68	21	66	37	61	62

By using the related t test for the BSI and the BDI, differences were calculated between the two conditions $t1$ and $t2$. In detail, these were as follows:

- BDI: n=15, t=5.925, $p < .0005$;
- BSI: n=15, df=14; TGSI: t= 5.426, p < .0005; TPST: t= 4.074, $p < .0005$; TPSDI: t= 5.906, $p < .0005$;

Overall, by the end of therapy, the severity of depression, as measured by the BDI, and the client's psychological distress, as measured by the BSI, had improved significantly.

Movement Analysis

The movement analysis of the 16 clients was subdivided into the five categories Body, Effort, Shape and Bipolar Shaping, Space, and Tension Flow Rhythms. The most relevant and noticeable observations were as follows:

Body: Between 14 and 16 clients showed high rigidity in body parts. This was particularly noticeable in the core (breast) and periphery (arms, head). Furthermore, they demonstrated shallow breath, evasive eye-contact and sequential sequencing of movements[13]. By the end of therapy, the rigidity only remained in two women. Seven women still had shallow breath. All clients were able to keep eye-contact.

Effort: The most characteristic finding was the initial absence of directness and strength. At the beginning, 13 women used little directness, and 15 clients little strength. At the end of therapy, only one woman showed the continuous absence of these elements. All the others were able to fluctuate between the efforts according to the context.

Shape & Bipolar Shaping: All clients were very vertical, and seemed very sensitive with their backs. This showed in convex changes when touching on emotionally difficult themes. Furthermore, there was low intensity narrowing and hollowing. 14 cli-

---

[13] Note: there are three variations of sequencing: simultaneous, successive and sequential (Lamb & Watson, 1979)

ents were rigid on the vertical axis, appearing stuck in the shrinking phase of bipolarity. At the end of therapy, the shaping of 15 participants fluctuated well on the horizontal and vertical axes, and nine women were able to bulge and hollow well.

Space: At the beginning, 15 clients had a very near personal reach space, one woman a very wide personal reach space. Movements were exclusively on a high level. This changed significantly at the end. The personal reach space was medium for all except for one whose was still near. Only one woman moved on the high level only, seven moved on the high and middle level, and eight clients could use the three levels high, medium and low.

Tension Flow Rhythms: The predominant rhythm of 15 clients was the biting rhythm in the periphery (hands, head/face). Toward the end of therapy, all participants had developed a preference for more indulging rhythms but were able to utilize fighting rhythms when necessary.

Self-Report Questionnaire on DMT

All women reported positive experiences in DMT sessions. They particularly emphasized that they had learnt to notice and name their own feelings, had felt accepted and respected, and had learnt to perceive and set own boundaries.

Furthermore, the presence of the therapist and her nonjudgmental commenting had inspired the women to think further than they had done before. In addition, all the women that had participated in the group found the group setting very supportive, in particular the realization that they were not alone with their experiences. This alleviated them from feelings of shame and guilt.

The therapeutic interventions had the following impacts: all the women reported that they were now able to see their bodies as fulfilling functional and emotional tasks which helped them become more sensitive towards moving in a healthier way, or how to become calmer and more self-confident in the body. In addition, the clients wrote that they were now able to feel and sense their bodies better, that they reflected more on their needs and feelings and that they were more sensitive and aware of their own boundaries and their body language.

For their own personal growth, almost all clients wished a continuation of therapy to stabilize and strengthen their new experiences.

Case vignette

Mrs S., 43 years old, mother of four children, aged 8, 12, 14, 16 years, with a long childhood history of physical, psychological and sexual abuse, had recently left her husband and had sued him for sexually abusing their youngest daughter. She came to individual therapy complaining of suicidal thoughts, depressive symptoms, anxiety, nightmares, panic attacks, loneliness and numbness in the body, leading to feelings of disembodiment. Mrs S. was obese, and did not seem to care about her physical appearance. This impression was supported by her overt rejection of her body, which, as she called it, 'was ugly and worthless'.

Initially, the goals she set were to sleep better at night and to regain her strength so that she could 'function better as a mother' during the day. She did not want to talk about the abuse, nor go into any in-depth analysis of her past. The first six therapy sessions were built on functional exercises, aimed at finding ways to become tired at night without medication. For this purpose, the therapist chose an environment that was natural to the client and went for outdoor walks with her. On these walks, the therapist taught the client some imagination techniques such as having a large lockable container in which she could put any negative thoughts, and hiding this container outside of the house in a place nobody else can get to, thus being able to return home alleviated of troublesome thoughts. Furthermore, the therapist started a nocturnal running programme with her, which was joined by her children, so that Mrs S. reached a neurophysiologically normal state of tiredness. In the therapy room, active imaginative exercises with props (fabrics, furniture, balls, etc.) were offered to strengthen her ability to create her own space, and to fill this space with positive thoughts and ideas.

The training of the body, the strengthening of imaginative, positive resources and the improved sleep at night encouraged Mrs S. to join a local sports club, which led to social contacts and to a heightened interest in her physical appearance. After ten weeks, she started to dress more colourfully, and voiced an interest in finding out more about how she could have contact to others without having her boundaries trespassed. The issue of boundaries was explored for five weeks on a sensory level by feeling and sensing the body boundaries in contact with the material world, and in contact with space and people within it. This led to a more intrapsychic awareness of how the body and ensuing reactions signal (past) experiences. In the following six sessions, the emphasis was on learning to say 'No' and to listen to body signals. By focusing on Shaping, and by offering exercises that combined Effort and Shaping elements, Mrs S. was able to move more freely and to voice her needs and wishes more clearly. After 25 sessions, free of medication, and with a positive outlook on life, the therapist and Mrs S. agreed to gradually end therapy.

DISCUSSION

The findings presented have to be understood as resulting from a complex research context in which Dance Movement Therapy is at the core. As the treatment was offered in an out-patient service, it was open not only for people with clinically relevant post-traumatic stress disorders but also for clients with subclinically relevant syndromes that, so far, have been the focus of only few clinically oriented studies. Thus, the setting also had a preventive character. Although many clients were in medical treatment, their difficulties and symptoms persisted as they were not seen as resulting from traumatic experiences. It can be assumed that the particular concept of the project helped greatly in addressing and supporting people who had experienced violence but had never dared to ask for help on this issue.

Seen from a post-project view, it is not justifiable to include only women, children, and adolescents in a support program. *For one*, from the 1204 total contacts[14] that were registered at the centre, about a fifth was made by men who had experienced diverse forms of domestic violence themselves, and who did not know where to go for support. This relatively high figure is surprising as men were not included in the project. *For two*, the psychotherapeutic work of Dance Movement Therapy pointed to the complex dynamics of adult partnerships and the difficulty to dichotomize between 'victim' and 'perpetrator'. If men seek help it should be offered to them, too.

The results of those clients that underwent therapy support the hypothesis that Dance Movement Therapy is very effective for the treatment of people traumatized by the experience of domestic violence. Due to the small sample, however, it is not possible to make general statements. In addition, as the movement analysis was only done by the therapist and not by external, independent raters, the results of this aspect cannot be seen as valid or reliable quantitative data but as qualitative case studies from a subjectively constructed view.

The particular attraction of Dance Movement Therapy is the merging of two levels: that of the body and that of the mind. By doing so, this approach can integrate the very aspects that all trauma theories have emphasized so far: the fragmentation of declarative/explicit and procedural/implicit memory processes after a traumatic incident. This

---

[14] This includes all types of professional and client contact, such as by telephone, or in person

does not mean that the memory of a traumatic incident needs to be exposed and worked through explicitly. Rather, it is a matter of helping the client become aware of the trauma-inherent fragmentation of body sensations and cognitions, and to find ways of non-threatening integration.

Besides working through aspects such as social isolation, boundaries, diffuse fears, anger and grief, partnership conflicts and the development of positive life visions (which can be done by other psychotherapies, too), it is particularly the psychosomatic syndromes and the fragmentation of body awareness and body image that Dance Movement Therapy can treat successfully.

In almost all cases, it was important to begin work with a slow, careful, not primarily dance-oriented approach. At the beginning of therapy, the majority of the clients in this project were not able to use the creative offers of either an experimental or a structured dance. As can be seen in the movement analysis section, most clients showed a lack of growing on all axes. The constant shrinking indicates extreme conditions of fear and insecurity. The women who had experienced violence usually viewed their bodies as 'non-existant', as lacking emotions or they rejected their bodies or parts of them and blamed them as 'the cause of all evil'. Therefore, as can be seen in the case vignette, the treatment process was focused on the client

- to become aware of the functional aspects of the body or body parts and to accept them and/or
- to become aware of her own movements and how these may be related to thoughts and feelings and/or
- in the course of therapy, to let the body express itself in improvised movements, thus finding a balance between the 'spoken' word and the 'moved' word and/or
- to express verbal and creative elements of the therapeutic process in movement with the aim to integrate and accept the emotional aspects of experiencing.

The therapeutic approach in this project was focused on letting the clients determine how they wanted to use their bodies and movements in the context of their themes. An important therapeutic intervention was the strengthening of the client's awareness of her bodily sensations and reactions. This awareness made it possible for the women to gradually move and expand in the three-dimensional space with more self-confidence than they had before.

To conclude, Dance Movement Therapy with its body-mind approach can positively influence the specific symptoms of abuse because the body is the central factor in the memorizing of traumatic incidents. To substantiate according findings, a larger sample and independent raters for the movement analysis are essential. Furthermore, the question of which methodological elements of this approach may be more or less helpful for traumatized clients should be discussed within Dance Movement Therapy. The main focus of the treatment should be stabilization, and thus the strengthening of ego-functions, not the working through of traumatic memories. By offering traumatized clients the possibility of re-inhabiting their bodies, and of respecting their unique embodiment of experiences, fragmentation can gradually be diminished.

REFERENCES

Abrahams, C. (1994). *The Hidden Victims: Children and Domestic Violence*. London: NCH.
Bartenieff, I., & Lewis, D. (1980). *Body Movement: Coping with the Environment*. New York: Gordon and Breach.

Beck, A. (1995). *Beck-Depressions-Inventar: (BDI) Testhandbuch.* Göttingen: Huber.

Bundesministerium für Familie, Senioren, Frauen und Jugend (BMFSFJ) (2004a). Lebenssituation, Sicherheit und Gesundheit von Frauen in Deutschland. Eine repräsentative Untersuchung zu Gewalt gegen Frauen in Deutschland. Zusammenfassung zentraler Studienergebnisse. In Bundesministerium für Familie, Senioren, Frauen und Jugend (Eds.). *Broschüre zur Lebenssituation, Sicherheit und Gesundheit von Frauen in Deutschland.* Berlin: BMFSFJ.

Bundesministerium für Familie, Senioren, Frauen und Jugend (BMFSFJ) (2004b). Gewalt gegen Männer. Personale Gewaltwiderfahrnisse von Männern in Deutschland -- Ergebnisse der Pilotstudie. In Bundesministerium für Familie, Senioren, Frauen und Jugend (Eds.). *Broschüre zu Gewalt gegen Männer.* Berlin: BMFSFJ.

Child and Woman Abuse Studies Unit (CWASU) (2005). *Statistics & Information. Domestic Violence.* Retrieved March 24, 2005, from http://www.cwasu.org.

Damasio, A. (1997). *Descartes Irrtum. Fühlen, Denken und das menschliche Gehirn.* München: dtv.

Franke, G.H (1995). *SCL-90-R. Die Symptom-Checkliste von Derogatis -- Deutsche Version.* Göttingen: Beltz Test GmbH.

Hagemann-White, C. (1998). Violence without end? Some reflections on achievements, contradictions, and perspectives of the feminist movement in Germany. In R. Klein (Ed.). *Multidisciplinary Perspectives on Family Violence* (pp. 176-191). London: Routledge.

Kavemann, B. (2002). *Kinder und häusliche Gewalt -- Kinder misshandelter Mütter.* Retrieved March 24, 2005, from http://www.wibig.uni-osnabrueck.de.

Kestenberg-Amighi, J., Loman, S., Lewis, P., & Sossin, M. (1999). *The Meaning of Movement. Developmental and Clinical Perspectives of the Kestenberg Movement Profile.* Amsterdam: Gordon and Breach.

Lamb, W., & Watson, E. (1979). *Body Code: The Meaning in Movement.* London: Routledge and Kegan Paul.

Löbmann, R., Herbers, K., & Schacht, G. (2004). *Vorläufige Ergebnisse der Evaluation der Beratungs- und Interventionsstellen (BISS) für Opfer häuslicher Gewalt.* Hannover: KFN.

Mirrlees-Black, C. (1999). *Domestic Violence: Findings from a new British Crime Survey self-completion questionnaire.* Home Office Research Study, 191.

Nds. Ministerium für Soziales, Frauen, Familie und Gesundheit (2002). *Die wichtigsten Fakten zum Thema Häusliche Gewalt auf einen Blick.* Retrieved January 27, 2002, from http://www.ms.niedersachsen.de

Ogden, P., & Minton, K. (2000). *Sensorimotor Psychotherapy: One Method for Processing Traumatic Memory. Traumatology,* VI(3), 3.

Sachsse, U. (Ed.). (2004). *Traumazentrierte Psychotherapie. Klinik, Theorie, Praxis.* Stuttgart: Schattauer.

Saltzman, L. (2004). Definitional and Methodological Issues Related to Transnational Research on Intimate Partner Violence. *Violence against Women, 10,* 812-830.

Stephens, N., & McDonald, R. (2000). Assessment of women who seek shelter from abusing partners. In J. Vincent & N. Jouriles (Eds.). *Domestic Violence: Guidelines for Research-Informed Practice.* Gateshead: Athenaeum Press.

Sykes Wylie, M. (2004). The Limits of Talk: Bessel van der Kolk wants to transform the treatment of trauma. *Psychotherapy Networker, 28(1),* 30-41.

Taket, A. (2004). *Tackling Domestic Violence: the role of health professionals.* Home Office Development and Practice Report, 32, 26-32.

Van der Kolk, B. (1994). The body keeps the score: Memory and the emerging psychobiology of post traumatic stress. *Harvard Review of Psychiatry, 1,* 253-265.

Van der Kolk, B., McFarlane, A., & Weisaeth, L. (1996). *Traumatic Stress. The Effects of Overwhelming Experience on Mind, Body, and Society.* New York: The Guilford Press.

Walby, S. (2004). *The Cost of Domestic Violence.* London: Department of Trade and Industry Women and Equality Unit.

Williamson, E. (2000). *Domestic Violence and Health. The response of the medical profession.* Bristol: The Policy Press, University of Bristol.

GENDER AND LEADERSHIP AT WORK: USE OF RHYTHMS AND MOVEMENT QUALITIES IN TEAM COMMUNICATION

Sabine C. Koch[15]

This chapter examines differences in movement qualities between men and women, leaders and members in organizational groups at the workplace. Sixteen work groups were observed during their routine team meetings (n=71). In the context of investigated movement-related communicative behaviour, movement qualities were assessed with the Kestenberg Movement Profile, yielding rhythms data for team leaders, and pre-effort and effort data for all participants. Results suggest gender differences in the use of tension-flow qualities of leaders only: Female team-leaders used significantly more jumping rhythms (og), and significantly more indirect efforts than male leaders. These qualities in combination with other results of the project indicate more assertion, goal-direction, and more nonverbal consideration of the entire group from the part of female leaders. Male leaders used significantly more running-drifting rhythms (u; including movement pauses) and more mixed fighting rhythms, indicating lower expressiveness, and a higher potential for aggressiveness. In the entire sample, women showed higher expressiveness than men (they moved more overall). Some findings not in accordance with the predictions from KMP-theory, such as higher use of fighting qualities in women, were explained with gender-related double standards theories. Inter-rater-reliabilities of rhythms coders on an entire profile were good. Agreement of effort-coders was not satisfying for experts, while it was satisfying for experts compared to a lay coder.

Keywords: Movement analysis, gender, leadership, groups, Kestenberg Movement Profile, rater reliability.

INTRODUCTION

Men and Women at Work: Do their Movement Qualities Differ?

This study investigated gender differences in use of movement qualities in team communication at the workplace. It was part of a national research project[1] (Koch, Kubat, Kruse, & Thimm, 2001) that assessed a wide variety of verbal and nonverbal variables in order to examine gender differences and gender-construction in communication patterns of work groups. This project used methods from language, social psychology, linguistics, and movement analysis. Interaction processes in face-to-face communication, many of which operate under the threshold of conscious awareness, may contribute to the fact that there still is no gender equality in parts of professional life. Theory and empirical research point to power and support-related processes as playing an especially important role within the communicative construction of gender. In this study, we analyzed differences in movement qualities of team leaders and team members in interaction sequences containing power- and support-related behaviors. We tested differences in movement behavior of men and women in leading positions with the Kestenberg Movement Profile (KMP); (Kestenberg, 1975; Kestenberg & Sossin, 1979; Kestenberg-Amighi, Loman, Lewis, & Sossin, 1999), specifically rhythms, efforts, and pre-efforts; difference in use of efforts and pre-efforts of all participants; and interrater-reliabilities of the main coders for rhythms and pre-/effort coding.

Key research questions were: How does the communication of men and women in face-to-face team meetings in different work contexts differ (e.g., in same-sex teams vs. mixed-sex teams, under male and female boss, in male-dominated vs. female dominated

---

[15] Thanks to Stefanie M. Müller for help with data analysis and organizing results. Thanks to I. Bräuninger, I. Cleff-Häusler, B. Drexlmaier, U. Lang, and C. Petermann for ratings of the material.

teams, in token teams, under changing leadership, etc.)? How is the verbal and nonverbal actual behavior related to beliefs about gendered communication (construction aspect)? First results indicated that there were more gender differences in nonverbal than verbal displays, particularly, there were pronounced differences in affect display (Koch, 2005) and gaze behavior (Koch, Baehne, Kruse, & Zumbach, in prep). Specifically, the observed nonverbal differences were:

a. Affect: We observed *Evaluative Affect Display* (EAD); (Koch, 2005), i.e., nonverbal expressions of agreement or disagreement that signal support or non-support of a current speaker. EAD is conceptualized as the expressive component of an attitude. Research findings support the idea that in many cases attitudes are communicated nonverbally, particularly if they are negative and the target of evaluation has a higher status position than the actor, i.e. the signaling person (Mehrabian, 1971). Evaluative affect is an important source of communicating attitudes and support in face-to-face interaction (Koch, 2005). It is mostly communicated non-deliberately. In our study, female leaders received more positive and negative affect displays by team members. I.e., female leaders were evaluated more often on the non-verbal level. In addition, female (and female-dominated) teams were more expressive overall.

b. Gaze: *Gaze* is the most important signal of nonverbal dominance, particularly when related to talking mode (Dovidio & Ellyson, 1985). It has an important function in the regulation of social interaction as a correlate of dominance- and influence-related behavior (e.g., Schmid-Mast, 2000). Dovidio and Ellyson (1985) operationalize the influence of person A in a dyad as the ratio of the time A talks and looks at B (looks while talks); (lwt) and the time, in which A listens and looks at B (looks while listens); (lwl). This value is called the *Visual Dominance Ratio* (VDR). The higher the VDR of person A in relation to person B, the greater is the influence of person A over person B. Persons with relatively little power or status display a longer gaze duration while listening to their partner compared to their gaze duration while talking, whereas more powerful persons look approximately for the same amount of time both while listening and while talking. Overall, less powerful persons look longer at more powerful persons especially while in the role of the listener (Dovidio & Ellyson, 1985). In our study (Koch, Baehne, Kruse, & Zumbach, in prep.), the visual dominance ratio as a measure of influence in teams was highest for female team leaders, followed by male leaders, then by male members and female members. I.e., status had a more important effect on dominance-related gaze behavior than gender. A balanced gaze distribution in teams, however, was higher in women. Men tended to distribute their gaze among only a few team members and ignore others. Women distributed their gaze more equal among all team members. Gender had a more important effect on support-related gaze distribution than status.

c. Movement qualities: The measures for gaze and affect, however, capture merely quantitative information. In order to assess information about movement qualities of participants we used the Kestenberg Movement Profile (KMP) as a theoretical and methodological device (Kestenberg & Sossin, 1979; Kestenberg-Amighi, et al., 1999). The surplus value of the KMP was that in addition to the "What" of the interaction it also captures the "How". The Kestenberg Movement Profile (KMP) is a well developed movement analysis method and theory that was introduced 40 years ago by Dr. Judith Kestenberg, a psychoanalyst from Poland, trained in Vienna, who later emigrated to the US East Coast (Kestenberg, 1975; Kestenberg-Amighi, Loman, Lewis, & Sossin, 1999). It is widely used in assessment and intervention planning in dance/movement therapy. With its high degree of differentiation of movement parameters it lends itself to research in expressive therapies and body therapies. Further work on gender and movement quality has been carried out by Lamb (1992).

Gendered Professional Behavior

Results from an interview study by our research group (Koch, Kubat, Kruse, & Thimm, 2001) indicated that:

- professional women often felt the need to assert themselves more ("you have to be twice as tough as a man to get equally acknowledged"),
- men rated themselves as being more aggressive in communication ("I will yell at others and attack them"), and
- for both, men and women the most important thing on the job was to be viewed as professionally competent.

In accordance with these research results we expected that in our sample

(a) women leaders would feel the need to assert themselves more than men leaders and would therefore use more (pure) fighting rhythms overall (Kestenberg-Amighi et al. 1999), as *fighting rhythms* promote separation, assertion and analytic mode

(b) men would display more aggressiveness and would therefore use more mixed-fighting rhythms (Kestenberg-Amighi et al, 1999), as *mixed fighting rhythms* indicate heightened readiness for aggression and are often an alarm signal in patients behavior,

(c) men would use more direct and women more indirect efforts (Kestenberg-Amighi et al., 1999; and in accordance with the results on gaze behavior), as *direct* indicates dyadic focus, *indirect* indicates multi-focus, and

(d) women would use more fighting efforts than men, because they would feel the need to assert themselves more and in order to be viewed as professionally competent.

Further differences would be assessed in an exploratory analysis.

These expectations are counterintuitive to Kestenberg's original assumption that men generally will use more fighting and women more indulgent efforts. In Western societies, men hold more commonly agentic roles (e.g., bread-winner; successful professional, competitor) and women more communal roles (e.g., child rearing, caring for the larger community, communicative tasks) making them more inclined to the according use of movement qualities. Here, however, it is hypothesized that women in their role as professionals and particularly in leadership roles will tend to overcompensate this traditional inclination by displaying even more fighting movement qualities than men. The following hypotheses resulted:

H1: Women leaders (Frauen) will use more (pure) fighting rhythms than men leaders (higher display of assertiveness in women leaders)

H2: Men leaders (Männer) will use more mixed fighting rhythms than women leaders (higher aggressiveness in men leaders)

H3: Men will use more direct and women more indirect efforts in team communication (dyadic focus in men vs. multi-focus in women)

H4: Overall, women will use more fighting efforts than men (higher display of assertiveness in women).

METHOD

Participants and Materials

Our sample consisted of 71 sub-clinical participants with age ranging from 20-59 years (30 men, mean age 39.1, and 41 women mean age 36.3; total mean age 37.7 years). Participants were recruited from 16 teams in industry, public administration and training sectors. The sample consisted of 16 team leaders (8 men and 8 women) and 55 team members (22 men and 33 women) who formed part of nine mixed-sex and seven same-sex teams as follows: five mixed-sex teams with a male leader, four mixed-sex teams with a female leader, four all-women teams, and three all men teams.

Teams were videotaped during their routine team meetings. For the main analyses we then selected scenes of about 15 minutes duration using the following criteria: (a) good general visibility and audibility, (b) the typicality of the interaction for the meeting (no exceptional situations), and (c) the involvement of as many team members as possible. In total, 4 1/2 hours of the almost 15 hours of team material were selected for coding.

Observational Method and Procedure

We coded movement qualities with the Kestenberg Movement Profile (KMP; Kestenberg & Sossin, 1979; Kestenberg-Amighi et al., 1999). The KMP is a movement analysis tool with a high degree of differentiation in the assessment of nonverbal behavior. It takes into account more than 72 motion parameters, in 9 diagrams, each of which provides a different perspective in a psychological domain or meaning area ("linking movement and psychodynamics", Kestenberg & Sossin, 1979). For our analyses we used 3 quality-related out of 9 diagrams: rhythms, efforts, and pre-efforts.

Diagrams: *Tension-flow rhythms* are mostly unconscious repetitive movements that indicate certain present needs of a person. They are manners of alternation between relative degrees of free and bound flow reflecting unconscious needs. They are related to the tension a person holds in the body. They are actually constituted of the tension flow or fluctuations in muscle tension that are ever-present in animate functioning. Rhythms are notated via kinesthetic attunement continuously as a curve of these fluctuations around a base-level (neutral line). The higher the intensity of a movement, the higher the amplitudes on the curve or the frequency of reversals of the time line. There are ten recognizable pure rhythms that correspond to developmental psychosexual phases, following Anna Freud (1965), elaborated upon by Kestenberg (1975) and Kestenberg & Sossin (1979). These phases are: oral sucking (O), oral biting/ snapping (OS), anal twisting (A), anal straining (AS), urethral running-drifting (U), urethral starting-stopping (US), inner-genital swaying (IG), inner-genital birthing/surging (IGS), outer-genital jumping (OG) and outer-genital spurting/ramming (OGS). All phases are composed of an indulgent part (for enmeshing oneself into the movement quality) followed by a fighting part (for separation). The fighting part of the rhythms carries the abbreviation S for "sadistic", which was taken from the originally used Freudian terminology. The original language was anchored in psychoanalytic developmental theory, differentiating libidinal from sadistic drives (and sub-stages). Kestenberg-Amighi et al. (1999) no longer employ the terminology of the psycho-sexual phases but alternative descriptors that are less related to drive theory. Instead they use the functional expressions of the rhythms (sucking, biting/snapping, twisting, straining, etc.). Abbreviations remain the same.

FIGURE 1: RHYTHMS NOTATION OF A TEAM LEADER (EXTRACT)

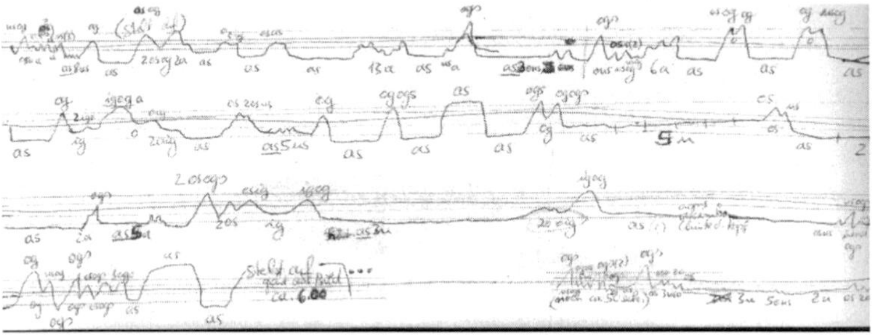

Note: interruption last line: actor left and re-entered room.

The prototypical movements are connected to physical locations prevalent in each developmental phase. In this study we only computed pure rhythms with the exception of mixed fighting rhythms (as one hypothesis related specifically to those). For an example of a rhythms notation see Figure 1.

Efforts are full movement qualities that indicate mastery of the environment in the dimensions of space, weight and time. The effort profile falls into the observational categories of *direct* use of space vs. *indirect* use of space, *strong* use of weight vs. *light* use of weight, *accelerated/quick* use of time vs. *decelerated/sustained* use of time (Kestenberg & Sossin, 1979; Laban, 1960). *Pre-efforts* are a pre-stage of efforts and signify attempts to cope with the physical environment by controlling tension. They mediate between the more inwardly focused tension flow attributes and the outward oriented efforts and are modes of adaptation, learning, and defense mechanisms (Loman, 1995). Pre-efforts indicate heightened self-consciousness such as in defense mechanisms, insecurity, learning, or problems with the environment. The sub-dimensions provide information about learning styles and ego-defenses. The pre-effort profile falls into the observational categories of *channeling* use of space vs. *flexible* use of space, *vehement/ straining* use of weight vs. *gentle* use of weight, *sudden* use of time vs. *hesitant* use of time (Loman, 1995). For both efforts and pre-efforts we also computed the total fighting qualities and the total indulgent qualities used. Raters coded all 12 sub-categories (six efforts and six pre-efforts).

Reliability: (a) Rhythms were coded for team leaders (n=16) by one main rater. An additional rater coded parts of the material for computations of inter-rater-reliability; both coded two entire profiles on a male and a female team leader; n=2).

(b) Efforts and pre-effort were coded for all participants (n=71) by two expert raters and one additional lay-rater. According to low reliability between the experts, we only included the values of the expert who agreed highly with the lay-rater.

Rater reliability for rhythms was very good (*r*=.83; *std. alpha*=.91; ICC, Ebel, 1951). For efforts and pre-efforts reliabilities were not satisfactory (*Kappa* <.45). However, rater 1 corresponded high to a lay rater, who coded the material in addition, with no training background in Laban Movement Analysis and merely a two hour introduction to effort-rating (*Kappa* >.70). We, therefore, decided to use only the ratings of rater 1 and not of rater 2 for computations of efforts/pre-efforts.

RESULTS

Results suggest differences in the use of tension-flow rhythms between male and female team leaders: women used significantly (statistics below) more OG (jumping), men more U (running-drifting; including pauses). Female team-leaders ($n=8$) used significantly more indirect efforts than men. Among team members ($n=71$) we found no significant gender differences. Additionally, women moved more overall than men (higher expressiveness: mastery-related but also defence-related).

The analysis of tension-flow rhythms of team leaders moderating a team session showed that participants used 5196 rhythms with 6909 elements overall. 2361 of them were indulgent and 1198 were fighting rhythms. It was hypothesized that female leaders (Frauen) will use more (pure) fighting rhythms than male leaders (higher display of assertiveness; H1); and that male leaders (Männer) will use more mixed fighting rhythms than female leaders (higher aggressiveness; H2). The author found that female leaders did not use significantly more fighting rhythms than male leaders ($M_F=1247$, $M_M=1114$ for indulgent and $M_F=651$, $M_M=547$ for fighting rhythms; H1 was rejected). However, male leaders used more mixed fighting rhythms. Of 52 mixed fighting rhythms 46 stemmed from men and 6 from women. However, the results (Kruskal-Wallis ANOVA $p<.05$, $eta^2=.24$) for H2 were only significant before the necessary Bonferroni-correction.

FIGURE 2: DIFFERENCES IN USE OF PURE RHYTHMS OF MALE AND FEMALE LEADERS

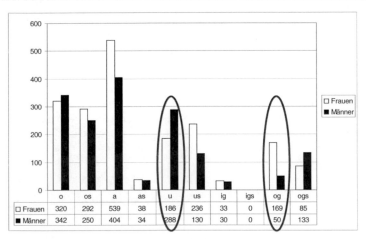

	o	os	a	as	u	us	ig	igs	og	ogs
☐ Frauen	320	292	539	38	186	236	33	0	169	85
■ Männer	342	250	404	34	288	130	30	0	50	133

The explorative analysis of gender differences in rhythms was also computed with a Kruskal-Wallis ANOVA. Female leaders used significantly more jumping (OG; $p<.05$, $eta^2=.56$) and that male leaders use more running-drifting (U; $p<.05$, $eta^2=.21$; see Fig.2). The rhythm is characterized by high intensity and abrupt changes with round reversals (in terms of tension-flow attributes). Male leaders do use more movement pauses and "drift" more (indulging in time) than female leaders. There is also ease and continuity of movement to this rhythm. In terms of tension-flow attributes, the running-drifting (or aimless running rhythm; u) is characterized by low intensity and very gradual drifts into either more bound or more free flow.

Analysis of Efforts and Preefforts of All Participants

We had hypothesized that men will use more direct and women more indirect efforts in team communication (dyadic focus vs. multi-focus; H3); and that women will use more fighting efforts than men (particularly in the leader condition; H4).

FIGURE 3: GENDER DIFFERENCES IN SPACE-RELATED EFFORTS

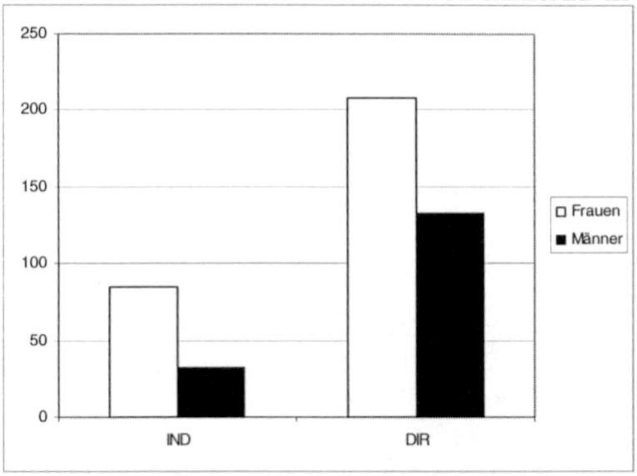

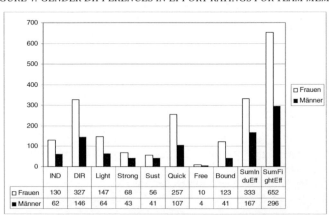

We found that women ($n=33$) used significantly more indirect efforts ($p<.05$, $eta^2=.29$; see Figure 3). Men did not use more direct efforts. That is, H3 was confirmed for women, but not for men. In the total sample, women used more fighting efforts than men ($M_F=1040$; $M_M=586$; $p<.05$, $eta^2=.13$; H4), however, this effect was only significant before the necessary Bonferroni-correction. A Kruskal-Wallis ANOVA showed only one significant difference between male and female team leaders: women used significantly more indirect efforts. This finding corresponds to the observation that in gaze behavior, women were more multi-focused, and men were more dyadically oriented. None of the specific effects for efforts or pre-efforts of team members was significant Bound reached exactly significance: $p=.05$, $eta^2=.11$ (see Fig. 4); women used more bound. The frequency analyses of efforts and pre-efforts revealed that women moved more overall (see Fig. 4 and 5). In unipolar shape-flow, coded only by lay raters, women used both more approach ($p<.05$, $eta^2=.13$) and more avoidance behavior ($p<.05$, $eta^2=.16$).

FIGURE 4: GENDER DIFFERENCES IN EFFORT RATINGS FOR TEAM MEMBERS

	IND	DIR	Light	Strong	Sust	Quick	Free	Bound	SumIn duEff	SumFi ghtEff
☐ Frauen	130	327	147	68	56	257	10	123	333	652
■ Männer	62	146	64	43	41	107	4	41	167	296

FIGURE 5: GENDER DIFFERENCES IN PRE-EFFORT RATINGS FOR TEAM MEMBERS

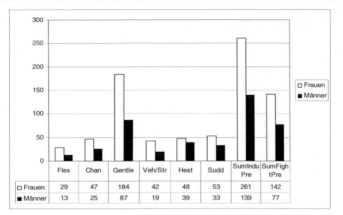

	Flex	Chan	Gentle	Veh/Str	Hest	Sudd	SumIndu Pre	SumFight Pre
Frauen	29	47	184	42	48	53	261	142
Männer	13	25	87	19	39	33	139	77

The Kestenberg Movement Profile (KMP) is one of the field's most advanced instruments for diagnostics and treatment planning in dance/movement therapy. Yet, reliability studies are rare. The few researchers reporting reliabilities are Birklein (2005), Birner (2004), Burt (1995), Koch (1999), McCoubry (1987), and Sossin (1987). Most of them find acceptable values (Koch, 1999, for an overview). Other improvement the KMP needs is normative data, standardization, and economization. Studies on a more economic coding method are presently conducted by Bräuninger. Mannheim works on aspects of standardized use, Sossin on normation and standardization. Lotan & Zipperman (1996) have contributed useful software as a shortcut for the calculations and the plotting. Next, reliability related results of the present study are reported.

Reliability

In this study reliability was assessed for two subsets of the data: (a) Rhythm-coders: On an entire profile for one female leader and one male leader and (b) Effort-coders: for 16 team leaders (8 men, 8 women). We computed Intra-class-correlations (ICC; Ebel, 1951) for all data and additionally Cohen's Kappas (Cohen, 1960) for the effort codings.

TABLE I: RHYTHMS CODERS: INTER-RATER-RALIABILITY OF THE TWO CODERS ON TWO ENTIRE PROFILES (MEANS)

Intraclass correlations for two main coders			
Profile	r	Std. Alpha	Agreement[a]
Rhythms	.83	.91	Very good
Attributes	.63	.77	Good
Pre-efforts	Neg. value	Neg. value	Cannot be
Efforts	Neg. value	Neg. value	computed due to
Bipolar	Neg. value	Neg. value	neg. values
Unipolar	.68	.81	Good
Directions	.76	.86	Good
Planes	.62	.77	Good
Total	.70	.82	Good

Note: n=2; p-values all < .001; [a]classification following Ebel, 1951, and Landis & Koch, 1977.

Rhythms-Codings: The two main coders of the rhythms analysis did two complete KMPs (all 9 diagrams) each (for the female leader of team C and the male leader of team G. We used intra-class correlations (ICC) and determined interrater-reliability on basis of the *frequencies of the time-corrected raw data*. We were able to compute reliability for five out of eight profiles, in the remaining four cases negative statistics resulted. Overall, reliability of the two raters was good. Particularly, their reliability on rhythms was very good with a standardized alpha of .91. Results are encouraging for the use of the KMP in research, diagnosis, and intervention (compare Table I). They could, however, also be due to target characteristics ($n=2$), i.e., the particular idiosyncratic patterns of the two leaders observed here.

TABLE II: EFFORT-CODERS: ICC BETWEEN EXPERT 1, EXPERT 2, AND LAY-RATERS FOR EFFORTS AND PRE-EFFORTS OF LEADERS

	Effort E1:E2	E1:L	E2:L			Preeff E1:E2		
	r	r	r	std alpha	Relia-bility	r	std apha	Relia-bility
Chef A	.60	.97	.68	.90	very good	.56	.72	Good
Chef B	.84	.85	.79	.93	very good	.16	.28	poor
Chefin C	.05	.74	.45	.68	satisf.	.38	.55	satisf.
Chef D	.23	.86	.41	.75	good	.38	.55	satisf.
Chef F/G			.69	.82	good	.	.	
Chef J	.77	.90	.87	.94	very good	.58	.74	good
Chef K/L			.14	.25	Poor	.	.	
Chefin M	.03	.46	.58	.62	satisf.	.79	.88	good
Chefin N	.29	.75	.65	.79	good	.29	.45	accept.
Chefin O	neg.	.69	.39	.56	satisf.	.49	.66	satisf.
Chefin P/Q	neg.			neg.	(poor)	.22	.37	poor
Chefin R	neg.			neg.	(poor)	.08	.15	poor
Chefin S	.38	.55	.75	.79	good	.40	.57	satisf.
Chef T1	.02	.42	.35	.52	satisf.	.23	.37	poor
Chefin X	.03	.72	.52	.69	satisf.	.74	.85	good
Chef Y	.31	.72	.65	.79	good	.83	.90	very good
Mean	*.32*	*.72*	*.57*	*.72*	sat. to good	*.44*	*.57*	*satisf.*
	poor	good	sat.	good		poor	sat.	

Note: N=71;E= Expert rater, L=Lay Rater; neg.= negative value resulted; [a]classification following Ebel (1951), and Landis & Koch (1977).

Effort-codings: The reliability analysis of effort codings gained particular importance, because of the missing data for pre-efforts, and efforts from the rhythms coders due to the resulting negative values. The two main coders of the effort analyses (one was also a rhythms-coder, all coders were female) showed an unsatisfying observer agreement in the one-on-one comparison of the raw data *across four teams* (with 72.7% and *Cohen's Kappa*=.14; Kappa was extremely low, partially due to asymmetrical margin sums, however, p was significant). The agreement on observed non-events was computed post hoc on the basis of the mean frequencies of the efforts. On average, we found one effort per 15 seconds.

Using ICC on a frequency basis for the leaders of all teams (8m, 8f) and additionally including lay-ratings of a female observer for efforts, results differed not much. Reliability of the two experts was not satisfying r_{Pre}=.32/r_{Eff}=.44 (possibly due to raters' heterogeneous training background), whereas reliability of Expert 1 and the lay-rater was good r=.72, and between Expert 2 and the lay-rater satisfying, r=.57; see Table II). Low values of effort-coders were probably partially due to a lack of criteria to determine the threshold between pre-efforts and efforts and the lack of models to compute partial reliabilities (Birklein & Sossin, this volume). All other categories were at least acceptable in terms of reliability. Generally, the KMP proved useful as a device for the assessment of gender differences in organizational group interaction.

SUMMARY AND DISCUSSION

Results suggest that similarities in movement qualities between men and women at work were bigger than differences. Some tension-flow rhythms were used with different frequencies by male and female *team leaders*. Female leaders used significantly more jumping (OG) which is an outer-genital rhythm (formerly called "phallic"). That is, female leaders used more of the "male" jumping rhythm than male leaders. They potentially wanted to demonstrate their "male" qualities, which in Western societies are often set equal to leadership qualities. Or, it may be especially those women with "male" movement qualities who reach leadership positions. Male leaders used more running-drifting (U), and more mixed fighting, that is, they made more movement pauses (u) and showed a higher potential for aggressiveness (mF). Women moved more overall than men. They showed a higher overall expressiveness, particularly in all-women teams. They expressed more mastery-related (efforts) but also more learning- and defense-related motions (pre-efforts). Women leading a team furthermore used more indirect efforts than men. Among *team members* we found no significant gender differences, yet, in the *total sample* women used fighting efforts significantly more than men. This effect points to the assumed overcompensation of professional women trying to be "particularly male". In the light of recent findings from gender research (e.g., Eagly & Karau, 2002) this strategy is dysfunctional, because it counteracts prescriptive role behavior: Gender researchers recommend that leading women mix agentic with communal behavior in order to be optimally accepted in their professional role (Eagly & Karau, 2002).

Interrater-reliabilities of rhythms-coders on two entire profiles were good. Agreement of effort-coders was not satisfactory. We attributed this lower Kappa to the higher number of categories used (12 instead of 10) and to the heterogeneous KMP training background of the two main raters. However, agreement between a lay rater and expert 1 was high (see Table II). We therefore decided to use the data of expert 1 for calculations. Pre-efforts and efforts seem to be the most difficult part to observe correctly. In fact, values below acceptability were merely the reliability of efforts and pre-efforts. This may be a problem of the threshold between the categories of pre-efforts and efforts. If the values for pre-efforts and efforts are aggregated the reliability for the new category rises to a higher alpha value. This finding could indicate that for raters there might be some confusion between efforts and pre-efforts (is it still a pre-effort or yet an effort?). While we agree that, conceptually, it makes a lot of sense to distinguish efforts and pre-efforts, this distinction may go at the expense of reliability. Overall, there are mixed results regarding reliability: some are encouraging, some are disappointing. One research necessity resulting from this study is to assess reliability and validity of the KMP more consequently and systematically. More studies are needed.

The value of the movement analysis for the entire project lies particularly in a closer investigation of the behavioral qualities. Movement analytic results underline many of the findings from corresponding quantitative (analysis of variance: gaze, affect) and qualitative studies (interviews: aggressiveness in men; assertion in female leaders). However, analyses of this study use a limited sample, particularly of leaders (n=16). Results should, therefore, be interpreted with caution. Gender and status related movement qualities need further investigation.

In sum, results in stereotypic direction were: Women were more expressive overall. They displayed more indirect, support-related gaze behavior, whereas men displayed more direct, dyadic gaze behavior and more potential aggressiveness (as measured by frequencies of mixed fighting rhythms). Results in counter-stereotypical direction were: particularly female team leaders showed more influence and dominance-related gaze behavior than men. They used more outer-genital jumping rhythm and tended to use more fighting rhythms. This finding potentially points to the *double standards* still valid for men and women in the working world: particularly women in leading positions seemed to feel the need to defend their status and assert themselves by being "maler than male", for example, by displaying more agency-related behavior than men.

REFERENCES

Birklein, S.B. (2005). *Nonverbal indices of high stress in parent/child interaction.* Doctoral Dissertation. New York: New School University.

Birner, B. (2004). *Reliability analysis of the Kestenberg Movement Profile. A study of novice and expert ratings.* Munich: Unpublished Thesis.

Burt, J.W. (1995). *Body, face, and voice: Nonverbal expressions of emotion in infancy.* Unpublished doctoral dissertation, MCP Hahnemann University, Philadelphia.

Cohen, J. (1960). A coefficient of agreement for nominal scales. *Educational and Psychological Measurement, 20,* 37-46.

Dovidio, J.F., & Ellyson, S.L. (1985). Pattern of visual dominance behaviors in humans. In S.L. Ellyson, & J.F. Dovidio (Eds.). *Power, dominance and nonverbal behavior* (pp. 129-149). New York: Springer.

Eagly, A.H., & Karau, S. (2002). Role congruity theory of prejudice toward female leaders. *Psychological Review, 109,* 573-598.

Ebel, R.L. (1951). Estimation of the reliability of ratings. *Psychometrika, 16,* 407-24.

Kestenberg, J.S. (1975). *Parents and Children.* New York: Jason Aronson.

Kestenberg, J.S., & Sossin, K.M. (1979). *The role of movement patterns in development, Vol. 2.* New York: Dance Notation Bureau Press.

Kestenberg-Amighi, J., Loman, S., Lewis, P., & Sossin, K.M. (1999). *The meaning of movement. Developmental and clinical perspectives of the Kestenberg Movement Profile.* Amsterdam: Gordon and Breach.

Koch, S.C. (2005). Evaluative affect display toward male and female group leaders. A replication and extension. *Small Group Research, 36,* 678-703.

Koch, S.C. (1999). *Reliability of the Kestenberg Movement Profile (KMP). Agreement of Novice Raters.* Stuttgart: Ibidem.

Koch, S.C., Baehne, C.G., Kruse, L., & Zumbach, J. (in prep.). *Visual dominance and visual support. Gender and status differences in task-oriented group.*

Koch, S.C., Kubat, A., Kruse, L., & Thimm, C. (2001). *Einfluß und Unterstützung in der Geschlechter-kommunikation am Arbeitsplatz. Entwicklung eines Kodierschemas und erste Ergebnisse* [Influence and support in gender communication at the workplace. [Coding scheme and first results]. Arbeitsbericht Nr. 2. Heidelberg: Universität Heidelberg. [Online-Document] http://workcomm.uni-hd.de

Laban, R. v. (1960). *The mastery of movement*. London: MacDonald & Evans.

Lamb, W. (1992). Gender and movement. In Loman, S. & Brandt, R. (Eds.), *The body-mind connection in human movement analysis*. Keene: Antioch New England Graduate School.

Landis, J.R., & Koch, G.G. (1977). The measurement of observer agreement for categorical data. *Biometrics, 33,* 159-174.

Loman, S. (1995). *Training Manual for the Kestenberg Movement Profile (revised edition)*. Keene, NH: Antioch New England Graduate School.

Lotan, N. & Yirmiya, N. (2002). Body movement, presence of parents and the process of falling asleep in toddlers. *International Journal of Behavioral Development, 26*(1), 81-88.

Lotan, N., & Zippermann, E. (1996). Lotan, N., & Tziperman, E. (1996). *The Kestenberg Movement Profile analysis program*. Available: http://www.weizmann.ac.il/ESER/People/Eli/KMP/home.html 11/17/04.

McCoubrey, C. (1987). Intersubjectivity vs. objectivity: Implications for effort observation and training. *Movement Studies: A Journal of the Laban/Bartenieff Institute of Movement Studies, 2,* 3-6.

Mehrabian, A. (1971). *Silent messages*. Belmont: Wadsworth.

Schmid-Mast, M. (2000). *Gender differences in dominance hierarchies*. Lengerich: Pabst.

Sossin, K.M. (1987). Reliability of the Kestenberg Movement Profile. *Movement Studies: A Journal of the Laban/Bartenieff Institute of Movement Studies, 2,* 23–28.

NONVERBAL INDICES OF STRESS IN PARENT-CHILD DYADS: IMPLICATIONS FOR INDIVIDUAL AND INTERPERSONAL AFFECT REGULATION AND INTERGENERATION TRANSMISSION

Silvia B. Birklein & K. Mark Sossin

The purpose of the present study is to examine correspondences between specific patterns of parent and child nonverbal behaviors and established indices of parental stress. These specific patterns, specifically tension-flow attributes, and bipolar- and unipolar-shape-flow factors, are derived from an encompassing theory-anchored system of movement notation and profiling called the Kestenberg Movement Profile (KMP; Kestenberg-Amighi, Loman, Lewis, Sossin, 1999). Comprising approximately one-third of the overall KMP, the chosen movement patterns are those most associated with affective experience, bearing conceptual linkage to nonverbal indices of high stress in parent-child interaction. These KMP patterns, conceived initially as potential stress indices, were examined in relationship to standardized life-, event-, parenting-, and overall-stress self-report scales through correlative study. Findings revealed that parents who are stressed are more likely to exhibit deanimated (neutral) abruptness. Children of stressed parents are more likely to show a mismatch between their safety/danger affects and their comfort/discomfort affects (which would otherwise offer structure through affinity). Furthermore, results indicate that when parents are stressed there is evidence for greater discordance between parent and child linking, stress with a decrease in attunement.

Keywords: stress; affect regulation; parent/child interaction; intergenerational transmission; nonverbal behavior/movement analysis.

INTRODUCTION

Nonverbal Patterns as Reflective of Emotional Statements

Nonverbal patterns (e.g. movement, paralanguage) are pivotal in the expression and regulation of an individual's affective and relational experiences. Many stressors, and certainly traumatic experiences, are particularly disruptive to both internal and reciprocally engaged regulatory processes (Fonagy, 2001). A large body of research has linked parental stress to decreased, engagement, playfulness, attunement, and sensitivity (e.g., Crnic, Greenberg, Ragozin, Robinson and Basham, 1983; Pianta & Egeland, 1990). Discussion of intergenerational transmission of stress highlights the idea that there are particular manners in which a parent encodes stress, and corresponding modalities through which a child decodes (and internalizes) stress as well. Can we actually observe such transmission in progress? Do we know which patterns of movement, for instance, communicate quantitative and qualitative aspects of stress? In this study, the authors examine correspondences in body movement indicators of stress in both parent and child, aiming toward the advancement of our knowledge regarding how stress is embodied, and how the adult's embodiment may likely be communicative to the child.

Anchored in Laban and psychoanalytic developmental theory, the Kestenberg Movement Profile (KMP) emerged as a psychologically- and developmentally-relevant means of appraisal, integrated into a systematic organization of codable patterns. Relative frequencies (and loadings) give indications about various psychic functions and their compatibility within an individual and between individuals (Kestenberg-Amighi, Loman, Lewis, & Sossin, 1999; Kestenberg, Marcus, Robbins, Berlowe & Buelte, 1975; Kestenberg & Sossin, 1979). By focusing on concepts such as empathy and mutuality, a basis was laid for the study of parent-child interaction through analysis of KMP movement patterns (Kestenberg & Buelte, 1977; Sossin, 2002).

Parental Emotions and their Transmission

Parental mood and behavioral style clearly influence children's psychosocial adjustment, attachment status, and emotional expression. Positive parental mood in parents is associated with greater positive affect and subjective experiences in children. Negative parental affectivity is associated with less nurturance offered to young children (Belsky, Crnic, & Woodworth, 1995). Regarding parental depression, Lyons-Ruth, Lyubchik, Wolfe, and Bronfman (2002) describe a set of studies that delineate two distinct parent-child interactive patterns. In the "hostile, self-referential pattern" (p. 113), parents are more negative, intrusive, and role-reversing. In the "helpless, fearful pattern" (p. 113), parents show reduced rates of positive structuring behaviors though they are not more negative; each corresponds to different types of disorganized behavior demonstrated by the infant. Similarly, Tronick and Weinberg (1997), calling on the Mutual Regulation Model, demonstrate that maternal depression disrupts the establishment of a dyadic infant-mother system, often forcing the infant into problematic self-regulatory patterns. Employing the concept of 'dyadic states of consciousness,' Tronick and Weinberg also describe how the infant and parent can establish intersubjectivity in such a way that the infant incorporates a state of consciousness that mimics the depressive elements of the mother.

Models have emerged that bear on the transmission of negative emotional states (e.g. emerging from Holocaust trauma) from parent to child (Bauman, 2003; Sagi-Schwartz et al., 2003). Parental stress corresponds to greater disorganized/nontraditional attachment in young children (Lyons-Ruth, Alpern, & Repacholi, 1993). This correspondence did not pertain in a study of parents of toddlers with neurological problems (Barnett, et al., 1999), perhaps, the authors suggest, because of differences in socioeconomic and psychiatric status of the families sampled.

Effects of Stress and Trauma

High stressors involve experiences wherein a significant degree of control has been lost: i.e. contingent expectations have been breached. The special case of trauma pertains to the most severe stressor(s), threatening physical integrity and compromising psychological functioning. Trauma involves the creation of emotional memories. Typically, the more direct exposure to the traumatic event, the greater the emotional effect (March, Amaya-Jackson, & Constanzo, 1997).

However, there is far from a one-to-one correspondence between objective indices of the magnitude of an event and clinical indices of the psychological experience of stress and trauma. Individuals appear to differ in their processing of events, and in their relative vulnerability and/or resilience to potentially traumatic events. Traumatic experience alters the regulation of physiological arousal and attentional processes, and it further compromises the early acquisition of a sense of security in relationships, as well as the attainment of mentalization capacities. Fonagy, Gergely, Jurist, and Target (2002) have integrated developmental research in articulating how an individual's attachment system mediates trauma, such that acquisition and use of the reflective function heightens resilience. Fonagy et al. suggest that by activating templates of early relationship patterns, trauma can be expected to have powerful consequences on the parent-child relationship.

Regulatory Processes in Real-Time

Microanalytic studies require nuanced attention to detail in cataloguing and quantifying nonverbal behaviors (Cohn & Tronick, 1988; Trevarthen, 1993; Stern, 1995), including their complex temporal nature. Multi-level time-series analyses of co-constructed relational behaviors, attempting to identify interactive contingency patterns characteristic of psychological state (e.g. maternal distress) have evolved (Jaffe, Beebe, Feldstein, Crown, & Jasnow, 2001).

Consideration of those nonverbal indicators/signifiers that are to be incorporated into operationalizations of stress-related experiences finds that differentiated gaze, vocal qualities, head orientation, and infant self-touch and mother-touch patterns are reliably notated (Beebe, Lachmann, & Jaffe, 1997) toward the capture of engagement- and regulatory-qualities that are further examined in terms of coordination and contingency patterns. Such qualities are predictive; Beebe et al. report findings linking higher maternal depressive symptoms with lowered infant gaze and vocal-quality self-regulation, as well as lowered maternal self-regulation in gaze, face and self-touch. Interactive analyses include the findings that higher maternal depressive symptoms correspond to greater time looking at the other for both mother and infant, yet dyadically, showing lowered gaze coordination. Moreover, Beebe et al. found that maternal distress corresponded to both heightened and lowered interactive regulation and fairly consistently lowered self-regulation.

While such dyad-framed time-series methodologies have clearly proven rich, the question remains as to whether there are other nonverbal features in parent and infant that correspond to stress and its influence upon the relationship. Clearly, it is posited in KMP theory, rooted as it is in the earlier conceptualizations regarding movement of Rudolf Laban (1966), that such patterns are evident in movement behavior. The KMP catalogues complex intrapsychic and relationally relevant patterns, and describes meaningful correspondences among these patterns. Identification of such stress-related movement behaviors would directly inform developmental and communicative theory building, clinical applications in parent-child therapies, and future interactively framed research.

Hypotheses

The current study was designed to explore relations among affect-related KMP movement patterns in each parent, each child, and each dyad. Measures of parents' stress-levels, gauged by self-report measures of life-stress, event-stress, and parent-stress were also employed. While the thrust of the study was exploratory, it was framed by general hypotheses anticipating positive correlations between stress levels in the parent (as reported on the self-report scales) and movement patterns associated with bound-flow and fighting tension-flow attributes, and with shrinking bi- and unipolar shape-flow patterns. Such correlations would follow directly for the adults, and through transmission processes for the children. It was further hypothesized that high stress would correspond to more intrapersonal mismatching between tension- and shape-flow patterns and to more interpersonal discordance between child and parent patterns across each movement cluster measures of parent's stress-level, gauged by self-report measures of life-stress, event-stress, and parent-stress.

METHOD
KMP Diagrams

In this study, three out of nine KMP clusters were calculated from movement notation: Tension Flow Attributes (TFA), Bipolar Shape Flow (BShF), and Unipolar Shape Flow (UShF). In the KMP literature (Kestenberg-Amighi et al., 1999), these clusters are all related to affect. Specifically, TFA is linked to experiences of safety/danger, and to pleasure/displeasure; BShF is linked to comfort/discomfort experiences, and UShF is linked to approach/avoidance. The TFA's belong to System I in the KMP literature while Bshfl and Ushfl belong to System II in the KMP. System I is thought to express internal dynamics while System II is thought to express more structural aspects of the psyche. Both systems complement each other and in this sense movements in the TFA diagram indicate affect dynamic while Bshfl and Ushfl provide the structure for these dynamics. These clusters were chosen because of their inherent correspondence to stress, i.e. higher stress would correspond to those intrapsychic and interpersonal patterns within each individual indicative of displeasure, discomfort, avoidance, and disharmony.

Tension Flow Attributes

TFAs are mood-regulating mechanisms, and are not themselves affects (Sossin, 2002). They reflect manners of change in the rise and fall of tension (elasticity); these temperament-related mechanisms are differentiated across the dimensions of level (even-adjustment), intensity (high-low), and time (abrupt-gradual). TFAs are a medium for affect expression, specifically of pleasure and displeasure. "Fighting" attributes (affined to bound flow) are differentiated from "indulging" attributes (affined to free flow). TFAs are patterns of ongoing regulation that are evident within a broad range of elasticity: animated flow patterns (more elastic) are differentiated from neutral (more inanimate, less elastic) flow patterns. Attunement in tension-flow in the dyad provides the basis of empathy (Kestenberg & Buelte, 1977).

Bipolar Shape Flow

As manifestations of changes in breathing (kinesic plasticity), bipolar shape-flow refers to symmetrical expansions and contractions in body shape. These are linked to feelings of comfort (growing and exposure) and discomfort (shrinking and reduction of exposure). One's sense of self in the world, alongside feelings of trust, stability and confidence, are served by bipolar shape-flow.

Unipolar Shape Flow

Unipolar shape-flow patterns involve asymmetric expansions and contractions. Such patterns are linked to approach-avoidance. The nature of the stimulus is relevant, as it is more likely one would approach an attractive stimulus and withdraw from a noxious stimulus. Unipolar shape-flow patterns pertain to affective experiences, especially to feelings associated with attraction/repulsion that might be reflective of responsiveness within the dyad. Both bipolar and unipolar shape flow patterns are catalogued across horizontal, vertical, and sagittal dimensions.

Intersystemic Correspondences Between the TFA's and Uni-Polar Shape Flow

Theoretical propositions of the KMP, anchored in Laban's original work (1960), and elaborated by Kestenberg (1975) and others (e.g. Kestenberg-Amighi et.al.1999), suggest that shape-flow patterns give structure to tension-flow patterns. Dynamic affect-elements (expressed in TFAs) can have, or lack, the support structure of relational affect-elements (expressed in BShF and UShF patterns). In prior KMP work (Kestenberg-Amighi, et al, 1999), there has been an overall tendency to link similarity of pattern distribution (between tension and shape flow) to intrapersonal (in the profile of one individual) or interpersonal harmony (comparing two individuals). Work in progress, such as research generating KMP normative data (Sossin, 2002), may alter this expectation. However, in the absence of more specific referential data, (e.g. population-specific norms), it was hypothesized that higher stress would correlate to less intraindividual matching of tension-flow/shape-flow patterns, and to less interpersonal concordance between parent and child across each of the three affect-related KMP clusters.

Matching and Concordance Variables Developed for Analysis

Our investigation led to refinements in methodology (Birklein, 2004). In order to compare the tension flow and shape flow diagrams, we developed new variables that would mathematically operationalize intrapsychic matching/mismatching and interpersonal concordance/discordance between two affined clusters. Rather than comparing frequencies of individual patterns, the newly developed variables *Beta (β)* and *Mu (μ)* compare each polarity (as a total) with each polarity within the shape flow diagram and describe whether the lines are skewed in the same direction, i.e. toward indulgent or fighting. *Beta* and *Mu*, were developed for related but slightly different purposes: Each Beta describes the direction and relative skew of a continuum line (e.g. Beta of TFA (flow adjustment -- even flow) and Beta of Bi-polar (widening-narrowing). Mu compares two Betas of two affined diagrams. When the Betas between two associated diagrams within one person are similarly inclined (i.e. demonstrating a higher correspondence, or affinity), then the associated Mu is lower, indicating what we termed a *matching* condition. In a like manner, when the Betas of two associated diagrams within one person are dissimilarly inclined, then the associated Mu is higher, indicating a *mismatching* condition. The Beta variables also allow comparison (via their associated Mu's) between the same diagrams of two different people. In this case, a balanced condition between parent and child is termed *concordance,* while an imbalanced condition is termed *discordance.* Thus, these variables help to identify relative matching or mismatching between each individual's diagrams, and between children and parents.

Sampling and Procedures

Participants included 26 parent-child dyads (*N*=52), experiencing subclinical stress, from the New York metropolitan area with children ranging in age from 11 to 53 months. Parents were administered three standardized self-report stress scales pertaining to life-, event-, and parenting-stress to assess their stress levels in a non-invasive procedure: The Social Readjustment Rating Scale-Revised (SRRS-R) (Hobson et al. 1998) taps life-stress through categories pertaining to family, income, occupation, and health. The Impact of Event Scale Revised (IES-R) (Weiss & Marmar, 1997) is comprised of subscales pertaining to reactions to stressful events, such as avoidance, intrusion, hyperarousal, and hypervigilance. The Parenting Stress Index-Short Form, 3rd Edition (PSI-SF) (Abidin, 1995) measures perceived stressors that are thought to affect parenting, e.g. "My child is so active, that it exhausts me." In addition, a fourth 1-item

Likert-scale measure, an "Overall Stress Rating" (OSR),[16] was included. As a measure of social support, we used the Multidimensional Scale of Perceived Social Support (MSPSS) (Zimet, Dahlem, Zimet, & Farley, 1988), including categories of family, friends and significant others.

Filming followed procedures recommended for use of the Parent-Child Early Relational Assessment Scale (Clark, 1985). A space was available with a table, specific toys (the same across dyads), and two chairs. Each dyad was filmed for a total of 15 minutes in each of three specific contexts, free play, structured play, and feeding. In the free pay section, the parent was told; "play with your child as you would at home"; in the structured play section the task was to build a tower (using blocks) with the child; in the feeding section, a snack was provided and the parent was instructed to feed the child. The researchers did not require specific seating arrangements or otherwise constrain movement. Movements patterns were notated with regard to the three clusters, discussed above, for both parent and child in each video, then calculated in accordance with KMP procedures (Kestenberg-Amighi et al., 1999), Frequency-derived KMP plot points (see Kestenberg-Amighi et al., 1999 for procedures) were then correlated with scores on the life-, parenting-, event-, and overall stress.).

Acceptable interrater reliability has previously been reported regarding the KMP (Sossin, 1987; Koch, 1999). In the current study, two raters coded TFAs of both children and parents, and three raters coded Bshfl and UShF of children and parents. Viewing reliability through the lens of percentage-agreement, reliability findings in the current study are mixed, as agreement met criteria (set at .70) for some, but not all, variables, such as parent even flow animated (.90), child flow-adjustment neutral (.90), child flow-adjustment animated (.80), child low-intensity neutral (.70), and child high-intensity animated (.70). Amongst others, child gradual animated (.10) was not as reliably coded. Reliability varied across individuals and across movement factors.

PRINCIPLE RESULTS

The first analyses were guided by the question, "do the parents' relative expression of specific Tension Flow Attributes and factors correspond to reported stress levels on the scales?" In this study, we initially expected to see more bound flow and more fighting patterns (i.e. even flow, abrupt, high intensity) corresponding to higher stress. The results are described below. For descriptives see Table I (Appendix).

Parental Expressions of Stress in Tension Flow Attributes

Parents who experienced higher (although subclinical) life stress showed a higher number of abrupt movements, specifically within the zone of neutral flow ($r=.39$, $p<.05$)[17][18] and a higher number of flow-adjustment movements, also in neutral flow (r

---

[16] Most studies choose a single stress measure to correspond to parent-child behavior. We argue that parents may embody different types of stress, and hence, we applied multiple measures. In addition to the standardized measures of Life Stress, Event Stress, and Parenting Stress, a simple one-item measure was also incorporated into the study. Parents were asked to identify, on a scale from 1 to 5, "How much would you say, your overall level of stress has been in the past year?" 1) not at all, 2) a little, 3) somewhat, 4) quite a bit, and 5) extremely (Adams & Birklein, 2003). This scale demonstrated a mean of 3.10, and a standard deviation of .97. Though caution should follow from the lack of complexity and standardization, of this scale, there is clear face-validity to its question and it seemed advantageous to include such a simple measure.

[17] The complexity of the KMP, and of the training required for coding, has long challenged researchers regarding the consistency of reliability findings. Issues pertaining to cinematographic factors, operationalized differences

=.40, p<.05). In movements indexed as animated, the initial correspondence was reversed, with higher life-stress corresponding to fewer abrupt movements (r=-.42, p<.05).

Children's' Expressions of High Parental Stress in Tension Flow Attributes

Children of parents who reported higher levels of stress on the OSR were found to exhibit *less* high intensity (r=-40, p<.05) and *more* free flow, relative to bound-flow (r=.48, p<.05), all in animated flow.

Examination of Potential Relationships among Parent Stress Levels and Bipolar and Unipolar Shape-Flow Patterns

Analysis of the hypothesized relationship between parent-reported stress and shrinking patterns of Bipolar and Unipolar Shape found no support in children or in parents.

Parent's Results in Terms of Intrapersonal Matching Between Tension Flow and Shape Flow

We did not find support for the hypothesis that greater parent-reported stress would be reflected by greater degrees of mismatching between affined TFA and BShF patterns and between affined TFA and UShF patterns.

Children's Results in Terms of Intrapersonal Matching Between Tension Flow and Bipolar Shape Flow

As predicted, less matching was evident between the child's tension flow cluster and shape flow cluster in the event of high parental life stress. Specifically, higher parent-reported life stress correlated to higher mismatching in the child between TFA and BShF (r=.41, p<.05)[19], and this same correspondence between TFA and BShF was also demonstrated for parent-reported overall stress (r=.48, p<.05).

Children's Results in Terms of Intrapersonal Matching Between Tension Flow and Unipolar Shape Flow

Children of parents experiencing high life stress also showed less intrapersonal matching between their Tension Flow and Unipolar Shape Flow clusters across several associated polarities. Child mismatching between TFA intensity factors and shape-flow vertical dimension factors showed the strongest correspondences to varied indices of parent-reported stress. In the intensity/vertical dimension analyses, higher parent-

---

between related movement factors (i.e. relative degrees of difference in notation), applicability of proper statistical approaches to measure reliability, and the extension of generalizability theory to movement notation, all pertain to future applications of the KMP. Current approaches to training and certification in KMP notation are beginning to address the skill factors that apply to the attainment of satisfactory inter-rater reliability. While these issues were not all addressed in the current study, it was deemed that raters agreed sufficiently to proceed with data analysis, and further study of differences will inform future attempts to increase KMP reliability.

[18] All correlations reported in the text were Bivariate Pearson correlation coefficients. In all analyses, social support, as gauged by the Multidimensional Scale of Social Support (Zimet, Dahlem, & Zimet, 1988), was partialled out.

[19] In all cases wherein relative degrees of matching or mismatching were appraised, the μ, ranging from 0 to 1, captured the degree of similarity of inclination of the β, which assessed the skew of each dimensional polarity line within the diagrams. In addition, the same analyses were done using the sum of difference variable and the cumulative-μ variable. Hence, for each examination for concordance or for matching, there were three distinct μ's (per polarity), somewhat expanded in the case of unipolar shape-flow, and one cumulative μ for the diagram comparisons (e.g. one cumulative μ for two clusters examined for affinity).

reported life stress corresponded to higher mismatching between the μ of the TFA low intensity/high intensity continuum and the Unipolar Shape Flow cephalad balance (lengthening/shortening up) (r =.44; p<.05). A similar correspondence appeared between the μ of TFA low intensity/high intensity and Unipolar Shape Flow growing/shrinking vertical (lengthening up/down; shortening up/down) continuum (r=43, p<.05). Higher parent-reported life stress corresponded to greater mismatching between the μ of TFA gradual/abrupt continuum and the Unipolar Shape Flow posterior balance (bulging/hollowing backwards) (r=.40, p<.05),20 and to the cumulative μ of TFA /Ushfl (r=.46; p<.05). Also, both parent-reported parenting stress and parent-reported overall stress were positively correlated with the child's sum of difference scores for TFA- Unipolar Shape-Flow (PSI r=.42, p<.05; OSR, r =.43, p<.05). Notably, higher parent-reported Event Stress was also linked to greater differences between the TFA intensity and UShF cephalad-caudal dimension (r=.49, p<.05).

Child and Parent: Interpersonal Concordance and Discordance

Tension flow attributes. Parents who experienced high Event Stress (IES) showed greater concordance in graduality with their child (r=-.49, p<.05).[21]

Bipolar shape flow. Findings indicated that parents who experienced greater Life Stress showed a greater discordance with their children in bipolar lengthening (r=.47, p<.05).

Unipolar shape flow. As a function of parent-reported Life-Stress (SSRS), similar discordances arose between parent and child factors of lengthening up/down (growing vertical) (r =.59, p<.05), lengthening up by itself (r =.49, p<.05), and bulging/hollowing front (anterior) (r=.42, p<.05). Furthermore, parents who experienced high Overall Stress (OSR) showed more discordance with their children within the dimension of posterior balance (bulging and hollowing back) (as per μ, r=.40, p<.05). Parents reporting higher Parenting Stress (PSI) demonstrated higher discordance with their child in unipolar widening (r=.41, p < .05), in sagital-shrinking (hollowing front/back) [22] (r =.41, p<.05), and in hollowing-back (r=.45, p<.05). Significant correlations also appeared between the parent-reported Event Stress (IES) and parent-child difference score of Uni-

---

20 We can only highlight these results in this chapter, as many complexities pertained. For instance, analyses incorporated dual polarity, and cumulative, μ-variables, and sum-of-difference variables. Moreover, analyses were conducted using cephalad-caudal and anterior-posterior, as well as growing-shrinking vertical and growing-shrinking sagittal variables. Full results are reported in Birklein (2004).

21 The minus value of the correlation reflects correspondence of high stress (IES) with smaller difference scores in graduality between parent and child.

22 We organized the movement factors in Uni-polar shape flow so that they could readily compare with the TFA elements. For this purpose, we combined elements in several ways: Because Unipolar Shape Flow is the precursor to Shaping in Directions on the KMP profile, lengthening and shortening up (cephalad), and lengthening and shortening down (caudal), as well as bulging /hollowing forward (anterior), and bulging/hollowing backward (posterior), were combined as they reflected similarly-directed patterns. Combining these elements according to their directions poses a challenge in defining matching and concordance variables: in this traditional arrangement, growing and shrinking elements are added together, obscuring any apparent tendency a subject may have toward growing or shrinking. Therefore, in this study, growing and shrinking vertically as well as growing and shrinking sagittally were alternatively combined to arrive at plot points that are purely growing and purely shrinking. However, this led to a large number of possible analyses. In the future, these variables need to be reduced and their overlap with bipolar variables factor-analyzed. Alternatively, the vertical sides of each diagram were compared. This was done by adding the indulging/growing (TFA/Shape flow) sides of each diagram, and then comparing these with the fighting/shrinking (TFA/Shape flow) sides of the same diagrams. This procedure aimed to capture their overall tendencies in clusters, i.e. whether they tended more towards indulging/growing or fighting/shrinking. The cluster tendencies could then be compared.

polar Shape-flow growing-sagittal (bulging front/back) $(r = .40, \text{ p} < .05)$ and the μ of cephalad-caudal patterns $(r = .40, \text{ p} < .05)$.

DISCUSSION OF RESULTS

Parents

Higher stress levels corresponded to higher frequencies of neutral abrupt and neutral flow adjustment, as well as to a lower level of animated abruptness within Tension Flow Attributes. This link between neutral flow and stress is consistent with psychological features attributed to neutral flow in the literature, e.g. inertia, deanimation, and disconnection. This finding regarding the time-dimension may reflect heightened uncertainty (under stress) and it may predict less efficient decision-making (which a further study of Effort patterns may examine). The diminution of animated abrupt flow captures the lack of resources for dynamic, spontaneous and reciprocal responsivity in the adult under higher stress, replaced perhaps, by greater anticipatory anxiety, hypervigilance and rumination.

Children

Children show a *decrease* of high intensity and an *increase* of free flow in relationship to a stressed parent. This may reflect the child's attempt to self-regulate, and to dyadically-regulate tension in the interaction with the parent, decreasing the demand on the parent by signaling more calm and less assertiveness. It appears that children who are in contact with stressed parents learn to tone-down their response-styles and intensity levels, perhaps as a way of managing the likely lowered response-thresholds of their stressed parents. By employing less high intensity and more free flow, a child of a stressed parent may not only decrease the amount of demand on the parent, but may also function for the parent by demonstrating more ease themselves, risking less negative attention from the parent. Such a finding, however, speaks to the complexity of transmission. Children are not only absorbing and internalizing parent stress, it appears that they are also adapting to it, and participating in the regulation of it. When interpersonally framed, stressed children may become regulators of the parent's stress, and in this regard, the use of low intensity is adaptive.

Children of parents demonstrating higher stress also appear to show higher *mismatching* between the safety/danger affects (TFA'S) and approach/avoidance affects (Unipolar) as well as comfort/discomfort affects (Bipolar). Though research validation would be required, it may be that TFA-BShF matching and TFA-UShF matching each reflect types of harmony linked to self-cohesiveness and security, both of which may be disrupted by the parent's stress. The child of a more stressed parent has a dynamic affect expression (reflected in tension-flow) that is not fully supported by affect relational structure (reflected in shape-flow), and vice versa.

Dyad

In general, there seems to be strong evidence of parent/child discordance in both Bipolar and Unipolar lengthening. In the KMP literature, lengthening in bipolar shape flow refers to feelings of elation or pride. In Unipolar shape flow, lengthening is linked to growing towards a pleasant stimulus, or object, or to the expression of authority. It may be that the meaningfulness of this finding lies in relation to tension-flow, specifically the tendency of children of stressed parents to demonstrate less high, and more low, intensity in their TFA's. If, for example, low intensity is not well structured by lengthening, then safe, calm feelings expressed in low intensity may not be accompanied, or structured, by comfortable pride and self-regard.

Discordance likely reflects a disruption in the interactive process of mutually growing and shrinking towards and away from each other, compromising parent-child relations. In stressed dyads, this mutuality and intimacy may be hindered. Future investigations into developmental and relational aspects of movement-anchored empathy and trust can build on the theoretical template of Kestenberg and Buelte (1985) and advance into real-time methodologies.

Further, the discordance may indicate that the stressed parent does not or cannot help the child in structuring or containing affective experiences. As a consequence, it is possible that the child may become under, or over-regulated, and either track the parent closely (hypervigilance), or try to keep stress out by withdrawing from the world (deactivation) (Bowlby, 1973). Without an adult helping the child to modulate and organize inner experience, the child may find emotions overwhelming and confusing. The discordance between parent and child in Unipolar Shape Flow may be one specific way in which intergenerational transmission of stress operates.

Limitations

The current attempt to link stress to movement patterns, while bearing findings and prompting new questions, is nonetheless restricted by the fact that the sample did not include adults with clinical degrees of stress. Hence, these results can be generalized only to a subclinical population. It may be that clinical stress levels (e.g. PTSD) would correspond to the movement factors linked here even more strongly, or it could be that different movement factors and relationships among intrapersonal and dyadic movement factors would emerge as meaningful linkages.

Methodological Contributions

This study incorporated new manners of operationalizing intrapersonal matching and mismatching, and interpersonal concordance and discordance of patterns, introducing the statistical constructs of beta (ß) and mu (μ). These lay the bases for further investigations, such as future KMP studies of parent-child relations that incorporate clusters not included herein (e.g. Effort, Shaping), and to real-time analyses that would follow moment-to-moment interaction sequences.

CONCLUSION

Parents reporting more stress showed more neutral-flow abruptness and flow-adjustment, and less animated abruptness. These basic tension-flow patterns may be pivotal in the conveying of stress from parent to young child, and if this holds true in clinical samples, these stress-markers may take on special meaning in therapeutic contexts.

The results generally supported the overall hypotheses that stressed parents and their children are more disjointed, showing less attunement and more discordance in their relationship. In general, findings support the existing literature, implying that stressed parents are less attuned, and less mirroring of their child (e.g. Osofsky, 2004). The present study specifically identified specific those affect-related movement patterns related to the parent's stress in the parent, the child, and in the dyad. For example, the discordance between parent and child in Unipolar shape flow, may be one way in which intergenerational transmission of stress operates.

As is well known, stress is a complex variable, and individual stress-reactions are variable. Nonetheless, in the pursuit of understanding general tendencies, differences in stress scales clearly matter. Different types of stress relate to different movement factors in the parent, the child, and the dyad. Not surprisingly, the relationship between stress and movement is also complex, and does not follow simple correspondences to fighting- or shrinking-patterns.

This study offers one window into possible modalities of stress-transmission, as specific movement patterns (e.g. greater low intensity) of children corresponded to parental stress, as did dyadic discordances. Such findings may be best understood in terms of mutual regulatory processes.

Methodological contributions, especially pertaining to the analysis of matching/mismatching and concordance/discordance were developed for this investigation. These operationalized dimensional variables, for use in both intrapersonal and interpersonal comparisons, offer a level of statistical analysis commensurate with theoretical conceptualizations in the literature. These are likely to prove invaluable in future time-series studies.

REFERENCES

Abidin, R. R. (1983). *Parenting stress index SF manual.* Charlottesville, VA: University of Virginia Press.

Appleyard, K., & Osofsky, J. D. (2003). Parenting after trauma: Supporting parents and caregivers in the treatment of children impacted by violence. *Infant Mental Health Journal, 24,* 111-125.

Barnett, D., Hunt, K., Butler, C., McCaskill, J., Kaplan-Estrin, M., & Pipp-Siegel, S. (1999). Indices of attachment disorganization among toddlers with neurological and non-neurological problems. In J. Solomon & C. George (Eds.). *Attachment Organization.* New York, NY: Guilford.

Bauman, T. (2003). *The intergenerational transmission of trauma symptoms in children of Holocaust survivors.* Doctoral Project, Pace University.

Beebe, B., Lachmann, F. M., & Jaffe, J. (1997). Mother-infant interaction structures and pre-symbolic self and object representations. *Psychoanalytic Dialogues, 7,* 133-182.

Belsky, J., Rosenberg, K., & Crnic, K. (2000). The origins of attachment security "classical" and contextual determinants. In S. Goldberg, R. Muir & J. Kerr (Eds.). *Attachment theory: Social, developmental, and clinical perspectives.* Hillside, NJ: The Analytic Press.

Birklein, S. B. (2004). *Nonverbal indices of high stress in parent/child interaction.* Unpublished doctoral dissertation. New School for Social Research, New York.

Bowlby, J. (1969). *Attachment and Loss.* London: Hogarth Press and the Institute of Psycho-Analysis.

Camras, L., Meng, Z., Ujiie, T., Dharamsi, Sh., Miyake, K., Oster, H., Wang, L., Cruz, J., Murdoch, A., & Campos, J. (2002). Observing emotion in infants: Facial expression, body behavior, and rater judgments of response to an expectancy-violating event. *Emotions, 2,* 1528-1542.

Clark, R. (1985). *The Parent-Child Early Relational Assessment instrument and manual.* Author, Department of Psychiatry, University of Wisconsin Medical School, Madison, WI.

Coates, S., Rosenthal, J. L., & Schechter, D. S. (Eds.). (2003). *September 11: Trauma and human bonds.* Hillsdale, NJ: The Analytic Press.

Crnic, K. A, Greenberg, M. T., Ragozon, A. S., Robinson, N. M., & Basham, R. B. (1983). Social interaction and developmental competence of pre-term and full-term infants during the first year of life. *Child Development, 54,* 1199-1210.

Ekman, P., & Rosenberg, E. (Eds.). (1997). *What the face reveals: Basic and applied studies of spontaneous expression using the Facial Action Coding System (FACS)*. London: Oxford University Press.

Fonagy, P. (2001). *Attachment theory and psychoanalysis*. New York, NY: Other press.

Fonagy, P., Gergely, G., Jurist, E., & Target, M. (2002). *Affect regulation, mentalization, and the development of the self*. New York, NY: Other Press.

Hobson, C. J., & Delunas, L. (2001). National norms and life-event frequencies for the revised Social Readjustment Rating Scale. *International Journal of Stress Management, 8,* 299-314.

Holmes, T. H., & Rahe, R. H. (1967). The Social Readjustment Rating Scale. *Journal of Psychosomatic Research, 11,* 213-218.

Kestenberg, J., & Buelte, A. (1977). Prevention, infant therapy and the treatment of adults 1. Towards understanding mutuality, 2. Mutual holding and holding oneself up. *International Journal of Psychoanalytic Psychotherapy, 6,* 339-396.

Kestenberg-Amighi J., Loman, S., Lewis, P., & Sossin, K. M. (1999). *The meaning of movement: Developmental and clinical perspective of the Kestenberg Movement Profile*. New York, NY: Gordon & Breach.

Kestenberg, J., Marcus, H., Robbins, E., Berlowe, J., & Buelte, A. (1975). Development of a young child as expressed through bodily movements. In J. Kestenberg, *Children and parents: Psychoanalytic studies in development*. New York, NY: Jason Aronson.

Kestenberg, J. & Sossin, K. (1979). *The role of movement patterns in development*. New York, NY: Dance Nation Bureau Press.

Koch, S.C. (1999). *Reliability of the Kestenberg Movement Profile (KMP). Agreement of Novice Raters*. Stuttgart: Ibidem.

Jaffe, J., Beebe, B., Feldstein, S., Crown, C., & Jasnow, M. (1999). *Rhythms of dialogue in infancy: Coordinated timing and social development*. Submitted to the Monograph Series of the Society for Research in Child Development.

Laban, R.v. (1960). *The mastery of movement*. London: MacDonald & Evans.

Laban, R. (1966). *The language of movement: A guidebook to choreutics*. Boston, MA: Plays.

Laban, R., & Lawrence, F. C. (1974). *Effort: Economy in body movement*. Boston, MA: Plays. Originally published in 1947.

Lyons-Ruth, K., Lyubchik, A., Wolfe, R., & Bronfman, E. (2002). Parental depression and child attachment: Hostile and helpless profiles of parent and child behavior among families at risk. In S. Goodman & I. Gotlib (Eds.). *Children of depressed parents: Mechanisms of risk and implications for treatment* (pp. 89-120). Washington, DC: American Psychological Association.

Lyons-Ruth, K., Alpern, L., & Repacholi, B. (1993). Disorganized infant attachment classification and maternal psychosocial problems. Predictors of hostile-aggressive behavior in the preschool classroom. *Child Development, 64,* 572-585.

March, J. S., Amaya-Jackson, L., Terry, R., & Costanzo, P. (1997). Posttraumatic symptomatology in children and adolescents after an industrial fire. *Journal of the American Academy of Child and Adolescent Psychiatry, 36,* 1080-1088.

Nelson, B. S., Waansgard, S., Yorgason, J., Kessler, M. H., & Carter-Vassol, E. (2002). Single- and dual- trauma couple: Clinical observations of relational characteristics and dynamics. *American Journal of Orthopsychiatry, 72,* 58-69.

Osofsky, J. D., & Fenichel, E. (1993). Caring for infants and toddlers in violent environments: Hurt, healing, and hope. In L. Leavitt & N.A. Fox (Eds.). *The psychological effects of war and violence on children* (pp. 1-48). Hillsdale, NJ: Erlbaum.

Osofsky, J. D. (1994). Participant in roundtable: Children and violence. *Scholastic Early Childhood Today, 8,* 46-48.

Osofsky, J. D. (2004). Young children and trauma: Intervention and Treatment. New York: Guilford.

Pianta, R., & Egeland, B. (1990). Life stress and parenting outcome in a disadvantage sample: Results of the mother-child project. *Journal of Clinical Child Psychology, 19,* 329-336.

Pynoos, R. S., Steinberg, A. M., & Goenjian, A. K. (1996). Traumatic stress in childhood and adolescents: Recent development and current controversies. In B.A. van der Kolk, A.C. McFarlane & L. Weisaeth (Eds.). *Traumatic stress: The effects of overwhelming experience on mind, body, and society*. New York, NY: Guilford.

Sagi-Schwartz, A., van IJzendoorn, M. H., Grossman, K. E., Joewls, T., Grossmann, K., Scharf, M., Koren-Karie, N., & Alkalay, S. (2003). Attachment and traumatic stress in female holocaust child survivors and their daughters. *The American Journal of Pyschiatry, 160,* 1086-1092.

Sossin, K. M. (1987). Reliability of the Kestenberg Movement Profile. *Movement Studies. A journal of the Laban Bartenieff Institut for Movement Studies, 2,* 22-28. NY Laban/Bartenieff Instiute for Movement Studies.

Sossin, M. K. (2002). Interactive movement patterns as ports of entry in infant-parent psychotherapy: Ways of seeing nonverbal behavior. *The Journal of Infant, Child and Adolescent Psychoanalysis,* 2(2), 97-131.

Sossin, K. M. & Loman, S. (1992). Clinical applications of the KMP. In S. Loman (Ed.). *The body-mind connection in human movement analysis* (pp. 21-55). Keene, NH: Antioch New England Graduate School.

Stern, D. (1995). *The motherhood constellation.* New York, NY: Basic Books.

Trevarthen, C. (1993). The Function of Emotions in Early Infant Communication and Development, in Nadel, J. & Camaioni, L. (Eds.). *New Perspectives in Early Communicative Development.* London: Routledge.

Tronick, E., & Weinberg, M. K. (1997). Depressed mothers and infants: Failure to form dyadic states of consciousness. In L. Murray & P. Cooper (Eds.). *Postpartum depression and child development* (pp. 54-81). New York, NY: Guilford.

Weiss, D., & Marmar, C. (1997). The Impact of Event Scale - Revised. In J. Wilson & T. Keane (Eds.). *Assessing psychological trauma and PTSD.* New York: Guilford.

Zimet, G. D., Dahlem, N. W., Zimet, S.G., & Farley, G. K. (1988). The Multidimensional Scale of Perceived Social Support. *Journal of Personality Assessment, 55,* 610-17.

APPENDIX: TABLE I

Means and Standard Deviations for Behaviour Observations on Selected Items (N=52)

Descriptives	Parents (N=26)		Descriptives	Children (N=26)	
Variable Stress	*Means*	*(SD)*	*Variable*	*Means*	*SD*
stressful events weighted (SRRS)	213.50	202.94			
overall stress rating (OSR)	3.10	0.97			
parenting stress (PSI) total	72.85	17.08			
impact of events scale (IES) total	24.08	14.98			
Variable KMP (Parent)			**Variable KMP (Child)**		
tfa flow adjustment -- total parent	1.65	0.40	tfa flow adjustment -- total child	1.26	0.34
tfa even flow total parents	1.74	0.41	tfa even flow -- total child	1.29	0.46
tfa low intensity -- total parent	4.91	0.77	tfa low intensity -- total child	5.14	0.82
tfa high intensity -- total parent	3.78	0.50	tfa high intensity -total child	4.14	0.48
tfa gradual -total parent	2.29	0.39	tfa gradual total child	2.35	0.45
tfa abrupt -total parent	2.13	0.35	tfa abrupt -- total child	2.27	0.45
bshfl widening parent	4.24	0.99	bshfl widening child	4.31	0.95
bshfl narrowing parent	3.74	1.00	bshfl narrowing child	3.90	0.84
bshfl lengthening parent	3.89	0.83	bshfl lengthening child	3.33	0.87
bshfl shortening parent	1.74	1.10	bshfl shortening child	2.48	0.93
bshfl bulging parent	2.08	0.63	bshfl bulging child	2.55	0.92
bshfl hollowingparent	1.74	1.16	bshfl hollowing child	1.65	0.70
Unishfl widening parent	3.43	0.87	unishfl widening child	3.50	0.81
Unishfl narrowing parent	3.11	1.05	unishfl narrowing child	3.31	0.96
unishfl lengthening up parent			unishfl lengthening up child	2.58	0.88
	3.02	0.86	unishfl lengthening down child	1.15	0.84
			unishfl shortening up child	2.07	0.75

Note: N=52; p<.05; SRRS: Social Readjustment Rating Scale Revised; OSR: Overall Stress Rating; PSI; Parenting Stress Index; IES: Impact of Event Scale; tfa = Tension Flow Attributes; bshfl = Bipolar Shape flow; unishfl = Unipolar Shape Flow.

DANCE/MOVEMENT THERAPY AND NONVERBAL ASSESSMENT OF FAMILY VIOLENCE -- A PILOT COMPARATIVE STUDY

Maria Gabriela Sbiglio

This is a pilot comparative study of two sets of families, one having a history of family violence and one not. The interactions observed for each group of families were evaluated using an adaptation of "Dulicai's Nonverbal Assessment of Family Systems". There were some evident differences, especially for the type of effort preferred for bonding, gesturing toward somebody and postural shifts. Families with a history of violence presented more blocking and bonding behaviors. Differences in the frequencies cannot be interpreted due to the nature of the sample; however, future research may allow testing the tool in larger multicultural samples. Nonverbal assessment is proposed here as a complementary tool for early detection of violence in families and ultimately secondary and tertiary prevention.

Keywords: Family violence, nonverbal interaction behavior, nonverbal assessment, DMT, Dulicai' nonverbal assessment of family system (DNAFS)

INTRODUCTION

In the present study, the aim was to investigate whether there are specific differences at the level of nonverbal interaction behavior between families with a history of violence and families without a history of violence. Family violence is defined here as a pattern of physical, sexual or emotional abuse by one member of the family group upon another. In the present study, family is considered from the systems theory standpoint. Systems theory stresses a comprehensive view of the family as a subsystem within a larger system (society). A system has been defined as a structure of elements related by various processes (Scherer, Abeles, & Fisher, 1975). Every element in a system is interrelated. Systems are organized in a hierarchical fashion. Within this framework, the nuclear family is a part of a larger family network, which, in turn, is part of a larger community and ultimately of society. Family violence represents a difficult topic for research for two main reasons: 1) incidence rates on family violence are difficult to estimate because many cases are unreported; 2) its cultural relativity, because of different norms. Some practices viewed as acceptable in one society can be considered abusive from the standpoint of another culture. However, each society and cultural group has criteria for identifying behaviors, which are outside the range of tolerance (Korbin, 1981).

Although the number of research in the area of domestic violence has increased in the last two decades, few of them truly met the criteria of having randomly and adequately sized sample. One of the most comprehensive studies concerning family violence has been conducted by Straus, Gelles and Steinmetz (1980). The study investigated the extent of violence in families living in the United States (U.S.). Data in this particular study was obtained trough interviews with a nationally representative sample of 2,143 families. This particular study established that several factors may be related to family violence, such as a history of violence, socialization for violence in the family, legitimacy of violence, marital difficulties, combination of low income, education and occupation, marital power and social integration (Straus et. al., 1980). Findings stated that minority racial groups tend to have the highest rates of violence (Straus et. al., 1980). Authors finally proposed that, in minorities; the roots of violence could be explained by the complex combination of stress, discrimination and frustration, factors these populations may have to face routinely. One of the minorities in U.S. with high rates of family violence is the Puerto Rican group. In considering the problem of violence for Puerto Ricans is important to take into account the impact of migration and the acculturation stress. The problems for Puerto Rican in the United States are more complex than for other immigrant groups. There seems to be a big difference between expectations and reality for Puerto Rican migrating to U.S. Actually Puerto Ricans has been used as temporary workers and not as citizens who have entitled rights (Puerto Ricans do not need a permission to be employed because Puerto Rico is considered an associated state to U.S.). Of the Latino male unemployment figures, Puerto Rican men represented the highest rate of unemployment at 15.9 % (Institute for Puerto Rican Policy, 1995). Fifty-five percent of the neighborhood in the Puerto Rican community in North Philadelphia was underemployed at the time of conducting the present research (Congreso de Latinos Unidos Records). The explanation of these phenomena in detail exceeds the purposes of this study, but a reference to socio-political factors is important here.

The present study represents a comparison between two groups of Puerto Rican families coming from the same class and social environment. Same criteria were applied in previous research on family violence in Puerto Rican families (Rodriguez, 1985). This study suggests that future research uses more detailed behavioral observations of the interactions patterns of spouses, parents, and children (Rodriguez, 1985). At the time of the development of the study, specific research combining family violence and the observation of nonverbal interaction behavior was not reported in the literature. Movement patterns and nonverbal interaction behavior has been described in a number of studies in the dance/movement therapy literature. Specific movement patterns correlated with acting-out violent behaviors were described in a previous research (Dulicai, 1973). Dulicai identified for these behaviors 1) phrasing that ranges from bound to very bound flow, 2) strength as a predominant or sole effort, and 3) retention of spatial clarity when moving, and sudden directness. A previous concrete application of nonverbal assessment of family interaction behavior was found in a study conducted by Dulicai researching family movement dynamics and creating an instrument for the collection of data on nonverbal interaction patterns. Dulicai (1977) devised an assessment scale, combining kinesic factors (Scheflen, 1967; Birdwhistell, 1963) and Laban's effort/shape analysis of body movement (Laban, 1950) adapted for family process (North, 1972; Kestenberg, 1975; Davis, 1968; Dulicai, 1975). The scale has 20 items that are scored by an observer from life observations or from videotape of any interaction, e.g. talking, playing a game. The items for observation are kinesic behaviors; unconsciously performed in face-to-face interactions and specific to the social context where it happens, such as gesturing, approaching someone, etc. Dulicai (1977) has found that sequences of the interactions between members of the families repeated themselves, as a pattern of behavior, yielding information of predictive value. Previous findings of the Dulicai' Nonverbal Assessment of Family Systems (DNAFS) include 1) statistical differentiation at the level of kinesics for biological and adoptive functional and dysfunctional families; 2) distinct and identifiable differences in effort qualities between normal and disturbed families (Dulicai, 1977; Webster 1987); 3) statistically significant differences in the blocking behaviors for men and women in family systems (Peterson, 1991).

The present research is an observation of the behavioral patterns of interaction conducted in order to prompt further inquiry into the possible relationship between nonverbal communication and family violence. This study constitutes the first application of the DNAFS for the research on family violence. As a pilot study, it attempts to generate new hypotheses about the potential of nonverbal interaction behavior for further studies related to nonverbal predictors. The use of some nonverbal predictors could facilitate the process of early detection of families at risk. Conclusions in this area could also benefit the treatment of family violence by the integration of a nonverbal approach. The field of dance/movement therapy (DMT) may contribute with its body of knowledge and methodological instruments (intervention tools) to the application of a nonverbal approach in early interventions in family systems affected by this problem and ultimately lead to secondary and tertiary prevention. Early interventions in a disturbed system can prevent future serious violence and interrupt the repetition of violence for the following generations.

METHODS
Setting

This research was done through the cooperation of Congreso de Latinos Unidos (CLU), a multicultural agency that provides social and financial support, and educational programs for the Latino Community of North Philadelphia. The study was mainly conducted at Julia de Burgos Family Center. The family center is located at the Julia de Burgos Magnet Middle School in the neighborhood of the families.[23]

Subjects

Four Puerto Rican families coming from the same culture and social environment, living in the same area of North Central Philadelphia, Pennsylvania, U.S.A. participated in the study. The Puerto Rican background was defined as having at least one parent of Puerto Rican heritage no further back than three generations. The types of parenthood considered were those with one biological parent, stepparent, paramour or foster parents. This study excluded any families having a member with problems of alcohol or drug abuse at present and also families having a member with a current major mental illness. Families having a history of violence were first identified by the Department of Human Services of Philadelphia and already had an open case at the family court for child foster care. Community leaders, social workers, and educators of CLU selected potential volunteers from two subject pools (1) families receiving case management services for reports of child abuse or domestic violence, and (2) families receiving services for housing, job training, or any other support. Families were selected according to safety in participation and availability. The participation was established on a voluntary basis. The potential risk for each family participating was evaluated with an emphasis on discerning the level of risk for any new violence or abuse potential in the family. Of all the families that met the inclusion criteria, the first three were recruited for each pool. Families appropriate for the study received a home visit from the researcher and the case manager. In the home visit, subjects were to read and sign a Consent Form. It was extremely difficult to get families involved in the study, especially those having

---

[23] This study was completed as a requirement for clinical internship and thesis work at the Dance/Movement Therapy Masters' Degree Program, School of Health Professions, Drexel University (former Hahnemann University), Philadelphia, PA, U.S..

an open case at the Family Court. Twelve families were asked to participate, but six finally accepted. One of the families, having a history of violence, withdrew at the last minute. The study became a comparison of four families: two families with a history of violence (Group A) and two families without a history of violence (Group B). Detailed information on demographics is not provided here for subjects' privacy.

ASSESSMENT PROCEDURES

Efforts were made to minimize risks and discomforts. The home visit was the first assessment point in which subjects completed a self-report scale -- the Conflict Tactic Scale (Strauss, 1989) that served also as a screening. The second assessment point was a structured interview that included a questionnaire designed for the purpose of obtaining clinical data (the same for both groups). Some methodological suggestions, made by Dulicai (1977) and Webster (1987), were included in the design of the present study. Those were as follows: having the same person conduct all the interviews, two or more observers to lessen the possibility of error or bias, the utilization of talking/sitting arrangement plus game situation (with props and toys). The videotaped interview had the following sequence: (a) verbal interview (questionnaire designed specially for this purpose) -- subjects were seated with the researcher (ten minutes), (b) observation of free play and interaction -- without active participation of researcher (ten minutes), and (c) facilitation of movement tasks by the researcher (ten minutes). A third interview was scheduled for any family interested in getting feed back on the observations made in the study. The researcher conducted all the interviews.

In preparation of the videotapes, a segment of ten minutes was excerpted from the middle of the tape for the purpose of rating. The middle of the session usually contains more about the relationship itself and less of the routine patterns in which most people engage anyway. This segment contained five minutes of the sitting arrangement and five more minutes of the free game with props part.

Assessment Design

An adaptation of the "Dulicai Nonverbal Assessment of Family Systems" (Dulicai, 1977) was used as a tool for the observation and evaluation of the nonverbal interaction behaviors. The nonverbal behavior demonstrated in the recorded interactions was rated on an observation sheet (Observational sheet is included in the appendix). The modifications to the original scale were made under the supervision of the scale developer (Dulicai). Modifications performed included: 1) the use of a selection of the items displaying affects, body boundaries, touch, and flexibility, 2) the additional notation of effort qualities in bonding behavior (any physical contact or touch between two people) and postural shifts and 3) the separated rating of postural shifts (toward/away from) for a better observation. Eye contact, shadow movements, body attitude, exploratory behavior, shared focus and partial or full body actions are items from the original scale that were not included in the present study.

Definitions of the kinesics observed

Gesture

A movement that does not imply weight change. Movement of a body part or combination of body parts

with the emphasis on the expressive aspects of the move. (Bartenieff & Lewis, 1980).
Postural shifts
Shape changes observed in a person moving that include the whole body or a shift of weight and position, simply to get a new configuration of limbs (Bartenieff & Lewis, 1980).
Postural shift toward/away from
The body (trunk) is moving toward/away from the person interacting with, in an inward/outward direction, always including a postural shift (Dulicai, 1977).
Blocking
Movement that covers or protects the centre of one's body. It is shown by the use of any part of the body (trunk, arms or legs) in a closed position toward the person interacting with. It may block the scope of view and space between the persons interacting. It does not include postural shift or touch (Dulicai, 1977).
Accommodating
Changes in posture and/or gesture in response to the interaction. This behavior does not imply any physical touch (Dulicai, 1977).
Separating
A person leaves the reach space of another (Dulicai, 1977).
Molding
Changes in the body attitude that compromise the structure of the trunk support and the limbs in the performance of shaping by the person interacting. This is a behavior in response to physical contact, which is often functional (mother may adapt the shape of her trunk to the child's shape) (Dulicai, 1977).
Bonding
Any touch behavior or physical contact between two people that defines the relationship whether for the positive or negative (Scheflen, 1973).

Rating

Raters (three graduate students having already completed three semesters in the same Dance/Movement Therapy Masters' Degree program) were trained in the use of the Dulicai's Nonverbal Assessment of Family Systems checklist, in a course taught by Dulicai. They also met with the researcher for one hour to practice and to clarify concepts, especially for the changes made to the original scale. One rater worked on four families, the other one worked on three and the third rater worked on one. Families were assigned randomly to each rater with two raters scoring each family. Raters, blind to the purposes of the study, independently rated the videotapes. They were allowed to view each videotape segment up to five times. Observations were made with the volume turned off. Raters were given the following instructions: 1) rate each time these behaviors (kinesics in observational sheet-see appendix) occur for each member of the family, 2) rate effort qualities for the specific items marked with (*), and 3) write any additional comment on relevant information considered important for the description of this family. Considering the fact that kinesics may happen in an interval that goes from 3 to 45 seconds, ten observational sheets for each member of the family observed were provided to the raters to facilitate the process. One observational sheet represented a time span of 60 seconds each. A numerical score for each kinesic observed for each family was obtained, summarizing each time the item was rated with an X for all members of the family. Some items included the specification of the member of the family towards the interaction behavior was directed (for example "gesturing toward") with initials (previously established on the observational sheet), like C1 for the older children.

The key for effort observation was established based on Laban Movement Analysis (LMA) (Laban, 1947) with a division in three ranges for each factor: low range (25% of the presence of effort), medium range (50% present) and high range (75%). The motion factors (Flow, Space, Weight and Time) were observed in a continuum between two opposites: indulging into and resisting (Bartenieff & Lewis, 1980). The effort elements in each extreme for the factors were established as follows from Laban (1947): for the flow factor, free and bound flow; for space, directness and indirectness; in relationship to weight, strength and lightness; and finally for time, quickness and sustainment.

Reliability

The raters were selected after a pre-test on Laban's effort analysis, taken by the director of the dance/movement program where the raters were trained and a specific test of reliability taken by Dulicai. The three raters were selected because they performed with high levels of agreement when identifying selected LMA elements (Efforts and Space aspects). Percentages of agreement indicate the rate at which each rater agreed with the 11 others trained in the same LMA observation course. Rater 1 had an agreement level of .85 with the others, Rater 2 had an agreement level of .84, and Rater 3 an agreement level of .87 with the others. For the present study, the scores of the two raters for each family were compared. There were just few discrepancies between the raters in the score of "molding" for the mother in one of the families of group A. One of the raters considered the behavior as "molding" and the other one as "accommodating". The other discrepancy was presented in the consideration of "lightness" for the scoring of "gesturing" in the mother of the other family of group A. One rater considered it as "bound flow" (restraint) and the other as "lightness". An additional meeting was performed for these two raters with the researcher to clarify these observations. After the clarification of the concept of "molding", both raters coincided in the consideration of the behavior as "accommodating" and, in the other case, after watching another time, they coincided about the presence of "bound flow" instead of "lightness".

Data Analysis

The researcher put together all the observation sheets. In this way a numerical score (a sum value) for each category of kinesic observed was obtained for each family. Then, following the time frame, for all members of each family, a pattern analysis of the interactions resulted ("what" and "how" a behavior is present in one of the family members and the resultant behavior of the others members at the same time frame).

RESULTS

The results suggested differences between the two groups compared at the level of:

1. Frequencies: families in group A (having a history of violence) presented more bonding, blocking and postural shifts away from; families in group B (without a history of violence) presented a higher frequency of accommodating, gesture and postural shift toward. Raw frequencies for the kinesics behaviors are presented in Table I. Statistical treatment was not performed.

2. Effort qualities rated for bonding, postural shift and gesturing were also different for both groups of families. In families with a history of violence, there was a higher presence of fighting efforts (rated as the 75% of presence in combinations of bound flow with strength and directness). Comparison at the level of efforts was limited just to the mother siblings interaction subsystems because in families from Group A was impossible to get male involvement. Data is presented in Table II.

Results on the self-reported data (C.T.S.) cannot be interpreted here. However is important to mention that mothers in group A (having a history of violence) rated 0 (almost never) for the items related to physical violence, while mothers in group B (having a history of violence) rated 2 (sometimes) or 3 (often) for some of the same items (for example in the item "slapped").

A qualitative pattern analysis sample has been performed for all families. For the purpose of this presentation the pattern of one family from the group B (without a history of violence) was selected and is included at the end of this section.

TABLE I:FREQUENCY OF KINESICS IN GROUPS A (HISTORY OF VIOLENCE) AND B

Kinesics	Group A			Group B		
	F #1	F #2	M	F #1	F #2	M
Blocking	3	4	3.5	0	3	1.5
Molding	3	4	3.5	5	5	5
Gesture toward	40	33	36	40	39	39.5
Bonding behavior	13	25	19	15	15	15
Accommodating	2	2	2	4	6	5
Postural shift toward	11	4	7.5	8	11	9.5
Postural shift away	5	6	5.5	2	5	3.5
Approach	11	11	11	16	11	11.5

Note: F #1= family number one, F #2= family number two; M= indicates the mean for each value.

TABLE II: PREFERENCES IN QUALITY OF EFFORTS IN KINESICS IN FAMILIES GROUP A (HISTORY OF VIOLENCE) AND FAMILIES GROUP B (WITHOUT HISTORY OF VIOLENCE)

Efforts	Family #1(A)	Family #2 (A)	Family #2 (B)	Family #2 (B)
Free flow			*	*
Bound flow	*	*		
Indirect space			*	*
Direct space	*	*		
Light weight		*	*	*
Strong weight	*			
Sustained time				*
Quick time			*	

Note: F #(1) = family number one, F #(2) = family number two, A (group A); B (group B); * and dark shade indicates the preference in efforts resulting from adding the combinations rated for all members of each family (more than 55%).

RESULTS

Pattern Analysis Sample-Family # 1 Group B

The following sequence resulted from the work of putting together all observation sheets for this family. This sequence repeated itself five times during the 10 minutes of the interview excerpted for rating. The whole sequence was divided in four subsequences like phrases as following:

1. Older daughter (C1) postures towards father, father reciprocates, mother bonds to the younger daughter (C2), C2 separates from mother and C1 separates from father, too.

2. Mother gestures toward C1 and father. Mother and father gesture toward each other (with some postural shift). C1 approaches father and bonds to him.

3. C2 approaches mother and mother bonds to and molds to C2, C2 bonds and molds in contact with father, father does not respond.

4. Father gestures toward C1, mother either bonds to C2 to separate her from father, or for holding her toward herself, and postures or gestures towards father.

5. The next sequence is a repetition, when C1 separates from father and mother and father gesture toward each other.

Integration of QualitativeData

Mother presented a big variety of gesturing toward C1 and C2. However the mother showed a preference of bonding and molding with younger child. The mother's preferred movement qualities were indirectness and some quickness. Father was more direct, light, and sustained in his movements. He seemed to be the center of attention because most of the kinesics performed by mother and the two daughters were directed toward him. Few interactions occurred between C1 and C2, but the kind of interactions were related to doing things together. The mother preferred movement qualities of indirectness and some quickness. Indirectness or flexibility allowed her to be able to pay attention to both children and father at the same time. In the context of the session, quickness permitted her to respond right on time to her children's needs. Father was more direct and light in his movements. His attitude seemed to be more stable. Raters commented on this family that the mother seemed to be more active, keeping things going, and the father seemed to be more passive. It was important to note that during the game with props, which last 10 minutes, the father did not move from the center (of the space) of the room. The family members moved around him in the different games they played. Additional information may shed some light to the observations made from the videotape. At the moment of conducting this study, the mother had a job and the father was unemployed. Considering the fact that being the "bread winner" is a very important task to achieve for Puerto Rican man, as reported in previous work (Salas, 1988); the father might feel frustrated by the fact he cannot fulfill his family's needs. It might be possible that the mother is trying to support the father's sense of centrality and hierarchy through directing all attention toward him. Family "centrality" has been described in the literature as one of the positives aspects of the prescribed gender role for Puerto Rican man (Torres, 1998). Considering this fact, it might be important for this father to keep the center of the space in order to have a sense of keeping the structure of the family (and being in control) even if he cannot fulfill financial support at this time. For this man, not being able to cover his family needs might be an area of conflict and a stress factor. The sense of authority of a man that cannot fulfill the expectations as the breadwinner and protector of his family is seriously challenged. It may leave him with the need to assert his dominance, and defend his sense of dignity, through the use of violence and physical force (Mizio, 1974).

As reported in the literature, in families exposed to high level of stress due to poverty and lack of social opportunities, members may release frustration through physical attacks (Gil, 1970). This family is probably exposed to stress and frustration, but fortunately, it seems they have developed ways of negotiating and problem solving. Observing the kind of nonverbal interactions for this family (without a history of violence), it seemed to show the ability of keeping boundaries, and establishing balance for the family structure. Perhaps in family systems affected by history of violence there is a disturbed way of setting limits due to a failing establishment of boundaries. It might be necessary for families with a history of violence to learn about different options to cope with anger and frustration.

DISCUSSION

The results revealed some differences between families with a history of violence and families without history of violence at the level of: (1) preferred interaction behaviors, (2) preferred effort qualities of the kinesics performed. Some of these differences, such as a higher presence of blocking, less molding, and less accommodating in families with a history of violence, were also presented for dysfunctional families in previous comparison between functional and dysfunctional biological and adoptive families (Dulicai, 1977; Webster, 1987). Blocking behaviors have been found to be an important cornerstone in defining family types (Peterson, 1991).

An unexpected difference observed was the presence of a higher frequency of physical contact "bonding" in families with a history of violence. Importantly though, almost 65% of the physical contact was a hitting, pulling, or grabbing type of bonding, especially in the siblings' subsystem interactions. In families without a history of violence the presence of pulling, grabbing or hitting corresponded only to 15% of the bonding behaviors and was not performed with the presence of "fighting rhythms" in high range. A consultation with the creator of the assessment instrument Dulicai, helped to clarify the concept of bonding to the purpose of the observation in the present study. In previous work this behavior was not rated with effort quality. It was rather considered as a positive interaction behavior, even as an indicator of functionality because of its higher frequency in normal families. Results in the present study being set forth, established a more differentiated view of physical contact in "bonding" as a category. Bonding was not necessarily positive. The discovery of this difference between the type of behavior (touching/bonding) and the kind of (the "how") came through observation of effort qualities. The main difference in terms of effort qualities present in "bonding," for the families with a history of violence, was the presence of "bound flow" combined with fighting efforts. The description of "how" the bonding behaviors were performed was relevant here to make a better description of the kind of touch behaviors in families with a history of violence. The use of the effort qualities in the nonverbal observation might serve to establish a differential diagnosis (for positive and negative bonding / physical contact, independent of shape/form). Depending on the effort qualities, physical contact needs to be either judged as positive or negative independent of the actual behavioral form. If pulling, hitting or grabbing is done with *lightness*, it might well be a positive bonding as in playful fighting. The comparison of the two sets of families, if weak to make final conclusions, may generate new questions for future research; especially about the role of bonding in families with a history of physical violence, the role of effort qualities for differential diagnosis of bonding behavior, and also about the features and frequency of bonding manifested in different cultural groups. Bonding behaviors might need to be tested in cross-cultural research with larger samples of families.

Another interesting finding was an important presence of postural shifts in the group with a history of violence. The researcher observed that the majority of the postural shifts away were performed with quickness and either extremely bound flow or strength. These postural shifts away were for example present in combination with gesture "blocking" performed by the mother as a reaction to child approach (the child being in foster care). Families without history of violence presented an important number of postural shifts as well, but mainly toward another person (in the interactions) and with a different effort combination (containing more or exclusively indulging elements). This information was confirmed by the additional comments of raters for these families. For future research it might be important to test for the presence of postural shifts in larger samples of families with a history of violence.

Specific acting out and self-harming behavior observed in the families with a history of violence presented similarities with the movement patterns observed in acting out (violent) behaviors in previous research (Dulicai, 1973). This behavior was performed by one child in either family of this group (group A). Integration with clinical data was important to understand this information. Both children performing acting out violent behaviors were the ones being in foster care. It is thus important in future studies to investigate whether this is a problem of families with foster care children in general.

The data of this study do not allow to compute any statistics due to the small sample size, yet results may suggest directions for future research. Based on the limitations of this present study, some suggestions can be made for the repetition of the study and further investigation. The author suggests 1) having the adequate resources to compensate participants and raters for the incredible effort and time spent in such a study, 2) normative data on nonverbal behaviors/kinesics to be established for this cultural groups, 3) matching the number of children and ages when applying the DNAFS, and 4) testing the correlation of movement pattern observed and violence in larger samples in this and other cultural groups.

The use of the nonverbal assessment of family violence could facilitate the use of more flexible settings where families are interacting routinely (family reunions at schools, playgrounds, etc.), being in this way a low cost and a non-invasive instrument. As an early intervention, it may help to prevent future serious violence and it may help to prevent the intergenerational learning and transmission process of violent behaviors from one generation to another. At the level of clinical applications for family violence, the use of nonverbal data may address the situation in a more acceptable way of intervention, because it is concrete and can be based on present actions being performed (facilitating understanding and learning processes). In this way, nonverbal interaction behavior could be used as a tool for a) feedback, b) relearning about body boundaries, c) learning different choices for bonding (physical touch) through experiencing different effort qualities, and d) exploring different ways to cope with anger and frustration.

In the assessment of families, both verbal and nonverbal approaches are important, but in the assessment of a potential for violence, it is generally difficult to rely on verbal testimony or self-reported data, as is demonstrated in the responses to the CTS by the participants of this present study. Considering the fact that victims are often children and woman, hesitant to report (or afraid of reporting) physical or sexual violence, a nonverbal tool to support clinical data may be relevant for health and social services. Finally, nonverbal behavior in interactions may provide data to support clinical hypotheses about family violence, without considering the data independent from the social context, structure (social or family), history of family, and individual aspects.

Besides the extensions to research and clinical work, the implications of the present study might also open new interest in sociological and cultural dimension of "movement", often absent in theory and research in the Dance/Movement Therapy field.

REFERENCES

Bartenieff, I., & Lewis, D. (1980). *Body movement: Coping with the environment.* Amsterdam: Gordon & Breach.

Birdwhistell, R.L. (1963). *The kinesic level in the investigation of the emotions. Expression of the Emotions in Man.* New York: International University Press.

Congreso de Latinos Unidos (1999). Unpublished flyer about records. Philadelphia, PA.

Davis, M. (1968). *Methods of perceiving pattern of small-group behavior.* Unpublished paper.

Dulicai, D. (1973). Movement therapy on a closed ward. *Journal of the Bronx State Hospital, 1*(4).

Dulicai, D. (1975). *Movement analyses in understanding family system.* Philadelphia: The Devereaux Papers.

Dulicai, D. (1977). Nonverbal Assessment of Family Systems: A Preliminary Study. *Art Psychotherapy,4*(2), 55-62.

Gil, D.G. (1970). *Violence against children.* Boston: Harvard University Press.

Kestenberg, J.S. (1975). *Children and Parents: Psychoanalytic studies in development.* New York: Jason Aronson.

Korbin, J. (1981). *Child Abuse and Neglect: Cross cultural perspective.* Beverly Hills, CA: University of California Press.

Laban, R., & Lawrence, F.C. (1947). *Effort.* London: Macdonald and Evans.

Laban, R.v. (1960). *The mastery of movement.* London: MacDonald & Evans.

Mizio, E. (1974). Impact of external systems on Puerto Rican family. Social Casework, 76-83.

North, M. (1972). Personality assessment through movement. London: MacDonald and Evans.

Peterson, D.S. (1991). *The kinesics of Family Systems: Distributional Features of Nonverbal Interactions.* Unpublished Doctoral Dissertation. Minnesota School of Professional Psychology.

Rodriguez, V. (1985). *Attitudes towards corporal punishment, social support system and conflict resolution techniques related to family violence in Puerto Rican families living in the United States.* Unpublished Doctoral Dissertation. Temple University.

Salas, R.A. (1988). A survey of a sample of Puerto Ricans living in the United States: family cohesion and *adaptability, acculturation and psychological impairment.* Unpublished Doctoral Dissertation, Indiana University of Pennsylvania, Pennsylvania.

Scheflen, A.E. (1967). On the Structuring of Human Communication. *American Behavioral Scientist,10* (8), 8-12.

Scheflen, A.E. (1973). Communicational structure: Analysis of a psychotherapy transaction. Bloomington, Indiana: University Press.

Scherer, K.R., Abeles, R.P., & Fisher, C.S. (1975). *Human aggression and conflict: Interdisciplinary perspectives.* Englewood Cliffs, NJ: Prentice Hall.

Straus, M.A., Gelles, R., & Steinmetz, S.V. (1980). *Behind closed doors: Violence in the American family.* New York: Anchor Books

Straus, M.A. (1989). *Manual for the Conflict Tactic Scales.* Durham: University of New Hampshire, Family Research Laboratory.

Torres, J.B. (1998). Masculinity and gender roles among Puerto Rican men: Machismo on the U.S. mainland. *American Journal of Orthopsychiatry, 68(1).*

Webster, J.C. (1987). *A comparison of functional and dysfunctional adoptive families: A nonverbal assessment.* Unpublished Master Thesis. Hahnemann University.

APPENDIX

Observational Sheet
Family:
Member:
Initials for other members:

Kinesics to observe (rate with an X and add the initials of the other members toward the behavior is directed to, following the specific time span)	Time span (60 sec.)
Blocking	
Molding	
Gesturing toward (*)	
Bonding behavior (*)	
Accommodating	
Postural shift toward (*)	
Postural shift away (*)	
Approach	
Separating behavior	

Note: (*) Means rate with effort qualities present adding range.
Key for range: High (75%), Medium (50%), Low (25%).

FROM CROCODILE TO WOMAN THE MULTIDIMENSIONALITY AND ENERGY DYNAMIC OF MOVEMENT SEEN IN LIGHT OF THE DANCE THERAPY FORM *DANSERGIA*

Helle Winther

This chapter focuses on movement as primary language, exploring the multidimensionality and energy dynamics of movement through the connections between the concepts of body and energy. A session from the dance therapy form Dansergia with a woman, here called Clara, is narrated, analysed, and compared to a daily life scene with the child Nina. These scenes are discussed in relation to phenomenological and energy theoretical aspects in order to open the research field for psychological themes, which include the body and yet do not exclude culture, history, and community. In order to respect the nonlinear movement language of the body, data and theory are in this chapter woven closely and organically together to follow the processes of Nina and Clara.

Keywords: Movement as primary language, energy and vitality, energy dynamics, multidimensionality of the body, the lived body

MOVEMENT IS THE BODY'S MOTHER TONGUE

Introduction

Nina is dancing in the living room with a little teddy bear in her hand. She is moving joyfully and quickly, up and down, up and down, up and then deep down, trying to jump and leave the floor. The intensity and excitement of the moment is shining from her brown eyes and her whole bodily presence. Then an older boy comes into the room. He enters her body space ruthlessly, trying to take the teddy bear out of her hands. Nina's reaction is brief and clear. Her mouth closes sharply; she bends her right arm across her breast while protecting the teddy bear in her left hand. Then she turns away from him and at the same time pushes him away with the back of her right bent arm. "UUUnnn" she says. As the sound comes through her throat and now half opened mouth, it is almost as deep as the sound of a small bear. She is only one year old and has not yet learned to say one single word. (Nina, July 2003)

Even if she is already imprinted by family, society and culture, nobody has yet taught my niece Nina how to behave, reflect, or not behave in a situation in which someone is going beyond her boundaries. Her reactions and the clarity of her movement communication grow spontaneously out of her moment-by-moment bodily sensations and feelings, without the reflectivity of the language level. Nina, only a small child recently born, already knows how to sense and speak through the body, how to be in contact with inner needs and senses and in dialogue with others. Every baby knows how to express the pleasure of being in contact with other warm bodies and how to express the painful experience of an absent mother, of basic needs not being met, or the frustration of the grown-up world not understanding simple signs in bodily communication. Life begins with the first cry, which is connected with vitality as Pierrakos writes (Pierrakos, 1986). A cry is a basic pulsatory movement of the entire organism of the baby. A strong cry indicates vigor, while a weak cry indicates lack of vitality (Pierrakos, 1986, p. 183). Vitality is the basic premise for life and movement is our primary language. We come into the world already moving and when we learn to move we do so on the basis of what is already there, an original kinetic liveliness or animation as Maxine Sheet-

Johnstone writes (Sheets-Johnstone, 1999). In fact we move already long before we are born: from conception until birth, the baby is moving in the mother's womb. Daria Halprin calls this primary movement language "the body's mother tongue":

"Movement is the body's mother tongue, a powerful and universal language. Made conscious and creative, movement is a language for the body and soul to speak through, a bridge to the interior world of self and between self and the world; it is a way to build bridges and begin dialogues with the separated parts." Daria Halprin (Foundations of Expressive Arts Therapy, Ch. 7, p. 134; Tamalpa Institute, 2005)

Focus and Background

This chapter focuses on movement as primary language, exploring the multidimensionality and energy dynamics of movement using connections between the concepts of body and energy. A session from the dance therapy form *Dansergia* with a woman, for confidential and ethical reasons here called Clara, is narrated and analysed compared to the above mentioned daily life scene with the child Nina. These scenes are discussed in relation to phenomenological (Merleau-Ponty, 1962; 1968) and energy theoretical aspects (Lowen, 1977; 1982; 1995; Pierrakos, 1990; Sabetti, 1978; 1986; 1989; 1992; 1993; 2001).

The background for the project is dance movement therapy with a fundamental focus on the relationship between inner movement and outer movement expressed in dance. Dance movement therapy has been developed by pioneers such as Marian Chace, Lilian Espenak and Mary Starks Whitehouse (Grønlund, 1999; Halprin, 2004). The most modern forms of dance movement therapy -- the use of dance/movement as a psychotherapeutic or healing tool -- are, as in the phenomenology of Merleau-Ponty (Merleau-Ponty, 1962) and Lowen's theory of Bioenergetics (Lowen, 1977; 1995), rooted in the idea that body, mind, and world are inseparable. This point of view was already practiced in tribal cultures, where dance has been a tool to establish and convey the relationship between the individual and the community, and the human and natural world (Halprin, 2004; Levy, 1992). To promote health and growth, and regain a sense of wholeness by experiencing the fundamental unity of body, mind and spirit, is the ultimate focus of dance therapy – regardless of particular forms, traditions or connections to psychological theories (Halprin, 2004; Levy, 1992).

Stèphano Sabetti (Sabetti, 1986; 1993; 2001) developed the concept of Life Energy Process through formal and informal research over more than thirty years, from which *Dansergia* evolved. The etymological meaning of the word Dansergia is dance and energy. Dansergia was developed using concepts of a holistic multi-level energy-based therapy (Sabetti, 1986, 1989; 1992, 1993, 2001). Life Energy Process is influenced by the Bioenergetics work of Lowen (Lowen, 1977; 1982) and Pierrakos (Pierrakos, 1986), the Gestalt therapy of Fromm and Perls, as well as concepts from Eastern cultures and medicine, martial arts, Shiatsu and acupuncture (Sabetti, 1986; 2001). In Dansergia there are two different approaches to the practice: one for personal development, bringing the issues and feelings of each individual into the present, giving him/her space to explore these issues in an experimental and creative way; and one for clinical therapy, including regressive movements and transference issues, in order to deepen the therapeutic process (Zoetler, Persson, Stühler, & Sabetti, 2001). Clara's process is a developmental process.

MOVING WRITING -- DATA FROM THE LIVED BODY
The Purpose of the Project

Most research projects in the dance movement therapeutic area focus on the *effect,* that is, the outcome of dance and movement therapy in relation to different groups. This chapter concerns the research project *Movement Psychology -- the Language of the Body and the Psychology of Movements based on the Dance therapy form Dansergia* which focuses on the moments of lived experiences in the *process. Effect* originally means "result" whereas the etymological meaning of process is "being carried" and "journey." With this article the author invites the reader on a dancing journey and enlightens the steps on the road.

Inspired by phenomenological (Merleau-Ponty, 1962; 1968), anthropological (Hastrup, 2003), depth-hermeneutic (Belgrad, 1997, Engel, 2001, Lorenzer, 1986) and autoethnographic narrative research methods (Bagley & Cancienne, 2002; Sparkes, 2002; 2003), the project explores the potentials of movement as personal development and therapy through the chosen dance therapy form Dansergia (Sabetti, 1992; 2001).

The aim of the project is to reveal new aspects of interrelations between the body and movement language, and emotional and psychological dimensions of the individual. From these aspects it might be possible to develop a theoretical and practical concept of" Movement Psychology," bridging energy psychological, phenomenological, and societal perspectives. The purpose is furthermore to research how these perspectives could grow into the movement pedagogical area as well, in order to open new development possibilities here. The approaches mentioned in this chapter could perhaps meet Samson`s and Sparkes` call for a need to establish a psychology which includes both body and psychology, but which does not exclude history, culture, and community (Samson, 1998; Sparkes 2005). As Sparkes writes about Sampson:

> *"For him the dominant position in psychology not only excludes history, culture and community, but the body other than the object body. Certainly phenomenology challenges this focus on the object-body by emphasizing the felt-body or lived-body, but it often does so in such a way that it ends up excluding history, culture and community from its sphere of understanding. Against this the emergence of social constructivism within psychology in recent years includes history, culture and community. However, according to Sampson for the most part it shares with the dominant tradition an exclusion of the body other than the same ocularcentric object-body" (Sparkes, 2005, p.34).*

In general, dance therapeutic work overcomes the here described dominant view of the body as an object body by working with body-mind approaches. From this point of view, dance and movement therapy coincides with the perspectives of Merleau-Ponty, who challenged the viewpoint of dualism and the separation of body and mind, subject and object, self and world, through the lived experience of the existential body and through his concept of the lived body (Merleau-Ponty, 1962). For Merleau-Ponty, intentional consciousness is experienced in and through our bodies (Merleau-Ponty, 1962). The challenge for dance-movement therapy as well as for phenomenological body approaches is to not only to overcome dualism, but also -- as Sparkes and Samson mention -- to find ways to integrate history, culture, and community into the sphere of understanding. This research project in dance therapy seeks an understanding of the multidimensionality of the lived existential body (Fraleigh, 1987; Merleau-Ponty, 1962). It further aims to explore socially, culturally, and spiritually embodied movement dynamics behind or beyond daily body language and culturally defined gestures.

Newer Narrative Forms of Writing

"Influenced by the Cartesian view of separation between body/mind, humanity/ nature, and objective/subjective "realities", western civilisation succumbed to centuries of dualistic thought. Although philosophers and mystics continued to honour paths of wisdom related to consciousness and spirit, the mainstream understanding of the human condition narrowed and was largely placed in the authoritative and controlling hands of specialists – clergy, scientists, and doctors who held to a mechanic view of human existence." (Halprin, 2004, p. 37)

The dualistic view of the body has been (and is) part of different scientific paradigms and ways of reporting research, even in the area of body and movement research. Dualism has not only created a split between body and mind; the split is also hierarchical: mind is more, body is less, theory first and then the findings. In order to fulfil the purpose of this project, a challenge of this view is needed.

In order to let the empirical work *move through* the individuals' bodies, this research project is based on a long-term field study and experience descriptions. Through scenic descriptions (Belgrad, 1997; Engel, 2001; Lorenzer, 1986) and poetic diary notes (Sparkes, 2002; 2003), developmental processes from Dansergia are described. The project explores the language of the body not only in the "what" that is researched, but also in the "how" the research is expressed in order to explore how to write in a bodily connected and moving language. As Andrew Sparkes points out, development in various scientific areas in recent years has opened a wide range of choices and is encouraging experimentation with novel, innovative forms of writing:

"In the wake of feminist, postmodernist, and poststructuralist critiques of traditional writing practises Richardson (2000) suggests that science-writing prose is no longer held as sacrosanct and qualitative work now appears in multiple venues in different forms. As such the ethnographic genre has been blurred, enlarged and altered to include poetry, drama, conversations, reader's theatre and many more." (Sparkes, 2003, p. 153; Richardson, 2000, p. 923)

The narrative focus gives the opportunity to work creatively with artistic inspiration, and let the empirical work be told, not *about* the body but *through* the body. This allows "moving writing" (Sparkes, 2002), a multidimensional writing process which entails moving away from *facts* toward *meaning*. Moving writing therefore provides an opportunity to give voice to the body (Sparkes, 2002). As this project is inspired by phenomenological, depth-hermeneutic and narrative based research methods, as mentioned, it is thus also approaching the post-modern scientific paradigm, which has other criteria and ways of reporting and evaluating research (Sparkes, 2003). These criteria could include perspectives which answer the questions: whether the piece succeeds aesthetically, whether the creative analytical practises open up the text, whether the text has impact and affects the reader, and whether the text gives a fleshed-out, embodied sense of lived experience (Richardson, 2000, p. 937; Sparkes, 2002, p. 209). The author of this chapter is subjectively involved in this work. The author is also present in the scenic description of Clara, whom you will soon meet, although because of the focus of the chapter, Clara is in the foreground. From a traditional scientific point of view, this could be critical because it affects the neutrality and possible objectivity and validity of the text. From a post-modern point of view, on the other hand, the author will always create and construct the text. Language therefore is seen as a constructive force that creates a particular view of reality (Sparkes, 2002, p. 12).

Experience-focused narrative research includes very conscious work, with the challenge of being subjectively involved as a researcher, balancing in a constantly *double
consciousness* (Bruner, 1986, p. 14; Hastrup, 2003), thus moving between an inside and
outside perspective, balancing between closeness and distance at the same time. The author uses the inside principle by expressively writing the scenes with Clara, and the outside principle to see the text "through the glasses" of different theoretical approaches.
Narrative approaches are furthermore often connected to aesthetic and artistic ways of
writing, or `dancing the data` performances (Bagly & Cancienne, 2002). Therefore, this
chapter will in form, content, structure and the language used differ from conventional
forms. As one of the purposes is to use "moving writing" respecting the non-linear language of the body, data and theory are through this double consciousness weaved very
closely and organically together following the Dansergia process. Let's now move further into the theme. Let's meet Clara.

Moving Into Clara's Spaces

*Clara walks into the room quickly -- very quickly. She seems stressed, coming directly from
somewhere else. The words almost pour out of her: how she has decided to leave her job, how
it is connected with a lot of other themes, with her husband, and the child who is not even her
own. About how she moves in between them, protecting the child against what she experiences
as the father's going beyond boundaries. Through this waterfall of words, she tells how she experiences that he is taking her space and how she slammed the door and left. "He is taking my
space -- and it is clear to me, that it is because I'm not able to create it myself," she says. "I
have only learned how to create my boundaries the hard way, but I can feel that there is something I have to learn, something about space.*

From the very first moments, everything Clara is telling through her words and bodily communication is about space. Her quick entry into the room, her telling about moving into the space between father and son, the experience of her husband taking her
space, and the statement of not being able to create her own space, all indicate -- as she
also formulates it herself -- a readiness to learn what this *something* about space is. At
this point it is already visible that the spaces Clara is talking about are different kinds of
spaces. These include the concrete and symbolic space with the slamming of the door,
the interpersonal space between father and son, her and her husband, and the inner experience of a space which can be *taken* or *created*. Clara has already defined space herself as having multiple meanings and touching embodied patterns of a lifelong, and perhaps also cultural, learning about space and boundaries. This may not only be connected to the solution of her actual problem. According to Merleau-Ponty, the human
body is an expressive space which contributes to the significance of personal actions.
The body is also the origin of expressive movement and a medium for perception of the
world. "Our body is not primarily *in* space: it is *of* it" as Merleau-Ponty writes (Merleau-Ponty, 1962, p. 171).

With the one year old girl Nina, we saw how quickly and focused she expresses her
frustration through movements and emotions, marking the boundaries of her personal
space in a social setting. Even if she has no words, she does have a connection to a clarity and unity in her communication, which most of us probably learn to move away
from as we grow up.

In Clara's case, on the contrary, *something* is disturbing the dynamic flow in her expressive space, and that is what she is going to inquire about and possibly change through movement. This *something* might be difficult to reach through words, and that is exactly the point at which movement may be a fruitful animator for the non-verbal sources and tacit knowledge of the body. Creative inner research about the connections between motion and emotion is actually in dance movement therapy the most fundamental vehicle through which an individual can engage in personal integration towards a clearer definition of self (Payne, 1992). Until now, we have met Clara primarily through the verbal communication, although the process is already moving through her body language as well. We shall now go further, exploring what is happening with her through a dancing journey with unity of inner and outer movement, motion and emotion, using the energy-based dance therapy form Dansergia.

Moving Down

As she is speaking, her hands are moving like knives in front of her, cutting in the air. Then her whole torso lifts up, while her arms and hands are moving softly to the sides." I have learned to move away from it" she says while lifting the shoulders. I invite her to stand on her feet and move slightly from side to side while feeling the contact to her center. After a while I ask her to research the dynamic of the two movements: the downwards cutting and the lifting and spreading out her shoulders, arms, breast and back. She continues with the up-and-down movement, going more and more into an inner research. After a while, the downward movement gets stronger, and her hands begin to pull together. She is moving more and more downward: down to the ground, down in the pelvis, down in the legs.

The cutting hands and the lifting torso are connected to Clara's daily body language although she is in the moment in a situation where she is going consciously into her personal dynamics. These apparently accidental signs of her body language are very intense and condensed movements. They are important resources in Dansergia for learning about possible embodied habits and patterns. Therefore, the cutting and lifting movements, together with the grounding and centering movements and awareness of the breath, create an organic continuation of the movement session, letting the body speak.

Dansergia has as mentioned a holistic approach and is inspired from both Eastern and Western energy concepts (Sabetti, 1986; 1992; 1993; 2001). Dansergia is developed from ancient traditions of world cosmology and healing. In almost every civilisation, modern as well as ancient, a concept of life energy understood as a universal force bringing everything in movement has existed (Sabetti, 1986 p.1). In early China, life energy was called *chi*, in India *prana*. The theory on which Dansergia is based furthermore balances current psychology and psychotherapy as well as modern physics, including connections to Einstein's believing in nature's wholeness (Sabetti, 1986; 2001). Energy is a complex phenomenon seen as the dynamic and vital expression of life in all systems. Every system, organic or inorganic, may be described by its quality of energy flow. Energy is basically *movement* (Sabetti, 2001; Zoetler et al., 2001, p.56).

As this dance movement therapy form is based on multilevel energy work, these first phases of grounding and centering are very important to ensure that Clara is really present and aware. Grounding is a well-known concept in electricity, for example for directing lightening to the ground. Alexander Lowen (Lowen, 1977) used the concept of grounding in an energetic and therapeutic perspective in order to describe the importance of channelling energy down to the ground. He realized that grounding supported the body with a reality base (Boadella, 1985; Lowen, 1977; Sabetti, 1978; 2001). Sometimes grounding is seen as a one-way phenomenon through which the body discharges energy into the ground. However, grounding, as Sabetti states (Sabetti, 1978), may be seen as a two-sided phenomenon. Just as the person is acting on the ground, so is the ground acting on the person. Furthermore, grounding is connected to the body's communication and contact points with the surrounding world. "Grounding can come through all of the contact points of the body, though the eyes, the feet, the hands and the skin appear to be the most important" (Sabetti, 1978, p. 14). Centering is done through contact to the core of the body, in the Orient known as "*hara*," in order to support the person in being able to effectively deal with the process in a focused and stable way (Sabetti, 1978; 2001). Physically, this center is located just below the navel and is manifest as a pulsating movement at the midpoint of the core of the body.

> *"Emotionally the hara is the seat of all deep feelings of anger, sadness, love and fear. Though other parts of the body are responsible for specific expression of emotions it is the hara from which the energy source of these emotions seems to derive. In dance, karate, T'ai Chi and meditation the hara is universally known as the lotus of balance, gravity and self-control" (Sabetti, 1978, p. 8).*

The center or hara might as such be regarded as the primal contact base of the body, balancing and stabilising the movement flow. If many people, including Clara, have learned to move away from this also very physical contact point, it might be important to re-connect in order to feel and express the connection between inner and outer movement.

The Crocodile Beyond the Cutting Hands

A sound comes. It's like an animal sound. Her hands are grabbing in the air, and I ask her to explore this. The movements are getting more powerful, the sound wilder, and soon she is moving on all fours. Her hips are moving back and forth, back and forth as in sexual movements. "I have to take care of my shoulder" she says, moving more down onto the floor. I ask her what is going on. She says that it is a crocodile. The wild sound continues. After a while, the crocodile moves onto two legs. Standing stable on her feet and moving slightly with her pelvis, Clara begins hitting with her hands in the air. The sound seems to go deeper, into her throat and stomach, "aaaargh".

As the body is seen as an expression of the person, it is possible to observe a compromise in the body in terms of movement and posture. Diagnosis in Dansergia is based on the view that every system is a whole. This diagnosis based on *holysis* is in contrast to analysis, which means to look at symptoms as isolated parts. A holysis view allows an identification of patterns of holding and possibilities for growth (Zoetler et al., 2001).

> *"In a holysis we look at many movements in a living system simultaneously. We observe how different parts fit together, how their connections affect each other, and what happens if a movement is changed in some way". (Zoetler et al., 2001, p.66)*

One aspect of a holysis is to observe both the static body as it stands, and the moving body in terms of a one-pointed focus in the center and any movement away from this point. "This can show for example how a person moves away upwards; lifting him/herself off the ground perhaps to avoid deeper contact issues connected with the earth" (Zoetler, 2001, p. 66). Each person tries to protect him/herself and his /her feelings, denying psychological themes, and these patterns may be visible in the body. In Clara's case it is obvious already from her body language in the verbal inquiry that she is moving away from something by lifting her shoulders, and saying "*I have learned to move away from it.*" Therefore, movement inquiry into this moving with the polarities up *and* down is important in order for her to feel what this *it* is beyond the cutting hands and the upward shoulder movement. Is she avoiding her own power? Actually, through this movement inquiry Clara is moving into a being, an animal, a crocodile. Being in contact with *animal qualities,* which are often visible also in daily habits of moving, eating and making sounds might give useful messages about e.g. resources or patterns of self-protection, such as in Clara's case (Zoetler et al., 2001).

Beyond the *hard* boundaries, Clara already knows, in her daily life -- perhaps expressed verbally or non-verbally by slamming the door -- are the resources and quality of a crocodile. This exploring of the inner powerful crocodile seems in Clara's case to be spontaneous movements coming to her. The continuity of her being in a stream of movements which just develop out of the first simple movement indicates that she is neither trying nor performing. The movement quality of a crocodile seems simply to be moving through her body.

LEVELS OF MOVEMENT
Increasing the Multidimensionality of the Body

Then her hands spontaneously begin shaking in very small quick movements. She is moving with it, letting her arms get more and more involved while her breath gets deeper. I ask her what it is. "It is the sauce" she says." All this sauce I'm filled with from all the others." I let her stay in this sauce for a while. The shaking grows to her shoulders, and her back begins moving. "How does it feel to be in this sauce" I ask, slightly confronting her. "Horrible" she says with a deep voice.

In the shaking hands and Clara's experience of being filled with the *sauce* of others, it is clearly visible that also in this part of the process, Clara's movements are not only connected to her object body as a physiological phenomenon, but to a body with multiple layers of movement and meanings. This *sauce of the others* that she is *filled with* also indicates that movement and influence can go on at very subtle levels. In Clara's case the *sauce* has inhabited her body and is now disturbing her own space. These meanings might be explained by increasing the multidimensionality of movement further, as something going on at different *levels.* Seeing movement in a broader perspective, again through the concept of energy, might answer some aspects of Samson's and Sparkes´ call for a psychology which include the body and yet does not exclude culture, history and community; a psychology which is overcoming dualism by perceiving the body as a unity.

From an energetic point of view, human beings are regarded as complex systems with a *multi-level* of energy processes. From this perspective, each individual is seen as the embodiment of a unique energy vibration, which includes the culture, history and lived life of the person. If the energy flow is interrupted, problems will evolve. These interruptions might, as seen from this perspective, manifest themselves at the body and movement levels, and will appear as disharmony in the body structure, hyper- and hypo-tensed muscles, and in the quality of movement as the body tries to balance itself (Sabetti, 1978; 2001) The body looses grace (Lowen, 1977). Simple movements in the body can be observed as being moved with ease or not. If somebody is using only the muscle tonus necessary for the movement, grace is there (Zoetler et al., 2001, p. 58). If grace is missing, this might indicate a disturbance manifested as a contradiction or pushing on the natural energy flow, a process which may have many reasons. Therefore, a very important principle in Dansergia is that every movement includes many energy levels: the *physical, mental, psychological, emotional, social, cultural* and *spiritual* (Sabetti, 2001; Zoetler et al., 2001, p. 58). These levels include the person's identity and life historical aspects and are connected to body, thought, being, feelings and emotions, social and cultural contexts and at the spiritual level the very essence of being, beyond the "I." Dissonant vibrations at any level will from this point of view affect all the other levels. Unexpressed feelings may create a conflict in the whole system. An outgoing movement which is repressed or suppressed manifests itself as a result in bound energy movements visible in the body (Sabetti, 2001). Letting movements move through the different levels at the same time is possible by being aware of the movement quality, directions, breath, space and time, as well as of body parts and their connections (Sabetti, 2001; Zoetler et al., 2001).

Dancing while deeply involved in one's own feelings is only possible when the dancing person is connected to his/her own healing possibilities. Returning to Clara's process, it is obvious that the spontaneous shaking movement with the hands experiencing the *sauce* of others, is a process moving at many levels at the same time. Physically it is moving in her body, psychologically she is conscious about what is going on and what the movement means, emotionally she is beginning to feel the internal *horrible* experience of being filled with the *sauce*, -- although she is not in the moment strongly expressing it externally as e-motion. Socially and culturally, she is saying clearly again that her experience is connected to the themes of space and boundaries. *The sauce of the others* might be seen as elements of the embodied socially learned patterns that she through her embodied life history has repressed in her body. She is no longer able to express the feelings or needs behind this. Could this *sauce* also involve *cultural* aspects of how to behave or not behave, how to react or not react, according to culturally embodied norms? The multidimensional body is seen through these "glasses" as a complex phenomenon, constantly embodying and expressing movements on many levels. The multidimensional body is a unity and not only body-mind. This body is in the here and now, as the case of Clara shows: it is "lived" in a very concrete way, and also wears social, cultural, and biographical traces.

Energy Dynamics in Embodied Space

"What does this sauce keep you away from?"" From following my need and lust," she says. "And if you follow that now?" Now a soft dance is evolving from the core of her body. Her breasts and hips are moving softly together. Her hands are exploring her face. They are softly grasping onto the skin of her cheeks and her half-opened mouth. Her hands float down to contact her stomach and thighs. Then she moves almost only the right side of her body. Her voice seems like it is coming from a place very far away. "It is my husband. I keep on feeling that he is taking my space and that I have to protect myself," she says, still moving only her

right arm. "Does he hear you?" I ask with a silent voice. "No" she says. "Are you aware that you are only moving your right side?" I ask. Silently she nods. "How would the boundary be if you involved also you left side?" I say. Her left hand begins slowly to move as if exploring totally new land, while tears stream down her cheeks. "The left is afraid of wizening" she says. "And if you continue?"" It would be a soft boundary with the heart," she says. Now she is dancing a very slow, intense and soft dance while her left and right sides are coming together. Melting tears are finding their own ways to flow down her cheeks. "Is it wizening, the left side?" I ask. She shakes her head. "No, it is only misused." She is now slightly moving forward. Her breath seems to flow more freely with a bigger volume. Calmness and release is filling the room. After a while, I ask her to find a way of rounding up. She is still standing. I sit down by the wall. After a while she says: "I feel that I just have to sit here with you for a while." Then she sits down just close enough so that we touch each other. She is touching me with her left side. She is breathing deeply. Then she takes my hand smiling through the tears with warm cheeks, now also decorated with black unlinear traces of mascara. "Thank you," she says. Now a pearling laughter comes. "What an adventure in space -- from crocodile to woman. (Clara, January 2005)

As Clara moves into this dance from the core of her body, also in contact with the emotional level, it becomes clear that it is not enough to protect her space in the old way -- from the right side. By letting more movement levels become involved, she is now able to feel the fear of wizening, and the misuse of the left side. This might indicate that Clara, even though she of course often moves her left side, has been holding it unmoved on other levels in order *not* to feel the fear and misuse. Getting in contact with it now and letting the left side move gives her a possibility to heal and change the pattern by exploring the *soft boundary with the heart*.

This left and right may be connected to the term *polarities* or *energy dynamics*. According to many understandings of energy, from physics to philosophy, energy does not seem to be content, but *process* -- moving in polarities from one pole to another, e.g. left and right, up and down, in and out (Pierrakos, 1990; Sabetti, 1978; 1993; 2001). This polarity or dynamic occurs on the physical level through balanced movements between for example upper and lower portions of the body and left and right sides; on the psychological level by balancing, for example power and softness, trust and distrust (Sabetti, 1978).

Being stuck in one polarity will, as seen from this perspective, prevent fluid movement, also in interaction with others. Regarding the emotional level, Sabetti writes that:

"Emotionally fluid polarity is achieved through a balanced expression of feelings, for example and openness of loving needs to be complemented by the protective quality of anger, when important" (Sabetti, 1978, p. 7).

Seen in the perspectives of Lowen and Sabetti, anger is an important emotion in the life of all creatures since it serves to maintain and protect the physical and psychological integrity of the organism (Lowen, 1995; Sabetti, 1989). The emotion of anger is part of the larger function of aggression, which literally means "to move toward." *Aggression* is the opposite of *regression*, which means "to move back" (Lowen, 1995; Sabetti; 1989).

The little girl Nina is balancing her openness and joyfully moving up and down, up and down with the clear boundary of anger -- her right arm. In Clara's case, the protective quality of *boundaries in the hard way* needs to be transformed into a constructive and protective power balanced by soft boundaries with the heart. She needs to learn to surrender to feelings without loosing her strength. Coming closer to this balance over time, not just in one session as described here, might give new possibilities in her space, with multiple layers of meaning -- some of them now more visible than before.

MOVEMENT AS PRIMARY LANGUAGE
Summary and Discussion

Hopefully this chapter has shown some of the potentials of narrative research, that "what" is researched came together with "how" it is expressed, and that the organic expressive moving writing style has been meaningful to the reader. In this chapter, movement as primary language has been explored through the examples of Clara and Nina. Using the phenomenological concept of *the lived body*, and concepts of energy, multilevel movements, and energy dynamics in relation to Dansergia it has been argued that movement is a multidimensional phenomenon of such variety that it has been possible to touch on only a few of its aspects here. Working consciously with the multidimensionality of movements, including understanding in terms of energy, adds new perspectives to the field of dance movement therapy. As movement may be considered the body's mother tongue, a future perspective may arise as well, transforming these approaches into the sphere of movement pedagogy. This opens possibilities in a wide range of professions, which might for example support children's identity processes, as movement -- as we have seen -- also is pre-reflective and can touch levels of meaning and identity issues before or beyond verbal language. Living in a global world has apparently given us, on the one hand, almost unlimited possibilities for making a lifelong issue out of creating and developing one's own identity. On the other hand, it carries the risk of developing rootless individuals. Being connected in a constant dialogue between inner and outer movements, staying in contact with the flow of fundamental vitality and life energy experienced in the body, may be helpful to many individuals, children as well as adults, when it comes to managing the challenges of living in a rapidly changing world.

REFERENCES

Bagley, C., & Cancienne, M. B. (Eds.). (2002). *Dancing with the data*. New York: Peter Lang.

Belgrad, J. (1997). Szenisches Verstehen als Grundlage tiefenhermeneutischer Interpretation [Scenic Understanding as Fundament for Depth Hermeneutic Interpretation], *Politisches Lernen, 3/4*, 7-26.

Bruner, E. M. (1986). Experience and its Expressions. In E. Bruner & V. Turner (Eds.). *The Anthropology of Experience* (pp. 3-30). Urbana: University of Illinois Press.

Boadella, D. (1985). Bio-Energie und Körpersprache [Bio-Energetics and Body Language]. In H. Petzold (Eds.). *Die neuen Körpertherapien* (pp. 14-51). Paderborn: Jungfermann Verlag.

Engel, L. (2001). Krop, psyke, verden [Body, Mind, World]. Højbjerg: Hovedland/Institut for Idræt.

Fraleigh, S. H. (1987). *Dance and the Lived Body*. Pittsburg: University of Pittsburg.

Grønlund, E. (Ed.). (1999). *Konstnärliga terapier. Bild, dans och musik i den läkande processen.* [Art Therapies. Picture, Dance, and Music in the Healing Process]. Stockholm: Natur og kultur.

Halprin, D. (2004). *The Expressive Body in Life, Art and Therapy*. Philadelphia: Jessica Kingsley Publishers.

Hastrup, K. (2003). Metoden. Opmærksomhedens retning [The Method. The Direction of Awareness]. In K. Hastrup (Ed.). *Ind i verden. En grundbog om antropologisk metode* (pp. 399-419). København: Hans Reitzel.

Levy, Fran (1992). *Dance/Movement Therapy: A Healing Art*. Reston, VA: The American Alliance for Health, Physical Education, Recreation and Dance.

Lorenzer, A. (1986). *Kulturanalysen, psychoanalytischen Studien zur Kultur* [Culture Analysis. Psychoanalytic Studies of Culture]. Frankfurt a.M.: Fischer Wissenschaft.

Lowen, A. (1977). *The Way to Vibrant Health.* New York: Harper Colophon Books.

Lowen, A. (1982). *The Language of the Body.* New York: Macmillan.

Lowen, A. (1995). *Den guddommelige krop* [The Spirituality of the Body].København: Borgen.

Lowen, A. (1995). *Joy. The Surrender of Body to Life.* New York: Penguin Compass.

Merleau-Ponty, M. (1962/2004). *Phenomenology of Perception.* New York: Routledge.

Merleau-Ponty, M (1968/2000). *The Visible and the Invisible.* Evanston: North Western University Press.

Payne, H. (1992). *Dance movement therapy: theory and practise.* London: Routledge.

Petzold, H. (1985). *Die neuen Körpertherapien* [The New Body Therapies]. Paderborn: Jungfermann Verlag.

Pierrakos, J. C. (1990). *Core Energetics.* Mendocino: LifeRhythm Publication.

Richardson, L. (2000). Writing. In N. Denzin & Y. Lincoln (Eds.). *Handbook of qualitative research* (2nd ed., pp. 923-943). London: Sage.

Sabetti, S. (1978). *Energy Concepts of Life Energy Therapy.* München: Institute for Life Energy.

Sabetti, S. (1986). *Wholeness Principle.* Sherman Oaks, CA: Life Energy Media.

Sabetti, S. (1989). *Expressive Energy 1.* München: Institute for Life Energy.

Sabetti, S. (1992). *Dansergia.* Sherman Oaks, CA: Life Energy Media.

Sabetti, S. (1993). *Waves of Change.* Sherman Oaks, CA: Life Energy Media.

Sabetti, S. & Freligh, L. (Eds.). (2001). *Life Energy Process, Forms -- Dynamics Principles.* München: Life Energy Media.

Sparkes, A. (2002). *Telling Tales in Sport and Physical Activity. A qualitative Journey.* New York: Human Kinetics.

Sparkes, A. (2003). Bodies, Identities, Selves: Autoethnographic Fragments and Reflections. In J. Denison & P. Markula (Eds.). *Moving Writing: Crafting Movement in Sport and Research* (pp. 51-76). New York: Peter Lang.

Sparkes, A. (2005). Reflections on an embodied Sport and Exercise Psychology. In R. Stelter & K. Roessler (Eds.). *New Approaches to Sport and Exercise Psychology* (pp. 31-55). Oxford: Meyer & Meyer Sport.

Tamalpa Institute (2005). *The Tamalpa Institute.* http://www.tamalpa.org/HTML/Home.html Retreived 04/20/05.

Zoetler, P., Persson, V., Stühler, V; Sabetti, S. (2001). Dansergia. In S. Sabetti & L. Freligh (Eds.). *Life Energy Process, Forms – Dynamics -- Principles* (pp. 55-73). München: Life Energy Media.

DANCE THERAPY AS PERSON-CENTRED CARE

Heather Hill

This chapter describes what has been learnt through a dance therapist's process of research in the field of dance therapy and dementia. This process began with a study of the experiential meaning of dance therapy for a person with dementia and moved on to the wider context of dementia care, specifically person-centred care. Coming full circle the author came to understand how dance therapy might be enhanced and expanded within a person-centred framework. Furthermore, she believes that the body wisdom of dance therapy may equally enrich the field of person-centred care in dementia.

Keywords: Dementia, person-centred care, DMT, aged care, phenomenology.

RESEARCHING THE DANCE THERAPY EXPERIENCE IN DEMENTIA

Introduction

There comes a time in the development of one's professional work, when it seems necessary to move outside the doing of the work and look more closely at the nature of what one is doing, to question, to sharpen understanding, to submit belief and conviction to rigorous scrutiny. After many years of working in the field of dementia as a dance therapist, the author embarked on a process of research over a period of 12 years, which included two research studies in dance therapy in dementia and a doctoral study of person-centred care.

In this chapter, the words "Alzheimer's Disease" and "dementia" will be used interchangeably -- following common usage -- although in fact there are at least 60 different forms of dementia, of which the degenerative dementias are the most typical form and Alzheimer's the most common.

Dementia: The Context for the Study

Dance therapists in the field of dementia work within a context dominated by biomedical perspectives on dementia. In this context, Alzheimer's Disease is viewed as an irreversible process whereby brain cells are progressively destroyed and for which there is no known preventative or curative method. More recently developed medications such as Aricept may preserve function a little longer, but cannot halt the process, which is progressive and inevitably impacts on all aspects of functioning. The person experiences a "slow downward course of mental, physical and social deterioration" (Snowdon, 2001, p.87). Bit by bit, the person with dementia is seen to lose all those aspects, which make him or her a person. This process is variously described as "loss of self" (Cohen and Eisdorfer, 1986), "death that leaves the body behind" (cited in Kitwood, 1997), "dissolution of the self" (Symonds, cited in Gidley and Shears, 1987). The person is no longer believed to be able to think or even feel, nor to be capable of intentional action. His or her behaviour is viewed as a symptom of the disease, to be controlled by behaviour management techniques or, as is more frequently the case, by medication. The self of the person with dementia, from a biomedical perspective, is most notable by its absence.

Since there is no cure, care is mainly custodial, ensuring the person is physically cared for and prevented from harming him- or herself, or others. While activities are now often a legislative requirement, they are still considered optional extras and are the first to be cut in hard financial times. For the person with dementia it is, all in all, a bleak picture offering little hope.

Aim of the Study

The purpose of this study was to understand the subjective experience of dance therapy for a person with dementia. Was the dance therapy experience meaningful for the person him or herself?

Methodological Considerations

Apart from the usual challenges of researching a complex and subjective human experience, there were additional methodological challenges due to the nature of dementia and the expressive and communicative difficulties of the person. The author selected a phenomenological methodology, which seemed appropriate to a topic concerned with understanding lived experience. "Phenomenological research aims to understand the meaningfulness of human experience as it is actually lived" (Barrell et al., 1987, p.447). In the phenomenological methodology, the researcher sets aside as far as possible preconceptions, theories, etc. (bracketing), and approaches the material through a cyclical process of description, reflection, progressive focusing and writing. Phenomenology seeks to explicate the essence, structure, or form of both human experience and human behaviour as revealed through essentially descriptive techniques including disciplined reflection. (Valle & Halling, 1987, p. 6)

Consistent with post-positivist approaches to research, the data was created through multiple perspectives and multiple modes of data collection. The presence of the researcher's perspective was overtly acknowledged and also worked with through a devil's advocate procedure, whereby the therapist had to verbally respond to the challenges to her findings made by her music therapy colleague. This process was documented as part of the final research report.

The author must admit here to sharing at that time a prejudice in the dementia field that it would be impossible to obtain coherent verbal feedback from the a person with dementia and anticipated that the data would be drawn solely from observation. Goldsmith (1996), in his study on opportunities and obstacles to "hearing the voice of people with dementia", notes:

> "The situation for people with dementia is that few people take either the time or the trouble to ascertain their views. This is presumably largely because they think that the nature of their illness means that self-reflection and expression are rarely possible and also because to attempt it is often a slow and laborious task. However, recognising that it is difficult is not the same thing as saying that it cannot be done." (p. 15)

Fortunately, on the advice of her supervisor, the author did attempt to collect the person's verbal material. The results in this instance were quite surprising. In moving beyond her own observations and reflections to the words and thoughts of the person with dementia, the author was able to access a whole other realm of meaning concerning the patient's experience.

Description of the Study

The study consisted of four individual dance therapy sessions with an 85 year old woman with moderate dementia, E., who was a patient in the assessment ward of a psychiatric/psychogeriatric hospital. The therapist -- the author of this chapter -- is an Australian-trained dance therapist who worked in this field for twenty years and had established the dance therapy position in the hospital. Each of the sessions was improvised, the dance therapist working solely with what occurred in the moment and a music therapist responding improvisationally to the dance/movement interaction. The sessions were videotaped. A few hours after the session, E. and the author watched a video of the session, and this in turn was videotaped in order to capture any verbal or non-verbal feedback.

Data Analysis

There were two major levels of analysis: On the one hand the in-depth analysis of the movement material in session 1 (that is, observational) on the other hand the analysis of the verbal transcripts (that is, the person's perspective through her words).

Session 1 Movement Material

Over many years of working in the field of dementia, the author had noticed that there were moments in a dance therapy session which "stood out", in which the person with dementia seemed to respond in a more integrated way. For this reason the author decided to identify and study in depth what she called "significant moments". She did not attempt to operationally define "significance". Rather, she selected from the video footage of the session those moments, which intuitively (based on her experience as a dance therapist) stood out for her.

The process of analysis of the movement material was adapted from Giorgi's phenomenological analysis of verbal transcripts (1985) and incorporated:

Naïve description. The movement material was described in as neutral terms as possible, that is not incorporating any dance therapy movement analysis tool such as Laban Movement Analysis (LMA).

Creation of Meaning Units: A separate meaning unit was created every time some change was noted in the description. The nature of the change was not defined in advance.

Focusing

Whereas Giorgi suggested certain psychological perspectives be applied in the rewriting and focusing, the author applied a dance therapy understanding to focus the material. The following aspects emerged as key foci in the material: movement quality (in relation to weight, space, time); flow of energy; interaction; affect. These aspects were studied individually, and comparisons among each of these were made across meaning units.

Music therapy analysis: An additional focus was the music, the analysis of which was carried out by the music therapist. His findings served as a comparison and validation for the dance analysis.

Indwelling: This was a cyclical process of "sitting with" the material, reflection and writing, which represented a progressive distillation of the data.

Making sense. It was only at this stage that the author began to draw on the literature, which would help illuminate the meanings emerging from the movement material. This literature came from writings on dementia, dance, dance therapy, Laban Movement Analysis, philosophy (embodiment), neuroscience, person-centred care, and on the self.

Verbal transcripts sessions 1-4: Perspective of the person with dementia

The author applied Giorgi's (1985) form of phenomenological analysis to the verbal transcripts.

Research Findings: Observational

Analysis of the Significant Moments of Session 1

E. moved during the significant moments in a more integrated fashion, which was very different from her confused and at times fearful state. She showed a marked preference for weight effort, particularly towards the strong end of the continuum. E herself confirms that the quality of strength for instance was very much part of her self-image ("I must have grown up with strength, Hill, 1995, p. 183). Her daughter confirmed that E. appeared to be more her old self on the video. These moments then appeared to represent an authentic expression of E.

An analysis of the movement descriptions based on Laban Movement Analysis, revealed increased complexity in the quality of movement and in the interaction, and an integration of movement qualities (weight, space, time), energy and affect in those moments. She seemed at ease within herself and conveyed a sense of personal mastery. If one takes Fraleigh's (1987) definition of dance as being characterised by heightened sensibility, expressiveness, aliveness, integration of body, mind, and feeling and an aesthetic quality, which go beyond the everyday and the merely functional, then E.'s movement in the significant moments could rightly be termed "dance".

Overview of session 1: Through the process of describing, focusing, indwelling and ongoing reflection and writing as noted above, the following overview of the session was created (Hill, 1995):

The first two significant moments introduced elements -- relationship, tiredness, bursts of energy, testing strength, humour -- which were explored more fully in the last significant moment. In the early stages, tiredness interfered with E.'s natural impulse to respond to humour, contact and strength. It was indeed the very acceptance of this tiredness by both H. and E., which seemed to liberate E. in some way from its power and which established the relationship on a more equal basis. Without this self-acceptance and trust in the relationship with H., it is doubtful E. could have undertaken the more risky testing out which occurred in the final significant moment.

In significant moment 3, she fully tested herself and H. and was very much in control of the action. E. revealed herself to be a person of high energy, strength, and humour, who enjoyed being in control but also felt confident enough to share power. The final resolution of the session comes in the scene of being friends, the emphasis resting on the word "being". No longer, is there a need to do, to act, to test out, to prove. There is simply acceptance and self-acceptance.

E. has made a significant journey in this session. No longer is she the tired, uncertain, unsure E of the early part of the session. Tiredness itself is no longer the enemy. It has been accepted and transformed into relaxation, ease of being. E. is no longer a patient, a follower, but an equal partner (p. 52).

The relationship established in this first session was a strong one, which underpinned all subsequent sessions despite each session being very different from the other. Indeed the relationship survived beyond the period of the research. When the therapist visited

E. on later occasions, she was always greeted as an old friend with whom she had experienced many things.

E.'s perspective of the experience as a whole (Analysis of the verbal transcripts)

Each of the sessions was quite different from the others. However, the transcripts revealed a process of continuous growth and change within E., a process which transcended individual sessions. This was most notable in her response to the videotaped "E.". In the first session, E. continually referred to "her" rather than "me" and despite assurances that it was indeed E. herself, she would not accept it. It may be argued that this is not unusual in a person with dementia. However, it seemed to the author that it was an existential, rather than a pathological, issue, that it was more about her being unable to identify with the strong, gutsy woman on screen. For example, while watching session 1, she commented: "Oh, that's not me...I'm not as good looking as that" (Hill, 1995, p.166). She certainly enjoyed watching this person and commented on the person's feelings and actions:

E.: "I think she's trying to pull him off the chair." (E identified the therapist on the video as a boy) Shortly after, E. in fact does so on the video. E. gives a hearty laugh and leans forward in her chair. Good on you mate (laughing). The boy wouldn't be able to believe he was beaten like that (Hill, 1995, p. 169).

By the time of the second video viewing session, she was sometimes using "I" and sometimes still "she". By the third video session, she was using "I" all the time, and indeed the "I" on the screen seemed mainly to have relevance to her as a reflection of herself and a path to reminiscence.

Over the course of the sessions, E went from lack of recognition of the woman in the video to recognising of herself and owning and reintegrating the positive qualities she saw. While watching the video, she said positive things about herself ("I'm glad I'm strong", Hill, 1995, p.179; "If my children see that, I don't think they'll recognise Mum", Hill, 1995, p.179), and it seemed to be only the prospect of ending the research sessions, which brought again some of her negative, fearful comments.

In between sessions, E. evidently was thinking about and reflecting on them with enjoyment. She started to think about the old times. "I've got together again. I talk about old times with myself now ...and I think it's brought me out...Wake up" (Hill, 1995, p.196).

Despite the limited time, a strong relationship was formed between E. and the therapist. E. was flattered to have been chosen for the research and very aware of her responsibility within it.

Conclusions on the Nature of the Dance Therapy Experience for E.

From the author's observations, it was clear that within the so-called "significant moments", E. functioned in a more integrated way, cognitively, emotionally, and bodily. However, E.'s own words gave a wider perspective on the experience as a whole, an experience which was about eliciting and affirming the self in the moment and facilitating a process of growth in her perception of self and self-worth.

Watching the video may have offered a way for E. to reflect on the movement experience and to re-integrate the qualities she saw on the screen with herself in the here and now. The therapeutic process for E. was therefore the actualisation of self through movement, the reinforcing of the self-image through watching herself dance, and further reinforcement and reintegration of the self through subsequent moving.

E. was very aware that things had changed for her through the dance experience and the relationship with the therapist. During the last viewing, she said: "Thank you for bringing me out of my shell" (Hill, 1995, p.193). It is interesting to note that in contrast to the first session where "I" was nowhere in evidence, in this remark, she not only uses the word "me" but emphasises it.

Bearing in mind the traditional wisdom that dementia is a progressive and irreversible disease, the challenge of the author's dance therapy study to traditional knowledge about dementia was twofold:

Firstly that a person with dementia who was confused, with cognitive and functional difficulties, could function at such an integrated level in the dance therapy session and, secondly, that a person with dementia could change and grow over a period of time.

STUDIES IN PERSON-CENTRED CARE IN DEMENTIA

It was in the course of the study with E., that the author became aware of the person-centred approach to dementia care, which seemed to be much more in tune with the author's professional experience and study in dance therapy, and her personal philosophy. The author's research findings were indeed quite consistent with a person-centred perspective on dementia. Subsequent doctoral studies in person-centred care have informed the author's understanding not only of dementia but also of the role of dance therapy in this field. These are discussed below.

Person-centred care as it has been developed in dementia, in particular through the pioneering work of the late Tom Kitwood, offers an alternative perspective on dementia care, in terms of an understanding of dementia, of the person with dementia, of the role of carer and the nature of care. This will be discussed in more detail below.

Understanding of Dementia

While the biomedical model understands dementia solely in terms of brain pathology, person-centred approaches view this as only part of dementia. According to their view, the experience of dementia is formed by many other factors. This can be expressed in the following formula: $D=NI+PH+P+BH+PE+SE$ (Moore, 2002), that is, the experience of dementia (and the resulting behaviour) is the result of Neurological Impairment, Physical Health, and Personality, Background History, Physical Environment and Social Environment. This means that every person's experience of dementia will be very different. Significantly, it also means that carers can have considerable impact on the person's experience of dementia and fulfil more than a custodial role.

Understanding of the Person with Dementia

Writers on person-centred care criticise the long tradition in the West of defining human beings by their cognitive, intellectual function and suggest a broader understanding of the self. While the cognitive aspects of a person's functioning are attacked in dementia, the feeling aspects remain and may indeed become more intense. "Dementia strips people down to the essence of their being and frees them to be in more direct touch with their emotions" (Gibson, 1998, p. 6). The person may be acutely sensitive to the non-verbal, feeling aspects of their relationships and environment. Furthermore, person-centred theorists emphasise the relational aspects of the self, which suggests that the self is formed and developed at least in part through relationship. We all need relationship, but the person with dementia needs it even more to maintain a sense of self. Garratt and Hamilton-Smith (1995) reject the traditional view of the person with dementia as passive victim, suggesting rather that the person with dementia remains a meaning-seeking person, who is actively trying to cope with the effects of brain pathology and to make sense of his or her world. The person is an active agent in the creation and maintenance of self.

The person with dementia, then, remains a person with a self, albeit a self under attack. The person still thinks, feels and acts intentionally, even if the resulting actions do not always make sense to others. From a person-centred perspective the behaviour of the person with dementia is not a symptom of dementia, but is meaningful in terms of his or her lived experience.

The Role of Professional Carer

Relationship is paramount in person-centred care. It should be what Buber (1965) calls an I/Thou, not an I/It relationship. People with dementia, threatened in their grasp on self (by dementia) and in their personhood (by the prejudice of others that they are no longer "one of us", i.e., a person), need to be in an affirming, trusting and above all equal relationship with other human beings. Kitwood (1997) contrasts I/Thou to I/It, the latter implying:

Coolness, detachment, instrumentality. It is a way of maintaining a safe distance, of avoiding risks; there is no danger of vulnerabilities being exposed. The I/Thou mode, on the other hand, implies going out toward the other; self-disclosure, spontaneity -- a journey into uncharted territory (p. 10).

More than in any other area of care, the human qualities of the carer are equally if not more important than their practical and theoretical skills.

The Nature of Care in Dementia: Maintenance of Personhood

Kitwood identifies the key psychological task in dementia care as the maintenance of personhood. Maintenance of personhood may be teased out further into two main tasks (Hill, 2004): An ethical task, which is to continue to value the person with dementia, and a psychological/emotional task, which is to maintain and strengthen the self.

A task relating to, indeed arising from the above, is the promotion of well-being. Kitwood emphasises the possibility of creating a sense of well-being in people with dementia and suggests four "global sentient states" which might serve as indicators of well-being: "a sense of personal worth", "a sense of agency", "a feeling of being at ease with others, of being able to move towards them of having something to offer to them"; "hope -- a sense that the future will be, in some way, good" (Kitwood & Bredin, 1992, p. 283). Hope need not be cognitive, but can be understood as "basic trust". Garratt and Hamilton-Smith (1995), draw on the wellness ("Sense of Coherence") work of Antonovsky (1987), suggesting that well-being for the person with dementia -- as for all human beings -- lies in having an internal and external environment which has some structure and which makes sense (comprehensibility); in having a sense of control, of being able to deal with demands placed on them (manageability); and finally, in being engaged meaningfully in life (meaningfulness).

Antonovsky, in his work on wellness, closely links emotional and personal resilience (Sense of Coherence) to a strong sense of self. Viewed in this light, the promotion of well-being itself must involve the maintenance of personhood. Kitwood uses the term "malignant social psychology" to describe actions which detract from personhood, such as ignoring, discounting, and infantilizing. He also identifies positive self- and life-enhancing actions, which he terms "Positive Person Work".

Further developments arising within the person-centred approach have been the suggestion of a role for counselling therapy for some people with dementia, an emphasis on communication and the role of the arts in promoting well-being (Killick & Allan, 2001; Gibson, 1998), increased efforts to listen to "the voice of people with dementia" (Goldsmith, 1996) on the kind of care and support they need, and efforts to bring them back into the community of persons (Hill, 2004). People with dementia, from a person-centred perspective, are human beings who need support rather than management, who need relationship rather than custodial care and who remain active participants in the creation of their own lives.

DANCE THERAPY AS PART OF PERSON-CENTRED CARE

Person-centred care offers dance therapists a useful framework for working with people with dementia. In the first place dance therapy and person-centred care share a similar ethic:

An overall humanistic and holistic approach, which works with people rather than diagnoses, and facilitates rather than manages and controls recognition and acceptance of the person with dementia as a creative individual regardless of cognitive abilities the valuing of presence and the use of self (relationship) to promote well-being and growth in others.

Person-centred theory also expands on dance therapy theory in dementia and can therefore clarify and focus practice. As noted earlier, Kitwood (1997) identified actions -- Positive Person Work -- which enhance personhood and well-being: recognition, negotiation, collaboration, play, timalation (working with the senses), celebration, relaxation, validation, holding, and facilitation. To these, he added creating and giving on the part of the person with dementia (Kitwood, 1997). This is a useful formulation of elements frequent in dance therapy and provides a common language for dance therapists and other carers who work in a person-centred way.

Kitwood's listing of basic human needs which are particularly under threat in dementia -- attachment, identity, comfort, and (meaningful) occupation -- along with Antonovsky's Sense of Coherence (comprehensibility, manageability and meaningfulness) provide an expanded framework within which to formulate the work of dance therapy.

In dance therapy, through relationship and the accompanying trust, the person with dementia has a touchstone for the self and a secure base to expand out into the world. (identity, attachment, and comfort). The therapist reinforces and affirms the person, meeting the person in their reality. The person is encouraged to come "out of (his or her) shell" (Hill, 2004, p.193). The holding created by the therapist, by the rhythms, the movement, the music, and the therapeutic space, all create a coherence, a space which is not fragmented, a space which enables rather than disables, a space which allows the person to be. Within this space, the person may be able, through words and movements to communicate, to enact who he or she is, to be creative, to find "a space to be myself" (Hill, 2003). The therapist encourages the inclusion of the person in the group, inviting the person to participate in whatever way he or she is able. Finally, the therapist seeks ways to engage the person in what is meaningful to him or her. All the time the therapist works with the person's mind, feeling, and body, a unified approach, which creates unity and coherence, rather than fragmentation and madness.

Situating her dance therapy work in dementia in a person-centred care framework has greatly strengthened the author's own work and her ability to advocate for the use of dance therapy in dementia. Within the biomedical context, dance therapy is viewed at best as a pleasant diversion for people with dementia. In contrast, viewed from a person-centred perspective, dance therapy lies right at the heart of care, sharing its ethic and purpose.

PASSING ON THE WISDOM OF DANCE THERAPY:
WHAT DANCE THERAPY CAN CONTRIBUTE TO PERSON-CENTRED CARE
Embodiment

Despite the rejection of a purely cognitive definition of "person" and a more holistic approach to care, person-centred care has yet to fully incorporate the notion of embodiment. Adams (2005) notes the lack of attention paid to the embodied experience of people with dementia: "Just as a person's understanding of themselves is generated by what they do: so too people with dementia experience personhood through their embodied interaction with the outside and non-discursive world."

For dance therapists, embodiment lies at the heart of their work. They always work with embodied persons. In more recent years, this rejection of Cartesian dualism has had support from neuroscience, within the writings of Sacks (1991) and Damasio (1996) who view the body as an integral part of the sense of self. Damasio (1996) indeed suggests that being precedes thinking "We are, and then we think" (p.248). "Thinking" itself need not be defined narrowly as a purely cognitive process. In describing the process of improvisation, Sheet-Johnstone (1981), a dancer, talks of "thinking in movement". Also relevant is the view of the self as process. The self is a "repeatedly reconstructed biological state" (Damasio, 1996, p. 226). For all human beings, the self is continually being reconstructed, though of course for the person with dementia this process is much more radical and overwhelming. This notion of construction of self is found also in the writings of Wigman: "Dance was a means toward self-knowledge -- not a disclosure of personality but a construction of it, not self-expression as self-indulgence but a creation of self in expressive action..." (Wigman, cited in Fraleigh, 1987, p. xxii).

Dance therapists, therefore, are perfectly placed to bring the body more prominently into person-centred care, through their work with people with dementia, which offers "embodied" ways of contacting and helping to strengthen the self of the person with dementia. The work on communication of Killick and Allan (2001) already addresses non-verbal aspects of communication, but dance therapy has its own theoretical framework for understanding and working with people in their bodies and its own special skills, which could greatly enrich this work.

Body Learning

Developing Non-Verbal Skills in Care Staff

While dance therapists can offer useful the training in arts activities in dementia, a more important (because more fundamental) area would be the developing of the non-verbal skills and awareness of carers in their day to day care of people with dementia. Relating to a person who has reduced verbal/cognitive skills and heightened sensitivity to the non-verbal and the feeling realms will involve sensitivity to one's own bodily presence, to the bodily presence of the person, to non-verbal interaction and to the non-verbal aspects of the physical, social and emotional environment.

Developing Empathy

Sheard (2002), a trainer in dementia care, notes that it is not enough to teach skills, but that care staff need to develop empathy, to be able to recognise the personhood of the person with dementia and the fact that the feelings and needs of people with dementia are not that different from their own. This difficulty in empathising with people with dementia is a major hurdle in training people for person-centred work. The author in her own research in person-centred care found that attitudes, in particular the difficulty of seeing people with dementia as people who are still basically the same as other people, was a major barrier to creating a person-centred environment. The use of dance/movement in offering learning experiences through the body offers a powerful way for people to "get into the skin" of the person with dementia and understand their experience not only cognitively but also physically and emotionally. Indeed current neurological research on mirror neurons (Gallese, 2003) suggests that, developmentally, empathy begins at a body level, thus supporting an approach which starts with the body.

CONCLUSION

Person-centred care developed in response to the limitations of a strictly biomedical view of dementia and its pessimistic outlook for the person. It advocates for the person as a "sentient, relational, and historical being" who continues to seek meaning even in the most challenging circumstances. Dance therapy -- literally -- embodies this approach, and as such should come in from the margins of care to the very heart of person work in dementia. For the future, dance therapists must promote by their work, research, writing and training of others, the idea that people live in through their bodies, and that it is by addressing embodied persons (mind, body, and feeling), that we ultimately maintain and strengthen the personhood of all.

REFERENCES

Adams, T. (2005). *Re-thinking person-centred care: The social inclusion of people with dementia and their carers within dementia nursing.* Unpublished paper. University of Surrey, Guildford.

Antonovsky, A. (1987). *Unravelling the mystery of health: How people manage stress and stay well.* San Francisco, CA: Jossey-Bass.

Barrell, J.J., Aanstoos, C., & Richards, A.C. (1987). Human science research methods. *Journal of Humanistic Psychology,* 27(4), 424-457.

Buber, M. (1965). *The knowledge of man: A philosophy of the interhuman.* New York: Harper & Row.

Cohen, D., & Eisdorfer, C. (1986). *The Loss of self: A family resource for the care of Alzheimer's disease and related disorders.* W.W. Norton: New York.

Damasio, A. (1996). *Descartes' error: Emotion, reason, and the human brain.* London: Papermac.

Fraleigh. S.H. (1987). *Dance and the lived body.* Pittsburgh, P.A: University of Pittsburgh Press.

Gallese, V. (2003). The roots of empathy: The shared manifold hypothesis and the neural basis of intersubjectivity. *Psychopathology, 36,* 171-180.

Garratt, S., & Hamilton-Smith, E. (Eds.). (1995). *Rethinking dementia: An Australian approach.* Melbourne: Ausmed Publications.

Gibson, F. (1998, October 29-November 4). Unmasking dementia. *Community Care, 6-7.*

Gidley, I. Shears, R. (1989). *Alzheimers. What it is and How to Cope.* Australia: Allen and Unwin.

Giorgi, A. (1985). *Phenomenology and psychological research.* Pittsburgh, PA: Duquesne University Press.

Goldsmith, M. (1996). *Hearing the voice of people with dementia: Opportunities and obstacles.* London: Jessica Kingsley.

Hill, H. (1995). *An attempt to describe and understand moments of experiential meaning within the dance therapy process for a patient with dementia.* Masters dissertation, Latrobe University, Bundoora, Vic, Australia. Australian Digital Theses. Available at: http://www.lib.latrobe.edu.au/thesis/public/index.html, retreived 11/7/2005.

Hill, H. (2003). A space to be myself. *Signpost to older people and mental health matters, 7(3),* 37-39.

Hill, H. (2004). *Talking the talk but not walking the walk: Barriers to person centred care in dementia.* Doctoral Dissertation, Latrobe University, Melbourne. Australian Digital Theses. Available at: http://www.lib.latrobe.edu.au/thesis/public/adt-LTU20041215.100826/index.html, retrieved 11/7/2005.

Killick, J., & Allan, K. (2001). *Communication and the care of people with dementia.* Buckingham: Open University Press.

Kitwood, T. (1997). *Dementia reconsidered: The person comes first.* Buckingham: Open University Press.

Moore, V. (2002, June). *Covering all bases.* Paper presented at the Dementia Services Development Centre Biennial Conference, Sydney, NSW, Australia.

Sacks, O. (1991). *Awakenings.* London: Pan.

Sheard, D. (2002). Beyond mechanistic dementia care training are real feelings and real life. *Signpost to older people and mental health matters, 7(2),* 10-12.

Sheets-Johnstone, M. (1981). Thinking in movement. *Journal of Aesthetics and Art Criticism, 39(4),* 399-407.

Snowdon, D. (2001). *Ageing with Grace: What the nun study teaches us about leading longer, healthier and more meaningful lives.* New York: Bantam Books.

Valle, R.S., & Halling, S. (Eds.). (1989). *Existential-phenomenological perspectives in psychology: Exploring the breadth of human experience.* New York, NY: Plenum Press.

DANCE/MOVEMENT THERAPY: A RESOURCE FOR ONCOLOGY
PATIENTS AND AN APPROACH TO COMPREHENSIVE PATIENT CARE

Maria Eugenia Lacour

This chapter describes a 3-year dance/movement therapy (DMT) work with adult cancer patients in two different phases of illness: (Part a) during medical treatment aiming to enhance quality of life, treatment compliance and immune function, and (Part b) after completion of treatment and in social recovery. Part (a) depicts a long-term intervention process of 3 years that involved for the most part newly diagnosed cancer patients and Part (b) assesses a special short-term 9-week-DMT program taylor-made to suit particular needs of social recovery which involved mostly breast cancer patients after mastectomy. This study suggests that DMT is an effective resource for oncology patients during and after treatment, providing enhancement of quality of life, of adherence to treatment and, in remission stage, of social recovery. A somatically and expressively oriented psychosocial intervention, such as DMT, provides an important rehabilitation tool for a program of comprehensive care of the cancer patient by a multidisciplinary team.

Keywords: Immune system, oncology patients, DMT, dancetherapy, breast cancer patients, tango, adherence to medical treatment, quality of life (QoL), mastectomy.

PART A: DMT AS A TOOL TO ENHANCE QOL, TREATMENT COMPLIANCE, AND THE IMMUNE FUNCTION IN ONCOLOGY PATIENTS DURING TREATMENT

On Dance/Movement Therapy (DMT)

Dance/movement therapy is the psychotherapeutic use of movement and dance to favour the processes of physical, emotional, cognitive and social integration (ADTA, 2005). Since DMT provides emotional support and enhances interpersonal relationships (Chaiklin, 1975) it is of great value in cancer treatment (Dietrich, 1991). Likewise, DMT allows for a smooth and gradual reintroduction of movement possibilities previously suppressed by illness and allows for feelings which maybe too overwhelming to be expressed and worked on a symbolic level.

It is logical to surmise that if phenomena and changes in the physical body are a source of pain, distress, anger, or isolation, then a somatically oriented method of psychosocial support and intervention will have meaningful impact (see Goodill, this volume).

On Psychosocial Interventions for Cancer Patients

Methods and disciplines, such as psychology, relaxation techniques, cognitive-behavioral therapy or meditation, are reported in studies with cancer patients to improve QoL, survival, and/or parameters of the immunologic system (Spiegel, Bloom, Kraemer, & Gottheil; 1989, Fawzy, Fawzy, Hyun, Gutherie, Fahey, & Morton, 1993). Moreover, in the first explicit meta-analysis, Meyer (1995) concludes that psychosocial interventions should not be considered as optional or extra, but as an integral part of the management program of the illness.

Hypothesis

DMT groups for oncology patients enhance QoL, adherence to treatment and immune system function in oncology patients undergoing medical treatment and are a useful resource in the integral treatment of these patients.

Background

A search on scientific studies on immunology and cancer patients, directed our work towards chronic stress and immunology. These studies, such as one that demonstrates the increased development of skin cancer in the frame of chronic stress (Parker, 2004), suggest an intertwinement of tumor activity and the immune system "status".

On Immunologic Defenses and Cancer

The immunologic system combats cancer via cellular immunology (Abbas, 2004), such as the activity of natural killer cells and of T lymphocytes.

Regarding immunologic indicators, scientific evidence shows that psychological stress (e.g., university exams or divorce) depression and bereavement are associated with depressed immunologic activity, such as a decreased response of lymphocytes to mithogens and less cytotoxic activity of natural killer cells (Greer, Morris, & Pettingale, 1979; Herbert & Cohen, 1993; Bartrop, Luckhurst, Lazarus, Kiloh, & Penny, 1977). Conversely, psychosocial support and an optimistic way of facing life are associated with enhancing the above mentioned cytotoxic activity and lymphocite response (Irwin, Daniels, Bloom, Smith, & Winrer, 1987; Andersen, Farrar, Kutz, & Glaser, 1998).

Regarding survival indicators, a study on survivors of cancer suggests increased survival in patients who expressed anger or will to fight than in persons who expressed hopelessness and depression or stoic acceptance (Greer, Morris, & Pettingale, 1979; Pocino & Castes 1999). Further scientific investigation is needed to verify these associations where the field of psychoneuroimmunology may have important contributions.

Regarding progression of cancer disease, researchers associated progression and recurrence of cancer with stress (Ramirez, Craig, Watson, Fentiman, North, & Rubens, 1989; Pocino & Castes 1999) and natural killer cells cytotoxic activity as a strong predictive factor.

Stress Alters Immunology in Two Different Ways:

1) Encouragement of conducts that alter immunity, such as smoking, inadequate diet or sleep, and, 2) Increase of hormones, such as steroids or epinephrine, which modulate the immune response with important effect on antitumoral activity cells, natural killer cells and macrophages (Lechin, Dijs, Vitelli, Lechin, Azocar, Cabrera, Lechin, Jara, Lechin, Gomez, & Rocha, 1990).

Cancer´s origin is based on an interplay of genetic and environmental factors. Environment involves carcinogen exposure, habits like smoking, and inadequate nutrition. These patients have been associated with a "Personality Type C", with reduced expression of negative emotions, especially anger, and with pleasing of external authorities (Morris, Greer, Pettingale, & Watson, 1981). If a Type C Personality does exist, then patients need to learn to express anger, take risks, and be authentic and not more compliant (Serlin, Classen, Frances, & Angell, 2000).

On Patient Adherence to Treatment and Cooperation with the Oncologist Physician

"Patients with chronic medical illnesses have higher rates of depression and anxiety and these ...are associated with poor adherence to medical regimens and adverse medical outcomes." (Katon, Unützer, & Simon, 2004; see Goodill, this volume)

It has been repeatedly shown that between 50% and 75% of the presenting symptoms brought to primary physicians are either amplified or caused by psychological factors (Wickramasera, 1998). "Dance therapists, working holistically with mind, body and spirit (also existential issues), are uniquely positioned to work with illnesses that become manifest in all three quadrants" (Serlin, Classen, Frances, & Angell, 2000).

METHOD

Sample

The sample consisted of 15 adult oncology patients (13 women and 2 men) with cancer in diverse locations under treatment. The age range was 39 to 62 years (mean=44.9 years old), all caucasian, argentinean and spanish-speaking. Recruitment was done through a hospital physician and a psychologist. An initial telephone interview was followed by a personal interview. The DMT group acceptance criteria were no medical counterindication for at least mild movement and being in newly diagnosed or chronically ill stage. This study did not work with terminally ill patients. Due to recruitment difficulties, it was not possible to develop a control group.

The majority of patients had previously or simultaneously participated in a psychotherapeutic group for cancer patients coordinated by a psychologist.

Materials and Methods

Methods for data recollection: Personal interviews at 0, 1, 2, 3 years and follow-up post program interview, a medical evaluation, a health review with routine questions about habits such as eating and sleeping, and participants' self reports and scales.

Group format: 2-hour-meetings on a weekly basis during 3 years (2002, 2003 & 2004) in Buenos Aires, Argentina. The meeting format was a 90-minute-DMT session preceded by 30 minutes of participant information and formation. The sessions involved a warm up, process or main part and a closing (Vella, 1998).

DMT sessions: DMT directives were designed with the goal to enhance the immune system and QoL in accordance to findings in scientific studies research. They included emotion expression (Chodorow, 2004), corporal supports, strengthening of authentic self, body awareness and integration, rehabilitation of movements (Fux, 2001), tension release, limits/boundaries and territoriality, resocialization and group network and belonging (Gonzalez, 2003).

Some Specific DMT Items

Emotion expression: Psychophysical expression of negative emotions was implemented (Chodorow, 2004) together with the complement of expression of affection (Gonzalez, 2003), caring for oneself and for others and working other positive emotions. Regarding negative emotions, not only individual but also social emotions were worked, such as the ones accompanying the economy disruption in our country during the study.

Stress reduction: The group explored relaxation techniques, sensoperception, grounding and centering. Fun, enjoyment and laughter were fostered.

Resilience: Worked through special DMT sessions with reading of special stories or testimonies plus posterior Authentic Movement. Readings of the Journey, Campbell's hero. The call, the outer or physical challenge, the inner or spiritual challenge and re-birth (Serlin, Classen, Frances, & Angell, 2000). It fostered identification of life stage, fading of the victim role. By becoming aware of the cyclical nature of process, relief and a sense of hope arose in some cases.

Cycle and Nature work: Awareness of the a.m. cyclical nature of process may be reinforced with DMT proposals inspired by nature, such as working the 4 seasons, or by working opposites

Being in charge and self-empowerment: It is useful to emphasize that each participant is in charge of his/her movement and that each one is in freedom to provide him/herself (e.g. movements or body supports only they know they need) and to regulate moving according to well-being.

Reframing the illness: As a dancetherapist and as a medical doctor, the process led the author to reframe illness to crisis, danger to opportunity, and victim to individual and dignity. For some participants this may help to facilitate hope and coping and undergoing exhausting treatments. It means not only enduring the crisis, but going for the fuel that the crisis brings and make changes in everyday life, in body movement, in self-efficacy, in love capacity. Cancer has some negative connotations that can be reframed, such as the mentioned "vital crisis" instead of only life-threatening illness, introducing meaning and getting away from unproductive ways of thinking and functioning. The author found that experiencing real pain or grief may be a relief, as opposite to the suffering of permanent victim roles or postures.

Projects: Personal project work was a good tool to accompany the phase of transition from patient status to healthy status.

Group: The group provided support and a sense of belonging, as a means for patients who anticipated little or no support from significant others (Greer, Morris, Pettingale, 1979).

Existential issues: They were planned for and arose in particular DMT sessions, such as death, renovation, meaning, freedom and isolation, (Serlin, Classen, Frances, & Angell, 2000) and were accompanied with movement and music with the addition of painting to favour further symbolic process, a space to share and referral for further discussion with personal psychotherapists.

One specific method: *Medicine scientific information was taken as an object to work through own experience and movement, and contribute to it.* Patients were eager to work this. Upon suggestion of Vella, the author constructed and implemented this working method during the 3-year-program. The method involves a theme presentation, such as quality of life or preventive health medicine, to the group and posterior movement with related proposals. The closing involves experience sharing and completing medicine knowledge with own experience, with a group synthesis in some cases. For example, the autonomous nervous system was presented and worked with the pair of opposites relaxation and tension.

Success experiences: Applause after dancing. Recognition for participants' steps forward and productions, celebration, and recognition for completion of treatment or control, also birthdays.

Adherence to medical treatment: During treatment, support was fostered and music was prepared to accompany chemotherapy, and, upon completion of treatment (or controls), celebration, support and emotional nourishment were issued. Significant others for emotional and practical support were included in occasional sessions.

The Following Parameters Were Measured

Quality of life parameters, illness evolution parameters, adherence to medical treatment and physiologic measurements.

Quality of life (QoL) involved:

Vigor, Sense of own strength (Self efficacy), Muscle tension, Depression, Psychological distress, overall sense of well-being.

Other parameters of QoL: Sleep, Nutrition, Work, Vocation and Personal project development, Relation to loved ones or support network.

Signs and symptom improvement report: Dyspnea, Pain, Adverse effects during Chemotherapy (Nausea, vomiting, and psychological resistance to treatment)

This work was started in the health house of Foundation Apostar a la Vida attached to hospital setting, going on in Caritas Argentina. Presently the author works in a Public Hospital in Argentina.

FINDINGS AND RESULTS

From the initial 15 participants, 4 dropped out (1 man, 3 women) because of personal preferences not because of illness evolution. Their evolution is not included here.

A) Quality of Life Parameters

Vigor: All 11 participants reported a moderate increase of energy, physical as well as psychic, feeling more active and willing to live.

Fatigue (non-related to chemo): All 11 participants reported moderate reduction. Fatigue is the most prevalent symptom experienced by patients with cancer. Some evidence exists that exercise interventions are of benefit in women with breast cancer (National Institute of Health Conference, 2002).

Sense of own strength (Self-efficacy) (see Goodill elsewhere in this volume): All 11 participants reported moderate improvement in sense of own strength and increased perception of ability to provide for own needs.

Muscle ache or discomfort: In this study, 5 patients experienced enlivened muscle pain or discomfort following the start of the DMT sessions. The pain was of non-oncology etiology, studied through x rays and nuclear medicine, among others, and referral to personal physician. After this study, finally, patients' discomfort was managed through the instruction to make only soft and mild movements during DMT sessions and referral to a personal physician for transitory pain relief, when necessary. As DMT sessions progressed, gradual and very good discomfort resolution was obtained with a slower integration of the specific body area.

The pattern that outlines in these patients is the following:

Initial report: Awareness of little or no muscle discomfort.

After 1st DMT session: Report of awareness of moderate muscle discomfort.

After 3rd to 5th D/MT session: Report of resolution or very little muscle ache or discomfort and patient satisfaction for better muscle awareness and relaxation.

These observations suggested a "Curve of Muscle Discomfort Awareness" (see Figure 1) that resolved in the above mentioned pattern.

FIGURE 1: CURVE OF MUSCLE ACHE AWARENESS

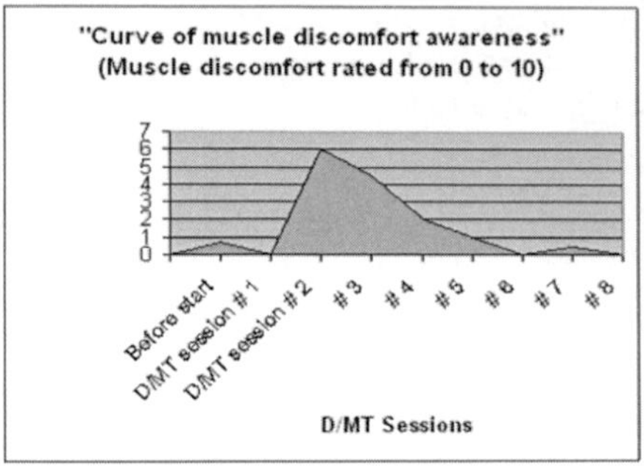

Depression: 0% (N=0) of new cases. We report 1 case of 10-year depression previous to diagnosis which ceased and personal projects flourished.

Psychological distress: 100% (n=11) participants reported moderate reduction of psychological distress, with less anxiety and worry (Dibbel Hope, 2000) and more daily life enjoyment.

Overall sense of well-being: 100% of moderate increase in well-being.

Other parameters of Quality of Life

Sleep: 73% (8 participants) gradually reduced and abandoned sleeping pills replacing them for other sleep hygiene methods. This happened after 6 months of DMT group and together with a module on Sleep, which was created because of participants' needs. It is to be outstantded that, in this sample, 100% of the participants reported in the initial evaluation daily sleeping pills prescribed by their physicians.

Nutrition: All 11 participants reported being able to acquire and maintain new healthy eating habits, reporting for example adding more fruit and fiber to diet.

Work: 9 participants kept their jobs, with license during oncology treatment.

Vocation and Personal project development: 6 participants reported starting previously blocked or completely new personal projects (1 in a new work project, 3 started new continuing education, 2 in starting a couple relationship). One observation in this group was an activation of things they never dared to do before in their lives, such as having a personal project.

Support network: All 11 participants reported ability to express their needs, to provide for themselves and more situations of love expression.

Signs and Symptom Improvement Report During Selected DMT Group Sessions

Dyspnea (breath difficulty): Case report -- Disappearance of dyspnea at the end of the DMT sessions, in 3 different cases of dyspnea of non-oncologic etiology.

Pain: Decline of pain perception to mild/moderate in a patient with moderate/severe bone pain of oncologic etiology on arrival to workshop. The participant displayed no intention to leave the DMT session despite repeated suggestions to go home and look for relief.

B) Adherence to Medical Treatment

All group participants have finished medical treatment as the pillar of health restoration and follow periodical medical controls.

Adherence to medical treatment: all participants

Adherence to medical controls: all participants

Adverse effects during Chemotherapy (Nausea, vomiting, and psychological resistance to treatment): Report of moderate reduction (from moderate/severe to mild/moderate) of symptoms.

Resistance to treatment: All 11 participants reported moderate reduction and acquisition of meaning and strength to undergo the treatment. However, when chemo was unexpectedly prolonged, strong resistance appeared. At last the participant resolved it and the last part of treatment was completed with more adverse effects than in the first part of treatment.

C) Illness Evolution Parameters

Evolution of Illness at the End of the 3-Year-DMT Program:

Partial illness remission in 1 participant

Total Illness remission in 8 participants: Six participants entered remission during the 3 years of the DMT groups and 2 maintained their initial remission. One of these patients had a metastasis diagnosis and treatment with posterior total remission at the time of end of the DMT program.

Stable disease in 1 participant. This participant had a recategorization from disease in progress to stable disease, but still serious because of metastasis in treatment.

Decease (casualties): No decease during these 3 years: As follow-up, 6 months after the end of the 3-year DMT group, 10 patients kept remission or stable illness status and one patient evolved to metastasis and rapid progression of illness.

D) Physiologic Measurements

Immunologic parameters: Due to the economic crisis in 2001, the costs of lab tests raised and were unattainable, the lab reactives were non available in the local market.

Autonomous nervous system (ANS) parameters: These one-time physiological measures were designed according to the economic possibilities, which required a registered nurse and equipment for measurement of *blood pressure* and *heart rate*.

TABLE II: HR AND BP MEASURES BEFORE AND AFTER INDIVIDUAL DMT SESSION

	Heart Rate before/after DMT Session (beats/min)		change	Blood Pressure before/after DMT Session (mm Hg)	
Participant 1	76	72	-4	130/80	120/70
Participant 2	64	64	0	**175/95**	**155/95**
Participant 3	72	64	-8	110/70	120/70
Participant 4	84	80	-4	**160/80**	**150/90**
Participant 5	80	76	-4	135/80	130/90
Participant 6	88	88	0	120/80	130/90

Note: Parameters were taken before and after a usual DMT session at the end of the 3 years DMT program.

Stress has an influence on the immune function and on blood pressure and heart rate (Benson H, Rosner, Marzetta, & Klemchuk, 1974; Hoffman, 1982). Acute and chronic stress should be differentiated and taken into account. Results see Table II and Figure 2.

FIGURE 2: HART RATE (HR) DURING DMT SESSION

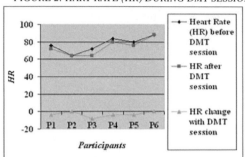

Heart Rate (HR): HR descended 4 to 8 beats per minute in most cases or remained the same. There were no increases.

Blood Pressure (BP): In the two cases of hypertensive registers, systolic BP decreased nearer to normal (Benson, Rosner, Marzetta, & Klemchuk, 1974). Normal systolic registers remained in normal range.

The two cases of hypertensive registers were from participants 2 and 4, who are over 60 years old. Both were instructed to do very mild movements and benefited after the DMT session with the a.m partial decrease. Both were referred to their personal physicians for antihyper-tensive diet and medication assessment.

Overall conclusion of ANS measurements: The reduction in HR and high systolic BP suggests that DMT modulates the activity of the ANS through stress reduction in the short term. However, a strong cautionary note needs to be added about this measurement, because it needs to be continued over longer periods of time and with a larger sample. At present, the author is carrying this out in a 1.5 month weekly DMT study in a public hospital with ANS measurements.

CONCLUSIONS OF PART A

This study suggests that DMT has a positive effect on cancer patients and their quality of life (QoL) and treatment compliance. Regarding physiologic measurements, there is a hint that DMT may decrease Blood Pressure in the case that a hypertensive register is found. It is important to further the objective demonstration of benefits of DMT for adult cancer patients (Cruz, 2001), where medical immunologic measurements have an important role together with control double-blind randomized studies.

Regarding immune system enhancement measures, they were provided in the frame of DMT and in accordance to scientific studies. Patients' self reports show stress reduction and the lab tests were not done because of unavailability of lab materials due the local economic crisis[24]. The contribution of the DMT group to treatment compliance

---

[24] Current Project = Fund raising for blood immune lab analysis. The raising of funds in Argentina is currently difficult. Interest to develop a multicentric and multicountry study, mail to author.

and psychosocial improvement was important in our teamwork contribution to the participant's physician.

The care of the oncology patient involves a multidisciplinary team, with a medical doctor, nurse, kinesiologist, family and friends, among others. In the first explicit meta-analysis, Meyer (1995) concluded that psychosocial interventions should not be considered optional or extra, but an integral part of the illness management program.

A somatically oriented method of psychosocial support such as DMT, has a valuable contribution to make. No two cancer survivors respond in exactly the same way (Abelof, 2000) nor have exactly the same needs. Thus, having different effective tools can be a good tool for caregivers. In the frame of an increasing world cancer patient population. More dancetherapists trained for this population, are needed.

Participant written testimony (translated and printed with consent of participant):

> *"At 34 years, when I believed I had my life organized, I was diagnosed with a pancreas cancer. It meant realizing that everything was not well controlled and that I did not have the propriety even on life. I fought my way through surgeries, rays and chemotherapies.*
>
> *But my more intense fight was the inner one.*
>
> *Knowing myself vulnerable, feeling hopelessness, fear, sadness. Learning to accept me, to love me, integrating hurts and joys. Walking a way of self-knowledge, recognizing the own body, with its changes, and identifying feelings, to start to express them moment to moment and stop accumulating and blocking them.*
>
> *In dance therapy I could integrate all of this. And give myself permission to play, opening the door to the girl I was. Enjoying the meeting and the communication with the group of dance therapy. Where I find the space to dream, create, dance, connect with the music, the group partners and all the pleasure that it moves in me. Each dance workshop is a party, where we share experiences and celebrate life.*
>
> *Today 7 years after diagnosis, I relate much better with myself and with others. Dance therapy contributed a lot to embellish my life, to grow and flourish, enjoying more fully my life". (Sandra D., October 2004)*

PART B: DMT AS A RESOURCE FOR ONCOLOGY PATIENTS AFTER TREATMENT IN SOCIAL RECOVERY

Cancer patients facing illness remission present new needs. In order to exit the strong vital crisis of cancer, tools equally strong are needed among which DMT with the additive of Tango seem to be a powerful one. In both approaches, body connection and sensuality can be retrained in an atmosphere of fun and trust. Furthermore, the safe and therapeutic environment provided by DMT allows working archetypes, trust, surrender and communion while dancing alone and together.

Issues of Cancer Patients after Illness Remission

Among oncology patients, as among other survivors of strong crisis, it is frequent to observe changes in the relationship to themselves and to others, such as their partners. Important question that arise often: "How are my relationships and my sexual relationships going to be? My needs are somewhat different now". Also there are specific needs according to cancer primary location and associated treatment. For example, breast cancer patients after breast mastectomy present specific challenges in this phase of return to social and couple life.

Experience as Dance Therapist

After 2-years of the DMT program described in Part A, the group entered a new phase, the stage of illness remission. New issues arised and awaited to be addressed. A specific extra DMT program was created and as an extra tool, Tango was introduced in a blend with DMT (Tango for cardiac patients, 2004; Varela, 2005).

About Tango: A Brief History

Tango is the product of cultural and identity issues of a vital time during the history of Argentina at the end of the XIX century (Abadi, 2001, Nau-Klapwijk, 2000). A time of immigrants, a time of living together with people of many different countries, a time of loneliness, a time of mostly immigrant young men. Tango was a cultural expression to meet their needs. Nowadays, Tango is changing under the influence of the XXI-century-society, with the phenomenon of an increasing divorce rate. A time of men and women newly single and returning to the dating arena. Tango has turned out to be an effective means to ease this way and a place to repractice interacting skills between men and women. Society presents new needs that are now slowly changing back Tango. For instance, a previous rigid role, such as the past tango men's macho-like role, is changing, encouraging men to become more integrated and genuinely open to the female world.

Hypothesis

Adult cancer patients in recovery, specifically breast cancer patients after mastectomy, will benefit from DMT groups with the additive of Tango when facing social recovery and the readdressing of couple.

Background

The field of Dance/Movement Therapy provides an opportunity and safe environment to work archetypes, emotion expression, body awareness and it enhances personal relations (Chaiklin, 1975). Tango provides its music, rhythm, dance, and philosophy, which are strong motivators of the forces of feminine and masculine archetypes. During the illness the body gains protagonism together with the task of looking for internal and external resources to go through this crisis, with remaining issues mostly being left aside. After the illness, issues of femininity and masculinity were reactivated.

If a Type C Personality does exist, then patients need to learn to express anger, take risks, and be authentic and not more compliant (Serlin, Classen, Frances, Angell, 2000). In face of social recovery these characteristics may gain importance.

Physical problems associated with cancer create psychosocial impact. For example, a perception of loss of attractiveness can diminish patient's overall sense of well-being (Abelof, 2000). This group phase was a call to provide an environment fostering activation and remaking of the female and male archetypes, with its strong inherent psychic energy.

METHODS

Sample

Eight cancer patients in illness remission (seven after treatment, one in stage of chronic stable disease with bone metastasis). The sample was composed of 7 women and 1 man (age range = 39 to 56 years; mean = 43.6 years old, all caucasian, argentinean and spanish-speaking). The cancer location and marital status was taken into account with the following data: There were 6 breast cancer patients (1 married in a long term relationship, 2 had short term couples, 3 were single) and 2 non breast cancer patients (both married in long term relationships), with non-Hodgkin lymphoma and with a neuroendocrine pancreas tumor.

Materials and Methods

Nine weekly 90-minutes DMT workshops were especially designed. Participants were recruited during 2004 in the DMT program for oncology patients described in part B of this chapter. One session was partially videotaped with participants' consent.

As mentioned, Tango was introduced in a blend with DMT, providing its music and some elements of its philosophy (Article: Tango for cardiac patients, 2004; Varela, 2005). The following issues were explored (Abadi, 2001, Nau-Klapwijk, 2000): Masculine and feminine archetypes, both in men and women

Surrender	Trust
Togetherness	Enjoyment
Seduction training	Leadership

Individuation process: Because tango dance requires two centered and grounded individuals to make a good couple. The above mentioned issues were developed with proposals such as a) dancing while surrendering body weight to the floor, to other surfaces, one hand in the other, to another person, following by b) dancing with closed eyes and been from time to time spatially moved by another person with whom a previous trust bond was promoted, among other directives. Part of this program was presented in a theoretic and experiential workshop at the 2005 ADTA Conference.

The female archetype, with all its inherent psychic energy, was particularly important for breast cancer patients after a breast mastectomy. This archetype was activated and called to surface through DMT proposals, Tango music and perfume as sensoristimulant. It was danced and explored together with recovering the enjoyment of the body regardless of form, enjoyment of its movement and of its sensoperception.

This was associated with working body areas integration, integrity and dignity. The group underwent a process involving the archetype of the warrior and the dignity of scars of living. Some words: "Yes, I am a survivor and this is the body of this survivor and warrior. War is over. I am worth to love and be loved. It's time to rest. I'm going home."

In the frame of studies' findings, the program design included optional participants' partners involvement in 2 specific sessions. The mentioned findings, conclude that spousal confidence ... constitutes a "fundamentally social protective factor" (Rohrbaugh, Shoham, Coyne, Cranford, Sonnega, & Nicklas, 2004; see Goodill, this volume).

The group format was the usual DMT frame: Warming up, Main part or Process and Closing. For patients with persistent concerns on body image and sexual function, also post-surgery, a referral to professionals trained in sexual rehabilitation was planned. This was not necessary in this group. The methods for data recollection were interviews and participants' written self report/scales.

FINDINGS AND RESULTS

A) Quantities

From single breast cancer patients after mastectomy: 2 out of 3 report to start dating and having later achieved successful couple relationships. One of them started sexual relationships in a very caring way and a steady relationship 6 months after. The other, who had reported no couple for more than 6 years before cancer diagnosis, started a steady relationship after illness.

From married patients: All 3 report to be satisfied in their relationships and report satisfaction and finding moderately helpful (4) the themes addressed in this program of DMT.

From participants with short term couples: 2 out of 2 report to be willing to look for better and more authentic bonds with their current partners or other.

All participants: Regardless from marital status, reported to have found the DMT workshops moderately (4) and extremely (5) helpful and to have started working relationship issues and choosing roles more in accordance with current personal needs.

B) Qualities

For married participants or couples with a strong bond, there was an opportunity for incondicional love, communion, for togetherness ("For holding a hand as they never held it before", "for looking the partners in the eyes with a depth they never had before").

For single participants, there was an opportunity for choice, choosing with whom, choosing how and reactivating their womanhood.

All participants, both married and single, reported to have chosen in a new way which role they want to play in their relationships tuned with their needs after illness remission. They also reported to have learnt new ways of how to be in touch with themselves and their personal needs.

C) Findings in Evolution of Illness
One Year After this Special DMT Program

Illness remission: conserved in 7 participants
Overall well-being: increased in 7 participants
Progression of illness: with metastasis and starting new treatment: in 1 participant

CONCLUSIONS OF PART B

A growing population of cancer patients in remission, who have successfully completed their cancer treatment, remain with a number of specialized needs. Timely recognition of arising patients' social and sexual needs is essential to comprehensive cancer care (Abelof, 2000). Unfortunately, health professionals often stress survival and control of the disease and disregard sexuality as an essential aspect related to the quality of life of the cancer patient (Abelof, 2000).

Vocational, spiritual, relational, sexual, emotional and psychological functioning are all affected to some degree. Thus, comprehensive health care should include services and professionals who can help patients and their families cope with the many attendant stressors and adjust to the inevitable changes (see Goodill, this volume).

Dance/Movement Therapy, in creative association with tools such as Tango, seems to be a complement and successful tool for patients that are getting out of a vital crisis as strong as cancer. It is important to further the objective demonstration of benefits of DMT for adult cancer patients (Cruz, 2001) with larger samples and a control group.

Tools to ease the way back to social life are very much needed in this population, moreover in breast cancer patients after mastectomy, together with trained dance therapists. Dance therapists are encouraged to specialize in this evergrowing population.

Participant written testimony (translated and printed with consent of participant):

> *"My name is Silvia Alejandra and I am 42 years old. Three years ago I underwent a breast surgery, which involved a mastectomy and a treatment which consisted in radiotherapy and 6 chemotherapy cycles. Currently I am in an excellent remission. I was invaded by anguish and fear, unable to feel again as a woman. I did not accept this new body with a mastectomy, losing my hair and with a temporary physical decay due to treatment.*
>
> *What could I do to love myself again? Which man was going to look at me? My self-esteem was almost nonexistent. They suggested to me to try Dance Therapy.*
>
> *At first I felt strange, and stopped going for some time. Afterwards I started to go more frequently and discovered what I could do with my body: simply dance, dance from my interior, dance my feelings, and from my girl essence and my womanly essence. Everything I had thought lost, I gradually recovered.*
>
> *Regarding the DMT and Tango Workshops, I really hooked up immediately with the 'Tango therapy' and the workshops on tango and Dance Therapy. I think that in a certain way it sped up the whole process that was developing in me, it gave me the way to reconnect with the external world, I started dating, using make-up and buying new clothes.*
>
> *Also, for almost a year now, I am learning to dance Tango, where I can relate again to men from another standpoint, feel secure, feminine, sensual and seductive and I allow the preparations to go to the tango-milonga to become a ritual.*
>
> *And in this way, I started to bet on love and a full life. It does not matter what we are lacking, discovering the valuable treasure that is inside of us, recover the self-esteem and come to good terms with one self, is a long and hard road that is worth walking."*
>
> *(Silvia A, September 2004)*[25] Note: This participant has currently a steady partner.

GENERAL DISCUSSION AND CONCLUSIONS

In recent years, there has been a strong movement to revisit non-comprehensive methods of science and medicine. Physical aspects of illness become only one part of a larger system that needs to be potentially targeted for multiple interventions. As medicine becomes more concerned with the overall well-being of the person, illness is being redefined to include not only the physical but the other three quadrants (mental, emotional, and spiritual) as well (Abelof, 2000). From a DMT point of view, the physical quadrant is much more than the description of the body parts and includes also body movement and its contribution to rehabilitation and recovery, the reintegration of silent or hurting protected parts, the body's sensations, its pleasure, its symbols.

Now, medicine is in a position to contribute to the restoration of health and the patient's overall sense of well-being. Regarding psychosocial interventions, a wider and richer range of interventions is suitable to different needs, personalities and life experiences. There are no two identical patients, in consequence there are no identical needs or ways to provide treatment to them. A somatic and expressive psychosocial interven-

---

[25] I would like to acknowledge Sandra D and Silvia A for their generous sharing of testimonies and Guillermo, Sandra D, Nancy, Amanda, Silvia A, Eva, Rosa, Sandra A and the rest of participants I have had the privilege to work with.

tion as DMT can be a positive addition, providing individual forms of outlet and recovery among others.

Health care providers who seek to treat the person comprehensively, i.e. to treat the whole illness as opposed to just the physical disease, must work in multidisciplinary teams and incorporate psychosocial rehabilitation into routine care. Physicians and treatment teams following a comprehensive care approach will find a valuable and readily available resource in DMT suited to enhance well-being, quality of life, and treatment compliance of the patient and social recovery after treatment. This comprehensive and unified approach to illness is presently gradually becoming the model of care in oncology (Abelof, 2000). The National Comprehensive Cancer Center Network (USA) is developing guidelines for the management of distress that feature psychosocial screening as a salient component of care (Abelof, 2000). It is recommended that a number of professionals with their unique expertise come together to provide the necessary care for each quadrant of the individual (Abelof, 2000).

Findings suggest that DMT interventions are a valuable resource for adult cancer patients. They can enhance quality of life and treatment compliance during treatment and enhance social recovery afterwards. It is of importance for the medical community to get to know all the resources that are available to contribute with the physician, to enhance well-being and satisfaction of patients together with promoting treatment compliance. Overall, this study suggests that DMT can be an effective resource for oncology patients.

REFERENCES

Abadi, S. (2001). *El Bazar de los abrazos*. Buenos Aires, Argentina: Lumiere.

Abbas, A., & Lichtman, A. (2004). Tumoral Immunology. *Celular and molecular Immunology,* Madrid, Spain: Elsevier, pp. 391-410.

Abelof, M.D. (2000) Psychosocial Rehabilitation. *Clinical Oncology,* Philadelphia:Churchill Livingstone, division of Harcourt Brace & Company, pp. 2845-2865.

Andersen, B.L., Farrar, W.B., Golden-Kreutz, D., Kutz, L.A., MacCallum, R., Courtney, M.E., & Glaser, R. (1998). Stress and immune responses after surgical treatment for regional breast cancer. *Journal of the National Cancer Institute, 90*(1), 30-36.

Bartrop, R.W., Luckhurst, E., Lazarus, L., Kiloh, L.G., & Penny, R. (1977). Deppressed lymphocyte function after bereavement. *Lancet, 16,*1(8016), 834-836.

Benson, H., Rosner, B.A., Marzetta, B.R., & Klemchuk, H.M. (1974). Decreased blood-pressure in pharmacologically treated hypertensive patients who regularly elicited the relaxation response. *Lancet, 23,* 1(7852), pp. 289-91.

Chaiklin, S. (1975). Dancetherapy. In S. Arieti (Ed), *American handbook of psychiatry,* 2nd ed, New York: Basic Books.Vol. 5 pp. 701-720.

Chodorow, J. (2004). *Seminar on DMT and Authentic Movement.* Argentina.

Cruz, R.F. (2001). Perspectives on the Profession of Dance/Movement Therapy: Past, Present, and Future, *Bulletin of Psychology and the Arts, 2*(2), pp. 74-78.

Dibbel-Hope, S. (2000). The use of dance/movement therapy in psychological adaptation to breast cancer. *The arts in psychotherapy: An international journal, 27*(1), pp. 51-68.

Dietrich, H. (1991). *The art of Healing: An integrative treatment approach to cancer using DMT and imagery.* Ross Hospital, Marin County, CA.

Fawzy F.L., Fawzy, N.W., Hyun, C.S., Gutherie, D., Fahey, S., & J.L. Morton, D. (1993). Malig-nant melanoma. Effects of an early structured psychiatric intervention, coping and affective state on recurrence an survival years later. *Archives of General Psychiatry,* pp. 681-689.

Fux, M. (2001). *Después de la caida, continuo con la Danzaterapia.* Argentina: Lumen.

Gonzalez, A. (2003). *Dance movement Seminar: Health, integration and prevention. Love energy as primary nourishment.* National Forum on theater and mental health, Argentina.

Greer S, Morris, T, & Pettingale, K.W. (1979). Psychological response to breast cancer: effect on outcome. *Lancet*,*2*, 785-787.

Herbert, T.B., & Cohen S. (1993). Depression and immunitiy: a meta-analytic review. *Psychology Bulletin. 113*(3), pp. 472-486.

Hoffman, W. (1982). Reduced Sympathetic Nervous System Responsivity associated with the Relaxation Response. *Science, 215*, pp. 190-192.

Irwin, M., Daniels, M., Bloom, E., Smith, T.L., & Winrer, H. (1987). Life events, depressive symptoms and immune function.. *American Journal of Psychiatry, 144*, pp. 437-441.

Katon, W.J., Unuetzer, J., & Simon, G. (2004). Treatment of depression in primary care: Where we are, where we can go. *Medical Care, 42*(12), pp. 1153-1157.

Lechin F., van der Dijs B., Vitelli-Florez G., Lechin-Baez, S., Azocar J., Cabrera, S., Lechin A., Jara H., Lechin M., Gomez F., & Rocha L. (1990). Psychoneuroendocrinological and immunological parameters in cancer patients: involvement of stress and depression. *Psychoneuroendocrinology. 15*(5-6), pp. 435-451.

Maunsell, E., Brisson, J., & Deschenes, L. (1995). Social support and survival among women with breast cancer. *Cancer.* 76(4), pp. 61-67.

Meyer, T.J, & Mark, M.M. (1995). Effects of psychosocial interventions with adult cancer patients: a meta-analysis of randomized experiments. *Health Psychology, 14*(2), pp. 101-108.

Morris, T., Greer, S., Pettingale, K., & Watson, M. (1981). Patterns of expression of anger and their psychological correlates in women with breast cancer. *Journal of Psychosomatic Research, 25*(2), pp. 111-117.

National Institute of Health State-of-the-Science. (2002). *Conference Statement: Symptom management in Cancer: Pain, Depression, and Fatigue.*

Nau-Klapwijk, N. (2000). *Tango, un baile bien porteño.* Argentina: Corregidor.

Parker, J., Klein, S., McClintock, M., Morison, W., Ye, X., Conti, C., Peterson, N., Nousari, C., & Tausk, F. (2004). Chronic stress accelerates ultraviolet-induced cutaneous carcinogenesis. *Journal of American Academy of dermatology, 51*(6).

Pocino Gistau, M., & Castes Boscan, M. (1999). "Psychoneuroimmunology: The IV tool in fighting cancer in an integral approach". Psychoneuroimmunology Laboratory. Immunology lecture, Medicine University, Venezuela. *Fundasinein, Fundación para el desarrollo de la Psiconeuroinmunologia. /www.psiconeuroinmunologia.org/articulos_3.html*

Ramirez, A.J., Craig, T.K, Watson, J.P, Fentiman, I.S., North, W.R., & Rubens, R.D. (1989). Stress and relapse of breast cancer. *British Medical Journal, 298,* 291-293.

Rohrbaugh, M. J., Shoham, V., Coyne, J., Cranford, J. A., Sonnega, J. S., & Nicklas, J. M. (2004). Beyond the "Self" in self-efficacy: spouse confidence predicts patient survival following heart failure. *Journal of Family Psychology, 18*(1), 184-193.

Serlin, I., Classen, C., Frances, B., & Angell, K. (2000). Symposium: Support groups for women with breast cancer: Traditional and alternative expressive approaches. *The Arts in Psychotherapy, 27*(2), 123-128.

Spiegel D., Bloom, J.R., Kraemer, H.C., & Gottheil, E. (1989) Effect of psychosocial treatment on survival of patients with metastatic breast cancer. *Lancet, 2,* 888-891.

Tango for cardiac patients (2004). *Clarín Argentine Newspaper.*

Temoshok, L., Seller, B., Sagebiel, R., Blois, M., Sweet, D., DiClemente, R., & Gold, M. (1985). The relationship of psychosocial factors to prognostic indicators in malignant melanoma. *Journal of Psychosomatic Research, 29*(2), 139-153.

The American Dance Therapy Association (ADTA), (2004). Dance/Movement Therapy Fact Sheet. Homepage www.adta.org. Retrieved: 20/07/05

Varela, G. (2005). On Tango. *Viva Newspaper Clarin.* Buenos Aires, Argentina. pp. 48-9.

Vella, G. *(1998). Seminar "Dancetherapy as a tool for education, art and health",* Argentina.

Wickramasera, I. (1998). Secrets kept from the mind but not the body or behavior. The unsolved problems of identifying and treating somatization and psychophusiological disease. *Advances in Mind/Body Medicine, 14*, 81-132.

HOW DO DANCE/MOVEMENT THERAPISTS BRING AWARENESS OF RACE, ETHNITICITY, AND CULTURAL DIVERSITY INTO THEIR PRACTICE?

Meg Chang

A workshop based on an ethnographic case study was designed to enhance clinicians' intercultural empathy with clients from diverse backgrounds. Critical reflection on the cultural, ethnic, and racial identity of the therapist was facilitated through the dance/movement therapy (DMT) process. Prior qualitative research in Seoul, Korea, examined whether theories and teaching methods of DMT were culturally congruent for adult students in East Asia and found that individual motivations to engage in DMT were congruent with those of students in the United States, but that education theories and approaches were conditioned by the habitus of each culture.

Keywords: Intercultural DMT, psychophysical habitus, qualitative research, aesthetic adult education.

INTRODUCTION

The majority of dance/movement therapists in the United States practice in racially, culturally, and ethnically diverse clinical settings. While such multi-cultural conditions apply particularly to the United States, in an increasingly interdependent world similar conditions are becoming more widespread. A corresponding circumstance occurs when non-North American DMT students travel beyond their home country for graduate school. Studying in the United States or Europe they are immersed in language and concepts that are foreign both literally and culturally. Upon returning home they import the theories, techniques, and modes of speech learned abroad for application in their local setting. Therefore, to provide effective treatment for all clients, inclusive of those from other cultures, ethnicities, or racial backgrounds, dance/movement and creative arts therapists need to be competent in multicultural interventions. Consequently, the American Dance Therapy Association (ADTA) has required that courses in multicultural psychotherapy be included in graduate education programs and training that grants the credential Dance/Movement Therapist, Registered (DTR).

In dance/movement therapy education, the body of knowledge and resultant learning methods that comprise the epistemology -- how we define and apply knowledge -- of DMT was developed over 30 years ago for treating culturally homogeneous psychiatric patients. Now considered traditional, such educational approaches and psychological theories continue to dominate many areas of clinical practice (Dokter, 1998). In the intervening years, demographic changes have led to cultural, racial, and ethnic diversity in educational and clinical settings. However, psychological concepts conceived under predominantly Western and middle class values remain the dominant diagnostic and treatment paradigm (Gilroy, 1998; Littlewood, 1992b). Coming from around the world, people with whom we work, patients and staff, speak languages that are mutually foreign or alien to each other.

Language barriers can only hint at the difference of perspectives regarding health and expectations of care for the mind and body. Different cultural and ethnic perspectives frame the therapeutic relationship. Concepts as basic as whether personhood is internally or externally motivated (Hoffman, 1998), or perceptions of whether the self is independent or socially embedded (Markus & Kitayama, 1991), are examples of cultural influence. Therefore we can not assume that patients will be familiar with psycho-dynamic theories on which dance/movement therapy protocols are often based.

Given such a globalized clinical environment, how are creative arts therapists educated to become culturally aware and culturally competent clinicians? Gender and class are also crucial factors in the identity of both therapist and client, which determine how race, culture, or ethnicity is experienced and perceived (Collins, 1990); as such, these issues merit a fuller discussion than is possible here. Examining how the theory of DMT is applied to clinical practices in multicultural settings can lead to *culturally congruent* (Kareem & Littlewood, 1992) treatment interventions for patients from a diversity of cultures, races, and ethnicities.

BACKROUND AND RATIONALE FOR THE STUDY

If applied uncritically, classically oriented DMT epistemologies can inherently reproduce racial bias and impede treatment with patients or clients from non-dominant cultures, or ethnic groups differing from the therapist's (Hanna, 2004). Instead of perpetuating what psychiatrist S. Acharyya terms "neo-colonial" attitudes and practices in psychiatry (Acharyya, 1992, p. 80), creative arts therapists must become *culturally competent* (Sue, 1981) in creating interventions to foster the bodymind[26] (Pert, 2002; Saltonstall, 1988) health of clients from non-majority cultures.

The social and cultural context in which dance therapy treatment and research occur is never neutral. Regardless of whether the therapist and patient are from the same *or* different cultures, races, or ethnicities, the particular history, culture, and political backgrounds of each one become the frame of reference for treatment interventions. When there is cultural congruence, both parties can agree that the original complaint or symptom for which the patient sought help has abated, and the patient feels helped with his or her problems (Kareem & Littlewood, 1992). Nonverbal communication cannot be assessed objectively without a thorough understanding of and respect for the client's lifestyle, communication style, and norms of emotional expression (Hanna, 2004).

Aesthetic values and artistic qualities are culturally determined; even something as basic to DMT concepts as assigning meaning to emotional expression in dance can be read differently depending on whose culture and cultural aesthetic is dominant (Hanna, 2004). These aesthetic elements of a society become embodied in each person as an unconscious "second nature" or *habitus* (Bourdieu, 1977) that is instilled pre-verbally and socially reinforced. This *habitus* mediates our perception of the world and functions as a pervasive and mutually reinforcing cultural sensor that rules the forms taken by symbolic expression. Advocates of the arts-for-healing commonly assert that dance, music, and art are universal languages. In fact, intercultural dance research suggests that each person develops a context and culture-specific *psychophysical habitus,* which operates to manifest racial identity, express ethnic inclusion, and reinforce cultural cohesion through movement and dance (Ness, 1992).

While the impetus to communicate symbolically may be a salient feature of human beings, the intentional use of the body in either improvised or choreographed dance/movement reflects and comments on the particular social, environmental, and

---

[26] Of the many terms that denote the interconnectedness of mind, body, and emotions, *bodymind* best indicates a holistic paradigm that supports the integrative and embodied praxis of DMT.

bodily belief systems of the dancer's community. In the Western tradition, dance and music are thought to be products of spontaneous creativity, but gesture and rhythm also come from and reinforce cultural values, along with reifying habitual movement styles and bodily presentation. Often local music and dance is associated with overtly ethnic forms and sensibilities by the dominant (non-ethnic) culture. However, these aesthetic elements are interpreted by each individual according to specifically encultured life experiences (Ling, Yamane, & Parker, 1991).

Dance/movement therapy is a 20th century form of healing through dance and movement that is taught and practiced as a means through which individual integration of body-mind-emotions takes place with the help of a specially trained professional who is proficient in both the non-verbal domain of dance-movement and knowledgeable in employing psychotherapeutic interventions. However, this recent form of dance-as-therapy is a modernist construct, in which the norms for mental health are derived from Western European conceptual models and psychodynamic theories. One such belief is the positive valance on autonomy. In the teaching and practice of DMT in the United States (Levy, 2005), the ubiquitous Marian Chace model of unison dance/movement in group therapy demonstrates American aesthetics that valorize the attributes of the autonomous pioneer.

Intercultural Dance/Movement Therapy Workshop

In order to critically examine the aesthetic premises and multicultural issues in Euro-American dance/movement therapy, a workshop format was developed to promote personal awareness of cultural, ethnic, and racial identity for the therapist as a component of enhancing clinical empathy with clients from various cultures. Clients from other races and cultures whose attitudes to healing seem foreign can be better apprehended by a therapist whose own cultural identity is secure.

Research findings from an *ethnographic case study* in Korea and Taiwan informed the design of the workshop that was presented at the First International Research Colloquium in Dance/Movement Therapy, in Hannover, Germany, 2004. The intention of these intercultural DMT workshops -- also taught in the United States and Finland from 1999 to 2004 -- was to enter into cultural congruence through experiential and creative movement exploration. Dance/movement therapy exploration of body attitude and breath, posture/gesture, time, and space allowed participants to discern how their *psychophysical habitus* -- personal culture and ethnic identity -- was embodied. Autobiographical dance investigations demonstrated the ways that norms of emotional expression are specific to each culture. Such kinesthetic information can serve as a reference point for interactions with patients from other cultures and races. Just as self-knowledge of movement propensities helps the dance/movement therapist adjust her movement to become synchronous with the patient's in dance therapy, externalizing one's own racial, cultural, and ethnic habitus develops psychophysical awareness. By bringing the psychophysical habitus to consciousness, the dance therapist has a frame of reference for unfamiliar behaviors or movement patterns that the client presents.

Using creative DMT to explore how the therapist's dance/movement aesthetics have been conditioned by culture clarifies the visceral reactions that arise in relationship with those clients whose use of the elements of dance, such as space and time, or touch, is diametrically different. For example, in therapeutic interventions is an urge to take hands with a client coming from the therapist's psychophysical impulse, or has touch been initiated by the client? Having knowledge of the client's culture is invaluable to understanding which interventions are culturally appropriate for a given person, time, setting, and relationship.

Qualitative Research Methodology

Qualitative research is an inductive and interpretive paradigm that begins with perception and observation to reveal general patterns of behavior, which makes it well-suited to DMT research (Berrol, & Cruz, 2004). The original research, on which the intercultural workshop was based, was an *ethnographic case study* of a 12-week dance/movement therapy (DMT) course (Chang, 2002). The purpose of the study was to discover in what ways dance/movement therapy was or was not an applicable and compatible intervention that was *culturally congruent* with the cultural and ethnic sensibilities of East Asian students. It was a representative case study, a discrete *bounded system* (Stake, 1995) that was situated in Seoul, Korea, for five months and was further bounded by purposive sampling. A qualitative research method was best able to convey the multiple dimensions of an intercultural education program in all of its interdisciplinary complexity (Creswell, 1998).

Because of the assertion that all research is based on an ideological position, and research design is not free of bias (Janesick, 1994), the researcher states his or her position and explicitly becomes the research instrument in much the same way that the dance/movement therapist uses her or himself in dancing with clients. This heuristic tradition is described as "the attribute of having insight, the ability to give meaning to data, the capacity to understand, and capability to separate the pertinent from that which isn't" through the personal quality and experience of the researcher (Strauss & Corbin, 1990, p. 42; Forinash, 2004). In keeping with the tradition of researcher involvement, the course was designed and taught, and the information was gathered and analyzed by the author, a Chinese-American dance/movement therapist. As qualitative research focuses on relationships and is influenced by humanistic values, there is a reduction of hierarchical relationships between the researcher and the researched (Forinash, 2004). For this reason, those involved are called participants rather than given the objectifying label of research subject.

The primary research method used was in-depth interviews. The secondary research method was videotape observation of classes and maintaining a fieldwork journal. Consistent with case study methods, extensive multiple sources of data were collected from participant interviews, videotape observation, and documents. These multiple sources of data were then coded, categorized, analyzed and compared against each other, or *triangulated*. A detailed descriptive narrative presented the information in terms of the problem, the context, the issues, and the "lessons learned" (Creswell, 1998).

Case study method is an emergent research strategy associated with ethnographic field research (Rudenstam & Newton, 1992). In the ethnographic tradition, weekly language study (of the author) began one year before the residency and continued throughout the research period in Seoul. To confirm interest in graduate level DMT education, a 16-hour weekend workshop in Seoul, Korea, had been previously conducted as a pilot study under the auspices of the Korea Dance Therapy Association (KDTA).

Participants

The study population was a purposeful network sample referred by the Korean Dance Therapy Association (KDTA). The 19 student members were mental health, education, dance education, or dance/movement therapy professionals whose background qualified them as competent key informants (Bernard, 1995) on the cultural fit of American DMT in Korea. These participants represented extreme case sampling; therefore, as a case study the findings and data analysis can only be valid for within-group similarities and differences. Even the participants described themselves as not having typical Korean characteristics. All were highly educated, many understood English, and most were at least socio-economically middle-class. All were highly motivated to learn DMT in a private studio setting. A summary of the class members follows.

FIGURE 1: SUMMARY OF MEMBERS BY GENDER, AGE, EDUCATION AND PROFESSIONAL BACKROUND

Gender	Women	17
	Men	2
Age	23 – 40 years old	All particip.
	20 – 29 years old	11
	30 – 40 years old	8
Education	Undergraduate degree	7
	Graduate degree	12
Profession **(some duplications,** **e.g. student can also be** **volunteer)**	*Disciplines by education major:*	
	Dance	12
	Social work, counselling	5
	Other (education, literature)	2
	Work, career, school experience:	
	Working in their chosen field	9
	Volunteer-psychiatric or community setting	5
	Full-time graduate students	5
	Recent graduates "thinking about being a dance/movement therapist"	2

Of the nineteen students in the class, seventeen agreed to participate in the research study and signed consent to participate in the study forms. To further safeguard confidentiality, only information that was public knowledge was included in participants' descriptions, and demographic information was aggregated into categories that could not be associated with any individual.

The participants' familiarity with, or prior study of DMT, ranged from the course comprising the person's initial exposure to dance therapy, to those who had four years of study and introduced themselves as dance therapists. Half of the class had studied or been involved with DMT for one year or less, and half had more than one year of experience studying DMT privately or in formal higher education.

12-WEEK COURSE CURRICULUM IN DANCE/MOVEMENT THERAPY

Design and implementation of the 12-week DMT course was modeled directly on the American Dance Therapy Association (ADTA) education curriculum for Master's level graduate education and advanced clinical training. The ADTA model was used because it has a well articulated educational canon, incorporates systematized standards of practice and ethics, and has maintained an internationally recognized credentialing process for over thirty-five years. It was also the education model most familiar to the (American trained) author. Further, the literature in international education specifically recommends that Western education not be adapted for Asian or African cultures, since that often implies a "watering down" and reduction of quality (Steiner-Khamshi, 1999). For these reasons, course content, reading materials, and teaching methods were not altered for teaching graduate-level DMT students in an East Asian culture. Teaching was conducted in English, with simultaneous translation.

Epistemology and pedagogical approaches used in the 12-week course represented both DMT education and *aesthetic adult education* principles. Aesthetic adult education was chosen for the educational framework because of the compatibility with DMT processes. Aesthetic adult education is a form of *emancipatory education* (Freire, 1970; Boal, 1985) that uses creative expression and psychological learning as a way to empower individuals and communities in naturally occurring affinity groups of shared interests (Jansen & Van der Veen, 1997).

Methods

Designing the 12-week dance therapy curriculum occurred in stages (Caffarella, 1994). Educational program objectives were developed. Experienced dance/movement therapy educators -- *subject matter experts* -- were interviewed to gather their observations of teaching East Asian students and to confirm that there were no major departures from American dance therapy education standards or norms during the delivery of the 12-week class. Interview guides for the first and second participant interviews were written, peer reviewed, and revised based on recommendations of subject matter experts in adult education.

Interview

The primary research method used was interview. Two in-depth semi-structured interviews of approximately 1.5 hours each were conducted with all of the participants in the study; all interviews were audio taped. Unless the participant preferred to speak English, a bilingual interpreter simultaneously translated all the interviews. Respecting Korean hospitality norms, snacks and coffee accompanied the conversation. In addition to the researcher and interpreter, other students and the President of the KDTA whose office we were using, were often present. As the participants told me, this was evidence of the "Korean Situation," a sociocultural code that covered any unexplainable social situation. Serendipitously, the interviews proved to be a culturally congruent strategy. The interview schedule was designed to collect demographic information and get to know the students better. In practice, it was an opportunity for student-teacher bonding, as well as a chance for students to impart private information away from the larger class.

Videotape

Each of the 12 classes was videotaped with a stationary Sony High-8 camera from before student-participants entered the classroom, throughout the class, and until they left the room. Videotape observation of the class teaching was used as a secondary source of data and as a visual record that facilitated accurate recollection of events discussed in the interviews (Eisner, 1998). A viewing log was developed to analyze the videotaped dance/movement explorations in class, in which all participants were referred to by pseudonyms to protect their confidentiality. The individual interviews were not videotaped to maintain confidentiality of the participants.

Documents

The researcher kept a field work and teaching journal throughout. More than a factual recording, the fieldwork journal was a repository of reflections on the experience of being immersed in a new culture. It contained examinations of the researcher's biases, prejudices, and cultural assumptions. Cultural missteps and miscommunications were included, such as when one of the bilingual interpreters resigned precipitously and very inconveniently, under conditions of her culturally unconscious *habitus* that were not comprehensible even to the researcher's (Asian) American logic.

Participants' homework or written reflections on a class exercise were informative as a non-vocal means of participant communication and self-disclosure. Students' comments confirmed their learning experiences, perceptions of the program, and understanding of the content during the 12 weeks of teaching. Similar to the videotape observations, these documents substantiated information reported in the interviews rather than providing new insights.

Analysis of Data

Each of the 17 participants was interviewed twice, once at mid-term and at the end of 12 weeks. These 34 two hour interviews were transcribed from the interview audiotapes and entered into Atlas.ti (Version 4.2), a qualitative data analysis software program (Muhr, 1997). From the transcripts, themes were identified, categorized, and analyzed using *open coding,* an interpretive procedure in the *grounded theory* (Strauss & Corbin, 1990) tradition. Thirty-six hours of class videotapes were observed by *open immersion* (Collier & Collier, 1986), logged onto a checklist, and analyzed for themes and contextual description. Documents were read and analyzed for content and corroboration of themes.

Interview

Open coding: Was the first step in analyzing voluminous interview transcripts. During open coding each line of the interview transcript was read multiple times and closely examined for the smallest bit of information relating to the research question, then grouped either by similarity or variation. Researcher preconceptions were acknowledged and then set aside, or *bracketed out* (Creswell, 1998) in reading so that themes common to all of the interviews could emerge from the text. Serving as both the researcher and remembering the teaching experience in Korea as a participant, the author experienced *bracketing* when listening to the audiotapes and transcribing the interviews. At first the information in the interviews sounded general and impersonal; but through the iterative process of re-reading the interviews many times, the texts revealed intimate information and privileged opinions that had been shared.

Codes: Were assigned to emerging themes in order to compare, conceptualize, and categorize the participants' responses to the interview questions, videotaped movement information, and documentary data. *Higher order categories* (Strauss & Corbin, 1990) were developed to correspond to each of the main research questions regarding individual feelings, teaching methods or educational concepts, and sociocultural influences. Finally, all of the interviews were coded with the ATLAS.ti qualitative software program (Muhr, 1997), which accommodates a heuristic approach based on *grounded theory* methods (Strauss & Corbin, 1990). *Grounded theory* is "inductively derived from the study of phenomenon…and provisionally verified through systematic data collection and analysis of data…one begins with an area of study and what is relevant to that area is allowed to emerge" (Strauss & Corbin, 1990, p. 23).

To insure inter-rater reliability, peer-review of a sub-set of interview transcripts with subject matter experts in aesthetic adult education, anthropology, and international education was conducted. Inter-rater reliability verified that themes were consistent, and that codes and categories were representative of the data.

Videotape Observation

Open immersion: (Collier & Collier, 1986) is a visual anthropology method that was used for observing videotaped images of the 12-week class. It is analogous to open coding for the interviews. Videotape observation was used as a secondary data source that supported the interview data and captured what actually happened, rather than the *espoused theory* (Schon, 1988) of DMT education. For example, often 40-60% of the class time was spent in verbal discussion rather than on experiential movement teaching.

All of the unedited videotapes -- 36 hours of classes -- were viewed four times in chronological order. Unusual or noteworthy segments were marked with footage markers corresponding to sections of the videotape. A *video observation log* (Schouten & Watling, 1997) was constructed that contained information on macro-level movement observations. Individual student comments on curricular content, their performance, or response to class material was noted as well as classroom group process. Categories that emerged from repeated viewing supported findings in the interview data (see Figure 2).

Along with categorizing entries from the field work journal as data, these multiple and different sources of evidence *triangulated* or verified the findings (Creswell, 1998). To further meet the requirement for trustworthiness in qualitative research, the videotapes were viewed by three subject matter experts for inter-rater reliability (Forinash, 2004). A Korean-American dance therapist, who was not a member of the 12-week class, corroborated hunches about cultural information and interpersonal classroom dynamics. Two American dance/movement therapy educators confirmed that the classes taught were consistent with dance/movement therapy graduate classes taught in formal education settings in the United States.

Levels of detail increased with each viewing, in a parallel process with interview transcription. The initial review (#1) immediately following field work served as a re-immersion in the material. During the second round (#2) of viewing, videotape footage was logged by second markers to capture basic class information about starting and ending, mood, activity levels, specific exercises, and salient interactions (Schouten & Watling, 1997). In the third round (#3) of video observation, patterns were identified that correlated with interview findings and clarified emerging code categories in the interviews.

FIGURE 2: VIDEOTAPE OBSERVATION LOG SUMMARY: EMERGENT IMERGENT INFORMATION FROM OPEN IMMERSION METHOD

Categories:	Class structure & Curriculum	Interactions	Dynamics	Researcher self-reflection
Viewing interval:	Creative dance exercises, improvisation, teaching interventions, etc. Human development through movement, ethnographic movement observation, etc.	Student -- teacher, teacher-student, student -- student. Range of participation level from little to all involved.	Individual or group; interpersonal, overall mood, energy level of class, dance/movements.	Learning and teaching process.
# 1 *One month* *post-field* *work*	Macro-level movement observation; overall impression of 12 classes. General context: classroom layout, space, light, gym mats on floor. Large group formations -- circles, lines, or small groups -- dyads, solos, etc.	Teaching interventions made; learning environment created.	Students surprised by actual appearance on videotape vs. self-perception.	Teaching errors and researcher's cultural breaches stand out vs. self-perception.
# 2 *Three* *months* *post-field* *work*	Participants' learning process and learning environment noted; curriculum content apparent.	Student performance & response to class material. Individual student's comments.	Students seen to resist or become involved with movement directives; engaged with each other.	Predominating mood for class is felt.
# 3 *Six months* *post-field* *work*	Observed difference in quality and intention in how movement assignments fulfilled.	One mental health professional joyfully announced, "I am a dancer!"	Mood -- trepidation in early classes, enthusiasm in later classes -- differentiated in class & week to week.	Role of the dancer corresponds to individual identity.
# 4 *One year* *post-field* *work*	Significant interactions; learning specifically mentioned in participant interview; exceptional movement events; students' response to directives.	Some absorbed in movement study, others with restricted, minimal range of postural movement looked "uncomfortable." Self-consciousness differs in dancing solo vs. group.	Students appear fascinated with each other's explanation of dance theme during verbal "sharing" and discussion of dance meaning.	Individualization and details observed: facial expression, alterations in feeling tone, capacity for the class to focus on experiential directives varies.

On the fourth viewing (#4), the variations in the tenor and progress within each class became more evident to the researcher. Also by the fourth viewing, each student's progress became clearer as characteristic individual movement preferences were differentiated from the group's cultural movement styles. Ways that the class as a whole had absorbed American dance therapy norms also became evident.

Since in this case study videotape observation was not the primary method; video data was only used to corroborate interview data. Promoting videotaped movement observation to a primary method would inform intercultural understanding of the dance/movement dimension. Comparing observations of participants from the local culture with observations of Western trained dance/movement therapists would highlight those areas of universal agreement and contrast it with the particular cultural or ethnic *habitus* of the local participants. In this way, delineating culturally congruent teaching theories and methods would be a step towards differentiating the universal aspects of dance-as-healing from the particular race, culture, and ethnicity of the individual.

Findings

Answers to the original research question, whether educational theories and practices of DMT were culturally congruent for these Korean students, were found in three interrelated domains: individual self-perception, educational systems, and socio-cultural context. In qualitative research, the perspective of the client is equally weighted with that of the researcher. Therefore whenever possible the student's words were applied as *in vivo* codes (Muhr, 1997; Chioncel, Van der Veen, Wildemeersch, & Jarvis, 2003). These code words and student/participant's quotations are *italicized* in the text.

Desire: At the level of the individual Korean student, the *desire* to study DMT was congruent with students in the United States and Europe. Over the 12-week course, discovering an autonomous identity, a *personal self,* took place for many of the participants. This desirable process of self-discovery or *self-finding* was the most often-stated reason for attending the 12-week DMT course. Students described themselves and other classmates as possessing a personality characteristic of either *openness* or *restraint.* For many of the students a kinesthetic identity, which they perceived as discrete, embodied, and sensorial, was highly valued by them as *genuine,* unique, and individually distinct from social aspects of themselves.

More of a science than an art: On the other hand, adult and higher education philosophies of student-centered learning were perceived as neither comparable nor culturally congruent. Classic DMT theories such as personality assessment using Laban Movement Analysis (North, 1972) or exploring theories of human development (Erikson, 1963) through reproducing stages of motor development (Mahler, Pine, & Bergman, 1975) were regarded by the Korean participants as *more of a science than an art.*

"In the USA, I think dance therapy is closer to psychology, but in Korea it is nearer to dance. This class is more like psychology, but it is better for dancers to teach dance therapy."

Verbal self-disclosure -- or *sharing,* as it is known in both countries from humanistic psychology -- was not perceived as culturally congruent by most members. Speaking in the large class especially caused the participants great social distress, by their own report.

"My education from elementary school to university, and even at the evening class (at a private institution), is the teacher giving lectures and student listening, just receiving information one way. Dance/movement therapy is totally the opposite. You make me do and find the answer. It is difficult. I have never had this kind of class before."

Paradoxically, participants interpreted student-centered dance/movement directives similar to those used in graduate programs in the United States to elicit learning about the self, as providing a chance for the student to *lead yourself.* At first these non-directive modern dance derived improvisations were *confusing* and interfered with students' learning because the teacher did not conduct the movement or prescribe an outcome. However, by the end of 12 weeks, these methods became valued as a change from more familiar teacher-centered models where there was *always a right answer.* Similarly, any dance explorations or written reflections that promoted self-reflection, were positively interpreted as a means of *looking back on myself.* These psychophysical movement exercises and *confessional* practices (Usher, Bryant, & Johnston, 1997) such as *sharing* led some of the students to believe that the class was a form of psychotherapy, which is also a common misunderstanding for beginning dance/movement therapy students in the United States.

Habitus: In the socio-cultural domain, when Korean students referred to cultural somatic states such as *nunci,* (literally "eye-measure,") meaning tact, a non-verbal social awareness (Martin, Lee, & Chang, 1967), an organizing historical structure (see Recommendations for future teachers, below), or pre-dispositions to time and space in the "embodied social and cultural world" (Kauppi, 2000, p. 9), it became evident that the application of dance/movement therapy in Korea was conditioned by the habitus (Bourdieu, 1977).

Western concepts of psychotherapy in 1999 (the year of the workshop) were still stigmatized for "normal" people, and marital or family counseling were not familiar to any of the students. Creative arts therapies were viewed as a popular therapy, similar to aroma therapy, or associated with psychotherapeutic interventions such as neuro-linguistic programming. Because structures for psychotherapy or counseling were not available outside of psychiatric facilities, most dance therapy occurred in hospitals, in a parallel development to the profession in the United States.

The students who were "volunteer" interns on psychiatric units indicated that one way to foster a culturally congruent practice of dance, as healing would be for the dance/movement therapist to perform for patients. For example, traditional Korean dance valorizes *Salp'uri,* a solo dance whose most respected performers are mature women. Dancers are held in high regard, and the best dancers personify and express emotions that are typically suppressed, such as bitterness and suffering (Loken-Kim, 1989). Another traditional Korean dance form recognized as healing, is participation in shamanic dance rituals, which are conducted by specially chosen individuals (Kendall, 1988). Since patients in psychiatric hospitals were more familiar with traditional Korean dance forms and motifs than with dance/movement therapy, performing a ritual dance or incorporating elements of shamanic dance were seen as efficacious forms of dance as healing in Korea.

Recommendations for future teachers. In the final interview the participants requested that future DMT speak Korean and have *knowledge of Korean history.* Learning about cultures through the structure of the language is a window that informs the researcher about local ontology, and sheds light on the operations of the habitus in daily life. Dance/movement therapists practicing in a multi-cultural environment require a thorough understanding and respect of core emotional values (Hanna, 2004).

"The Korean person is very different from American persons. Cultural things make a difference. In ancient history, so many other countries came into Korea [that is, a history of political dominance and/or occupation]; from that kind of situation, the Korean people are not very active, but patient. They have patience."

Even though the original research was a case study, which being unique precludes generalization, it is tempting to consider how these findings might reconcile future study of universality of dance/movement with the opposite assertion of dance/movement as race, culture, or ethnicity specific. According to the Korean study participants, their motivation for pursuing DMT as a form of embodied self-discovery and danced freedom of expression was identical to American and European students' reasons for studying DMT. In this case, the habitus of the field of DMT suggests that a universal model of dance-as-healing could underlie the profession. However, socio-cultural structures, such as the Korean educational system, dictate the forms through which DMT is experienced. It is common for Korean students to inactively receive a didactic lecture with 50-75 other undergraduates as their first exposure to dance therapy. Such formal and traditional rote learning is in contrast to the Euro-American emphasis on theory-driven participatory learning. In the case of Korean dance/movement therapists, there was friction between the researcher as educator when they were not taught a dance routine that they could apply in their hospital or school regardless of client age or diagnosis.

Next Steps

Members of the 2004 research conference in Hannover, Germany, took part in a DMT workshop presented to enhance cultural congruence between client and therapist. Guided psychophysical exercises assisted participants' self-reflection on how they embodied their own race, culture, and ethnicity -- including first languages, their "mother tongue." Sensitizing these creative arts and psychotherapists to their habitual bodily manifestation of emotions and symbolic dance movement engendered their discovering qualities of *flexibility* and *responsiveness* towards their clients or students who were members of non-Western cultures. Workshop participants agreed with the concept that once the therapist identified the roots of his or her own cultural stance, the development of a culturally congruent practice was more likely to occur. Intercultural case study research in Korea informed the ensuing dialogue of how understanding the socio-cultural context needs to precede therapeutic interventions with clients from different cultures, races, or ethnicities.

Creative arts therapy provides a safe context to explore such intercultural themes as alienation, individual and group identity, ethnic projections and Otherness, and cultural idealization. Further investigation is needed as to whether culturally embodied knowledge and indigenous forms of psychophysical healing can be learned across cultures, and requires a collaborative approach between local knowledge and the best practices in Euro-American DMT. The case study research found that an active and multidisciplinary method was compatible with traditional approaches to personal wellness and social well-being, as long as modes of experiential learning were appropriate to the local context, and movement observation systems considered Korean cultural aesthetics. As students, dancers, and psychotherapists from non-Western countries study in Europe and North America and apply DMT precepts in their particular milieus, movement observation systems and treatment options created in and applied to local cultures will expand dance therapy practices.

REFERENCES

Acharyya, S. (1992). The doctor's dilemma: The practice of cultural psychiatry in multicultural Britain. In J. Kareem & R. Littlewood (Eds.). *Intercultural therapy: Themes, interpretations and practice* (pp. 74-82). Oxford, England: Blackwell.

Bernard, H. (1995). *Research methods in anthropology: Qualitative and quantitative approaches* (2nd ed.). Walnut Creek, CA: AltaMira.

Berrol, C., & Cruz, R. (2004). *Dance/movement therapy in action: A working guide to research options.* Springfield, IL: Charles C. Thomas.

Boal, A. (1985). *Theater of the oppressed.* Theater Communications Group, Inc., 355 Lexington Ave., New York 10017.

Bourdieu, P. (1977). *Outline of a theory of practice* (R. Nice, Trans.). New York: Cambridge.

Caffarella, R. (1994). *Planning programs for adult learners: A practical guide for educators, trainers, and staff developers.* San Francisco, CA: Jossey-Bass.

Chang, M. (2002). Cultural congruence and aesthetic adult education: Teaching dance/movement therapy in Seoul, Korea. *Dissertation Abstracts International.* (UMI No. 9315947).

Chioncel, N.E., Van der Veen, R.G.W., Wildemeersch, P., & Jarvis, P. (2003). The validity and reliability of focus groups as a research method in adult education. *International Journal of Lifelong Education,* 22(5) pp.495-517.

Collier, J., & Collier, M. (1986). *Visual anthropology: photography as a research method.* Albuquerque, NM: University of New Mexico.

Collins, P. (1990). *Black feminist thought: Knowledge, consciousness, and the politics of empowerment.* New York: Routledge.

Creswell, J. (1998). *Qualitative inquiry and research design: Choosing among five traditions.* London: Sage.

Dokter, D. (1998). *Arts therapists, refugees and migrants reaching across borders.* London: Jessica-Kingsley.

Eisner, E. W. (1998). *The enlightened eye: Qualitative inquiry and the enhancement of educational practice.* Upper Saddle River, NJ: Prentice Hall.

Erikson, E. (1963). *Childhood and society.* New York: W.W. Norton.

Freire, P. (1970/1997). *Pedagogy of the oppressed.* New York: Continuum.

Forinash, M. (2004). Qualitative data collection and analysis: Interviews, observations, and content analysis. In C. Berrol & R. Cruz. *Dance/movement therapy in action: A working guide to research options* (pp. 125-143). Springfield, IL: Charles C. Thomas.

Gilroy, A. (1998). On being a temporary migrant to Australia: Reflections on art therapy education and practice. In D. Dokter. *Arts therapists, refugees and migrants reaching across borders* (pp. 262-277). London: Jessica-Kingsley.

Hanna, J. (2004). Applying anthropological methods in dance/movement therapy research. In R. Cruz & C. Berrol (Eds.). *Dance/movement therapists in action: A working guide to research options* (pp.144-165). Springfield, IL: Charles C. Thomas.

Hoffman, D. (1998). A therapeutic moment? Identity, self, and culture in the anthropology of education. *Anthropology and Education Quarterly* 29(3), 324-346.

Janesick, V. (1994). The dance of qualitative research design: Metaphor, methodolatry, and meaning. In N. Denzin & Y. Lincoln (Eds). *Handbook of qualitative research* (pp. 209-219). Thousand Oaks, CA: Sage.

Jansen, T. & van der Veen, R. (1997). Individualization, the new political spectrum and the functions of adult education. *International Journal of Lifelong Education,* 16(4): 264-276.

Kareem, J., & Littlewood, R. (1992). *Intercultural therapy: themes, interpretations and practice.* Boston: Blackwell Scientific.

Kauppi, N. (2000). *The politics of embodiment: Habits, power, and Pierre Bourdieu's theory.* New York: Peter Lang.

Kendall, L. (1988). *The life and hard times of a Korean shaman*. Honolulu, HI: University of Hawaii.

Levy, F. (2005). *Dance movement therapy: A healing art* (Rev. ed.). American Alliance for Health, Physical Education, Recreation and Dance, 1900 Association Dr., Reston, VA. 22091.

Ling, J., Yamane, J., & Parker, L. (1991). *The Asian American Experience*. Printed for use at the Claremont Colleges, California. Abridged version, 1998.

Littlewood, R. (1992b). *How universal is something we can call therapy?* In J. Kareem & R. Littlewood (Eds.). *Intercultural therapy: themes, interpretations and practice* (pp. 38-56). Boston: Blackwell.

Loken-Kim, C. (1989). *Release from bitterness: Korean dancer as Korean woman*. Doctoral dissertation. University of North Carolina.

Mahler, M., Pine, F., & Bergman, A. (1975). *The psychological birth of the human infant*. New York: Basic Books.

Markus, H. and Kitayama, S. (1991) Culture and the self: Implications for cognition, emotion and motivation. *Psychological Review, 98*, 224-253.

Martin, S., Lee, Y., Chang, S. (1967). *A Korean -- English dictionary*. New Haven, CT: Yale University.

Muhr, T. (1997). ATLAS.ti (Version 4.2) [Computer software]. Retrieved from http://www.atlasti.com

Ness, S. (1992). *Body, movement, and culture: Kinesthetic and visual symbolism in a Philippine community*. Philadelphia, PA: University of Pennsylvania.

North, M. (1972). *Personality assessment through movement*. Boston, MA: Plays.

Pert, C. (2002). The wisdom of the receptors: Neuropeptides, the emotions, and bodymind [From the Past]. *Advances, 18*(1), 30-35.

Rudenstam, K., & Newton, R. (1992). *Surviving your dissertation: A comprehensive guide to content and process*. Newbury Park, CA: Sage.

Saltonstall, E. (1988). *Kinetic Awareness: Discovering your bodymind*. New York: Publishing Center for Cultural Resources.

Schon, D. (1988). *Educating the reflective practitioner*. San Francisco: Jossey-Bass.

Schouten, D., & Watling, R. (1997). *Media action projects: A model for integrating video in project-based education, training, and community development*. Nottingham, U.K.: University of Nottingham.

Stake, R. (1995). *The art of case study research*. Thousand Oaks, CA: Sage.

Strauss, A. & Corbin, J. (1990). *Basics of qualitative research: Grounded theory procedures and techniques*. Newbury Park, CA: Sage.

Steiner-Khamshi, G. (1999). Transferring education, displacing reforms. In J. Schreiver (Ed.). *Discourse formations in comparative education* (pp. 155-187). New York: Lang.

Sue, D. (1981). *Counseling the culturally different: Theory and practice*. New York: Wiley.

Usher, R., Bryant, I., & Johnston, R. (1997). *Adult education and the postmodern challenge: Learning beyond the limits*. New York: Routledge.

Van der Veen, R. (1998). The transformation of community education. In D. Wildemeersch, M. Finger, & T. Jansen (Eds.). *Adult education and social responsibility: Reconciling the irreconcilable?* (Vol. 36. Studies in Pedagogy, Andragogy and Gerontagogy; pp. 1-25). New York: Peter Lang.

About the Editors

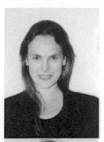

Sabine C. Koch, Ph.D., M.S.W., M.A., DTR, studied psychology at the University of Heidelberg, Germany, and Madrid, Spain (UAM). Dance/movement therapy training at MCP Hahnemann University, Philadelphia, PA, USA (Fulbright grant). DMT experience with diverse populations. Specialized in Kestenberg Movement Profiling (KMP), its use in research, and education. Ph.D. in microanalysis of verbal and nonverbal communication patterns in task-oriented groups. Currently at the gender and personality psychology department, University of Heidelberg. Research interests: embodiment, trans-disciplinary creative arts therapies, gender, personality and social psychology, movement rhythms, interaction patterns, diversity, groups.

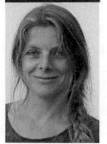

Iris Bräuninger, Dr. rer.soc. (University of Tübingen, Dept. of Clinical and Physiological Psychology, Germany), European Certificate for Psychotherapy (ECP), former board member and acknowledged DMT trainer of the German DMT association BTD, Dance Therapist Registered (DTR) of ADTA, M.A. in DMT from Laban Centre/City University London, KMP Notator. She is currently the deputy head of Physio-, Dance-, Movement Therapy Department at Psychiatric University Clinic Zurich, Switzerland. Research emphases: DMT efficacy studies, stress management, quality of life, Kestenberg Movement Profile (KMP) and movement analysis in relation to emotion, interaction, and psychopathology.